De pratica seu arte tripudii

GUGLIELMO EBREO OF PESARO

DE PRATICA SEU ARTE TRIPUDII

&

ON THE PRACTICE OR ART OF DANCING

EDITED, TRANSLATED,
AND INTRODUCED BY
BARBARA SPARTI

POEMS TRANSLATED BY
MICHAEL SULLIVAN

CLARENDON PRESS · OXFORD
1993

Oxford University Press, Walton Street, Oxford OX2 6DP
Oxford New York Toronto
Delhi Bombay Calcutta Madras Karachi
Kuala Lumpur Singapore Hong Kóng Tokyo
Nairobi Dar es Salaam Cape Town
Melbourne Auckland Madrid
and associated companies in
Berlin Ibadan

Oxford is a trade mark of Oxford University Press

Published in the United States
by Oxford University Press Inc., New York

British Library Cataloguing in Publication Data
Data available

Library of Congress Cataloging in Publication Data
De pratica seu arte tripudii = On the practice or art of dancing /
Guglielmo Ebreo of Pesaro ; edited, translated, and introduced by
Barbara Sparti ; poems translated by Michael Sullivan.
Includes bibliographical references and index.
1. Dancing—Italy—History. 2. Court dances—Italy—History.
I. Sparti, Barbara. II. Title. III. Title: On the practice or art
of dancing.
GV1655G8413 1993 792.8'0945—dc20 92-31812
ISBN 0-19-816233-2

Typeset by Rowland Phototypesetting Ltd,
Bury St Edmunds, Suffolk
Printed in Great Britain on acid-free paper by
Biddles Ltd., Guildford and King's Lynn

To my children David and Donatella

PREFACE

THE possibility of a translation of Guglielmo Ebreo's *De pratica seu arte tripudii* was first discussed in 1980 in the office of Genevieve Oswald, then Curator of the Dance Collection of the New York Public Library. Fifteen years earlier the Dance Collection had received a manuscript copy of *De pratica* as a gift from Walter Toscanini, who had purchased it in Florence in 1932. Mr Toscanini had devoted several years' research to unearthing information on the fifteenth-century dancing-masters and was planning, with Ms Oswald's help, an edition and translation of his (the 'Giorgio') manuscript. This project was never carried out, owing to Mr Toscanini's untimely death in 1971, and at the meeting I was asked if I would undertake the translation. Also present was Dr Julia Sutton, then Chairman of the Department of Music History and Musicology at the New England Conservatory of Music, and, afterwards, translator of Fabritio Caroso's *Nobiltà di dame* (OUP, 1986). Dr Sutton suggested that a translation of what is generally considered to be Guglielmo's first and 'basic' treatise (the *De pratica* now in Paris, Bibliothèque Nationale) would be a more appropriate choice, particularly as this copy—and not the Giorgio/Toscanini codex—includes the music for many of the dances. Besides the transcription and translation of the 1463 *De pratica*, signed and dated by the scribe Pagano of Rho, I decided to include Appendices containing the additional chapters, choreographies, music, and autobiography from the later copy of the treatise under the name Giovanni Ambrosio.

In the twelve years that have elapsed since that meeting, many more people have become involved in the reconstruction and performance of fifteenth-century dances; archival research has brought to light significant information about Guglielmo's life and work; and an international conference dedicated to Guglielmo was organized in his native town of Pesaro. The results of these endeavours have enhanced the introductory chapters and music transcriptions of this edition and translation.

I wish now to take the opportunity to thank Julia Sutton for her initial—and many subsequent—suggestions, her unlimited faith and encouragement, and her scrupulous reading of an early draft of the introductory chapters and much of the translation. To Genevieve Oswald goes my appreciation for her enthusiastic support and for her generosity in putting at my disposal all Walter Toscanini's correspondence and notes pertaining to the Jewish dancing-masters in Italy.

It would not have been possible, however, for me to have translated *De pratica* if, in 1976, Peggy Dixon of 'Nonsuch' had not directed my attention to the Italian dance sources, and if Dr Ingrid Brainard had not invited me, eight years later, to present a paper at the International Congress on Medieval

Studies in Kalamazoo, Michigan. And without the experience of recon-
structing and performing dances with the 'Gruppo di Danza Rinascimentale'
(which I founded and directed for twelve years), and without the experimenta-
tion and provocative questions of numerous students, musicians, and dance
groups in Urbino, Salzburg, England, Germany, and at UCLA, this work
would have been merely theoretical and infinitely poorer. To Professor Barbara Haselbach of the Orff Institute in Salzburg I am deeply indebted, first for
introducing me, in 1970, to the wonders of early dance, and then for inviting
me to teach at the Institute and urging me to complete this translation.

    Last but not least I should like to thank those who helped to bring a final
polish to the translation and edition. Michael Sullivan not only translated the
poems, but was an invaluable editor, contributing his experience as writer,
translator, and poet to both the translation and the introductory chapters.
Special thanks go to Professor Nino Pirrotta, who more than once spared me
a precious hour or two in an attempt to decipher musical ambiguities, and to
Professor Francesco Luisi, who graciously helped me solve some final uncer-
tainties. Véronique Daniels, as a specialist in early notation and Renaissance
dance, gave unstintingly of her time and expertise, patiently examining the
entire translation and Glossary, and shedding light on even the most obscure
musical concepts. I also wish to express my particular gratitude to her, and to
her friends and colleagues at the Schola Cantorum in Basle—Eugen M. Dombois, Karin Paulsmeyer, Crawford Young, and Willem de Waal, for the
enlightening suggestions and explanations which they generously shared with
me and which have greatly enriched my chapter on the *Balli* Tunes as well as
the musical transcriptions and commentaries. My appreciation also to my
friends Jehanne Marchesi and Linda Davidson, each of whom kindly and
painstakingly read over and improved drafts of the translation, and to Andrea
Marchesi, who helped to solve knotty problems in Italian and Latin. I am
grateful to Lieven Baert for his acute eye in proof-reading the Italian transcription. To Anna Ciolli, who eagerly translated the Latin poem and prose into
Italian, I am indeed much obliged. And as *De pratica* goes to press I must add to
these names that of Bonnie Blackburn, whose knowledgeable and scrupulous
editing went beyond the call of duty of a copy-editor, her many suggestions
greatly enriching this book.

    Fortunately, all these people have been compensated by Guglielmo himself,
for each found his story a fascinating one.

                                                                    B.S.

ACKNOWLEDGEMENTS

The illustrations are reproduced by permission of the Biblioteca Estense, Modena (Pl. 15), Biblioteca Nazionale Marciana, Venice (Pl. 12), Biblioteca Universitaria Alessandrina, Rome (Pl. 16), Bibliothèque Nationale, Paris (Pls. 1–4 and facsimiles from MSS fonds ital. 973 and 476 reproduced with the *balli* notations), Gabinetto Fotografico Soprintendenza per i Beni Artistici e Storici di Firenze (Pls. 8 and 9), Istituto Centrale per il Catalogo e la Documentazione (I.C.C.D.), Rome (Pls. 6, 7, 14 (E16225, E16226, E96789), Musées Royaux des Beaux-Arts de Belgique (Pl. 5), and Trustees of the British Museum (Pl. 11).

The preparation and publication of this volume was made possible by a grant from the Memorial Foundation for Jewish Culture.

CONTENTS

List of Illustrations   xiii

Abbreviations   xv

PART I. INTRODUCTION

1. Status and Description of *De pratica*   3
2. Guglielmo's Life   23
3. Dancing in Fifteenth-Century Italian Society   47
4. The Music in *De pratica*: Transcribing the *Balli* Tunes   63

PART II. *DE PRATICA SEU ARTE TRIPUDII*
ON THE PRACTICE OR ART OF DANCING

Notes on the Transcription and Translation   75

Ad Illustrissimum Principem   80
Dedication and Dedicatory Poems   81

Dal harmonia suave   84
Prefatory sonnet   85

Prohoemium   86
Preface   87

[*Liber Primus*/Book I]

  Capitolo Primo & Generale   92
    *Capitolo di Misura, di Memoria, del Partire di Terreno, dell'Aiere
    di Mayniera, di Movimento Corporeo*
  Introductory Chapter   93
    Chapters on Measure, on Memory, on Partitioning the Ground,
    on Air, on Manner, on Body Movement

  Experimentum   100
  Exercises [I–V]   101

  Capitulum Regulare   104
  Rules [I–IV]   105

  Capitulum Regulare Mulierum   108
  Rules for Women   109

Liber Secundus/Book II

  Argumentum Discipulorum [et] Responsio Guilielmi   112
  The Pupils' Contentions and Guglielmo's Rejoinders [I–IV]   113

Conclusio Guilielmi [et] Documentum Guilielmi   120
Guglielmo's Conclusion and Precept   121

Il bel danzar   122
Sonnet in Praise of the Dance   123

Tavola di Bassedanze   124
Table of *Bassedanze*   125

Tavola di Balli   124
Table of *Balli*   125

Bassedanze   126
Bassedanze Choreographies   127

Balli   146
Balli Choreographies   147

Canzon Morale di Mario Philelfo   172
A Moral Ode by Mario Filelfo   173

Scribe's Signature and Date   177

I Balli Notati   179
The *Balli* Tunes, with Commentary   182

PART III. CRITICAL APPARATUS

Biographical Notes   211

Glossary of Dance, Music, and Humanistic Terms   217

Appendices: Additions from the Giovanni Ambrosio copy of *De pratica*   229

    I. On Dancing   232

   II. Choreographies and Music   234

   III. Autobiography   248

Bibliography   255
Index   261

LIST OF ILLUSTRATIONS

PLATES

1. *De pratica*: first page — 2

2. *De pratica*: dedicatory page — 5

3. A trio dancing accompanied by a harpist. Miniature from *De pratica* — 8

4. Duke Galeazzo Maria Sforza and members of his court. Miniature in Girolamo Mangiaria's *Opusculum de impedimentis matrimoni . . .* , 1465–6. Bibliothèque Nationale, Paris — 10

5. Workshop of Rogier van der Weyden: Detail from *The 'Sforza' Triptych*. Musées Royaux des Beaux-Arts, Brussels — 28

6–7. Bonifacio Bembo (attributed to): Portraits of Francesco Sforza and Bianca Maria Visconti Sforza. Brera, Milan — 30

8–9. Piero della Francesca: Portraits of Battista Sforza and Federico of Montefeltro. Uffizi, Florence — 40

10. Details from a wedding *cassone* (anon., probably late fifteenth century, northern Italy). Hermitage, St Petersburg — 46

11. Detail from the engraving (anon., c.1460) *The Planet Venus*. British Museum, London — 47

12. Woodcut (anon., early sixteenth century) from *Opera nuova mai più vista . . . sopra le meretrice . . .* Biblioteca Marciana, Venice — 48

13. Benozzo Gozzoli: Galeazzo Maria Sforza and his uncle Sigismondo Malatesta. Detail from *Procession of the Magi*. Palazzo Medici Riccardi, Florence — 50

14. Benozzo Gozzoli: Lorenzo de' Medici as one of the Magi. Detail from *Procession of the Magi*. Palazzo Medici Riccardi, Florence — 50

15. Taddeo Crivelli: Miniature from Borso d'Este's Bible. Detail. Biblioteca Estense, Modena — 60

16. Frontispiece (anon.), *Canzone a ballo* (Lorenzo de' Medici, Angelo Poliziano, etc.). Florence, 1562. Biblioteca Alessandrina, Rome — 60

MAP

1. Italy, showing the towns Guglielmo worked in and visited — 24

ABBREVIATIONS

Rather than invent my own sigla for the fifteenth-century dance sources (thus adding to the many already in existence), I am using those devised by F. A. Gallo ('Il "ballare lombardo" (circa 1435–1475)', *Studi musicali*, 8 (1979), 61–84) and since utilized—with some changes—by scholars in Italy. It is hoped that sigla will be standardized in the near future, thus making them more accessible to all readers. Each abbreviation is made up of a capital letter which indicates the present location of the treatise (M = Modena). In the case of Florence, where codices are in two different libraries, a second capital letter specifies the library. For the three treatises in Paris, Bibliothèque Nationale, a small letter after P indicates whether it is Guglielmo's, Domenico's, or Giovanni Ambrosio's. So as not to confuse Foligno with Florence, its abbreviation is Fol.

FL	Guglielmo Ebreo, *De pratica seu arte tripudii*, Florence, Biblioteca Medicea Laurenziana, Antinori 13
FN	Guglielmo Ebreo, *De pratica seu arte tripudii*, Florence, Biblioteca Nazionale Centrale, Magliabecchiano XIX. 88
FN¹	Florence, Biblioteca Nazionale Centrale, Cod. Palat. 1021 (fragment of *De pratica*, Book I)
Fol	Foligno, Seminario Vescovile, Biblioteca Jacobilli D. I. 42 (*bassedanze*)
M	Guglielmo Ebreo, *De pratica seu arte tripudii*, Modena, Biblioteca Estense, ital. 82. a. J. 94
N	Nuremberg, Germanisches Nationalmuseum, MS 8842/GS 1589 (*balli*)
NY	Guglielmo Ebreo (Giorgio's copy), *De pratica seu arte tripudii*, New York Public Library, Dance Collection, ★MGZMB-Res. 72-254
Pa	Giovanni Ambrosio, *De pratica seu arte tripudii*, Paris, Bibliothèque Nationale, fonds ital. 476
Pd	Domenico da Piacenza, *De arte saltandi et choreas ducendi*, Paris, Bibliothèque Nationale, fonds ital. 972
Pg	Guglielmo Ebreo, *De pratica seu arte tripudii*, Paris, Bibliothèque Nationale, fonds ital. 973
S	Guglielmo Ebreo, *De pratica seu arte tripudii*, Siena, Biblioteca Comunale, L. V. 29
V	Antonio Cornazano, *Libro dell'arte del danzare*, Biblioteca Apostolica Vaticana, Capponiano 203
Ven	Venice, Biblioteca Nazionale Marciana, It. II. 34 (= 4906), *Il libro di Sidrach*, c.105 (fragment with choreographies)

ASL   *Archivio storico lombardo*

Crusca *Vocabolario degli Accademici della Crusca* (Venice, 1612; fac. repr. Florence: Licosa, 1976)

Florio   John Florio, *A Worlde of Wordes* (London, 1598; fac. repr. Hildesheim: Georg Olms Verlag, 1972)

Guglielmo *Guglielmo Ebreo da Pesaro e la danza nelle corti italiane del XV secolo*, Proceedings of the 1987 Pesaro Conference, ed. M. Padovan (Pisa: Pacini, 1990)

JAMS *Journal of the American Musicological Society*

Litta   Pompeo Litta, *Famiglie celebri di Italia* (Milan, 1819–83)

Mesura Patrizia Castelli, Maurizio Mingardi, Maurizio Padovan, *Mesura et arte del danzare: Guglielmo Ebreo da Pesaro e la danza nelle corti italiane del XV secolo* (Pesaro: Gualtieri, 1987)

New Grove Stanley Sadie (ed.), *The New Grove Dictionary of Music and Musicians*, 20 vols. (London: Macmillan, 1980)

PART I

❦

INTRODUCTION

GVILIELMI HEBRAEI PISA-

RIENSIS DE PRATICA SEV

ARTE TRIPVDII VVLGARE

OPVSCVLVM. INCIPIT :·

Dalharmonia suaue il dolce canto
Che per l'audito passa dentro al cuore·
Di gran dolceza nasce vn uiuo ardore:
Dacui il danzar poi uien che piace taro.
Pero chi di tal scienza uuol il uanto
Conuien che sei partite senza errore·
Nel suo concetto apprenda e mostri fuori
Si come io qui discriuo insegno. et canto.
Misura e prima. & seco uuol memoria.
Partir poi di terren con aire bella.
Dolce mainera & mouimento & poi
Queste ne dano del danzar la gloria.
Con dolce gratia a chi l'ardente stella
Piu fauoreggia con gli ragi suoi.
E i passi et gesti tuoi
Sian ben composti et destra tua persona
con lo intelletto attento a quel che suona.,

1. First page, *De pratica*, fo. 1ʳ (Bibliothèque Nationale, Paris)

I

Status and Description of *De pratica*

FIFTEENTH-century Italy produced the earliest known treatises on the art of the dance.[1] These treatises contain the choreographic descriptions and music of dances which were performed on public and private occasions. Furthermore, they provide the first formulation of a theory of the dance and set out its basic principles.

Nine of these treatises—plus assorted fragments—have survived, and others may yet come to light.[2] What is believed to be the earliest (*c*.1455) is an anonymous manuscript which includes twenty-three dances and their music as well as the aesthetic doctrine of the great innovator, meticulous choreographer, and brilliant theorist, Domenico of Piacenza, Knight of the Golden Spur and dancing-master (though this is only generally presumed) at the Este court in Ferrara.[3] Domenico, also known as Domenico of Ferrara, appears in Ferrarese records as early as 1439, and he named some of his early dances after people and places connected with the Este court. His position is never specified in any document except as 'familiaris noster' (of our household), and as 'specta-

---

[1] A manuscript containing seven *basse danses*, the property of Jean of Orléans, is dated 1445 by Frederick Crane and is therefore probably the earliest known document to record choreographies. (For an extensive list of sources of 15th-c. dance and dance-music, see Crane, *Materials for the Study of the Fifteenth Century Basse Danse* (New York, 1968). The ancient Greeks and Romans—for example, Plato, the rhetoricians Lucian ('On the Dance'), Libanius ('On the Dancers'), and Quintilian—discoursed on dance, seeing it in part as a representation of the movement of the heavenly bodies and in part as pantomime, gesture, and the expression of emotions. (See Lillian B. Lawler, *The Dance in Ancient Greece* (Middletown, Conn., 1964), and Mark Franko, *The Dancing Body in Renaissance Choreography* (Birmingham, Ala., 1986) for more information.) To date no attempt has been made to determine whether—or to what extent—the authors of the Italian treatises (or, for that matter, any European dance-treatise) drew on, or were even aware of, the writings of Greek or Roman theorists, though so far none appears to have been used—as was the case for many Renaissance treatises on other topics—as a model.

[2] A fragment, containing several choreographies included in other treatises, was discovered by A. William Smith in the Biblioteca Marciana, Venice, in 1987. See 'Una fonte sconosciuta della danza italiana del Quattrocento', in *Guglielmo*, 71–84, and below, n. 54.

[3] The treatise is written in the third person, by different hands (six, according to Edward Tuttle —see W. Thomas Marrocco, *Inventory of 15th Century Bassedanze, Balli & Balletti* (New York, 1981), 11, and D. R. Wilson, *Domenico of Piacenza (Paris, Bibliothèque Nationale, MS ital. 972)* (Cambridge, 1988), 2–3). The title, *De arte saltandj & choreas ducendj / De la arte di ballare et Danzare* ('On the Art of Dancing and Choreography'), was added later, together with the number MMCCCCXVI, thought to be an old catalogue reference (Wilson, *Domenico of Piacenza*). It is located in Paris, Bibliothèque Nationale, fonds ital. 972. Wilson's edition fortunately replaces the unreliable one by D. Bianchi (*La bibliofilia*, 65, 1963). It is not clear whether this treatise (the last folios of which are written with far less care than the rest) is a copy of a more elegant—now lost —version, or is simply incomplete. The initial letters of each choreography, as well as those of the introductory paragraphs, are missing, presumably awaiting the hand of an illuminator.

bilis eques' and 'spectabilis miles', titles of nobility bestowed, for the most part, only on gentlemen. His wife, a lady-in-waiting, was a Trotto, from the same family that served the Estes as courtiers and ambassadors.[4] In April 1455 Domenico was in Milan attending Beatrice d'Este's wedding to Tristano Sforza, and during the festivities he danced with the Duchess of Milan, Bianca Maria Sforza. His treatise, which—according to an inscription on the fly-leaf —belonged to the Duke of Milan, may have been a homage to Beatrice, or a gift to the Sforza library, for in October of that same year Domenico was again in Milan, attending the celebrations for Ippolita Sforza's betrothal to the Duke of Calabria.[5] Despite these visits, and a reference to him (by his disciple Antonio Cornazano) as Ippolita's 'bon servitore', there is no evidence that he was in the employ of the Sforzas. Indeed, his name appears in the Ferrarese accounts through 1475. It seems likely that he died in 1476 or 1477.

Another dance-manual is the work of Antonio Cornazano, humanist, poet, and courtier. Like Domenico, whom he calls his master in the art of the dance, Cornazano was born in Piacenza and was later at the Este court in Ferrara. In 1455, soon after entering the service of the Duke of Milan, Cornazano presented his *Libro dell'arte del danzare* ('Book on the Art of Dancing') to the Duke's young daughter, Ippolita Sforza, on the occasion of her betrothal to the Duke of Calabria. Another redaction[6] (probably an exact copy, thought to have been set down ten years later) was dedicated by Cornazano to Ippolita's half-brother, Sforza the Second, and it is this copy—still bearing the 1455 inscription to Ippolita—which survives.[7] It contains an important theoretical introduction, Cornazano's summary descriptions of eleven of Domenico's dances—including occasional comments which illuminate particular aspects of a choreography, and Domenico's music for the dances—with the valuable addition of three *bassadanza* tenors, and remarks concerning their interpretation.[8]

[4] This information comes from a letter of the Director of the State Archives of Modena to Walter Toscanini of 9 Nov. 1959, and includes references up to 1462, from records that register special payments only. Domenico's name appears in 1439, 1441, 1445, and 1450. I have myself found him in the list of salaries of 1456 as having received payment the previous year (unfortunately, no prior list is available), and regularly thereafter (some volumes are missing or incomplete) through 1475 (Camera ducale estense, Computisteria, Bolletta de' salariati, reg. 1–8). For further information on Domenico's treatise, see Gallo, 'Il "ballare lombardo" '.

[5] For brief biographies of illustrious personages mentioned in this and in the following chapters, see Biographical Notes.

[6] The term 'redaction' is used here and throughout this chapter to indicate a copy, but not necessarily a replica, of a treatise. In other words, a 'revised edition' of a treatise.

[7] *Libro dell'arte del danzare*, Rome, Biblioteca Apostolica Vaticana, Capponiano 203 (ed. C. Mazzi, *La bibliofilia*, 18 (1915); tr. M. Inglehearn and P. Forsyth). For information on Cornazano's life see C. Fahy, 'Per la vita di Antonio Cornazano', *Bollettino storico piacentino* (May –Aug. 1964); A. Pontremoli and P. La Rocca, *Il ballare lombardo* (Milan, 1987), 29–44; I. Brainard, 'Cornazano, Antonio', *New Grove*; as well as C. Poggiali, *Memorie per la storia letteraria di Piacenza* (Piacenza, 1989), i.64–130, and M. A. Silvestri, 'Appunti di cronologia cornazaniana', in *Miscellanea di storia, letteratura e arte piacentina* (Piacenza, 1915), 30–71.

[8] *Re di Spagna*, *Cançon de pifari dicto el Ferrarese*, and *Collinetto*. For a definition of the *bassadanza*

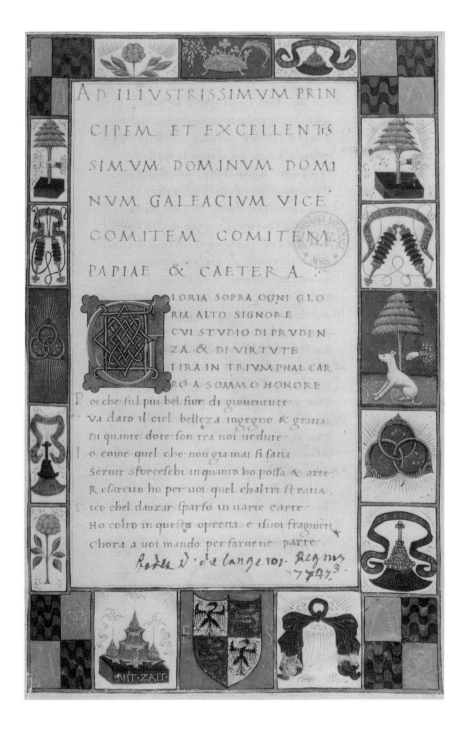

2. Dedicatory page, *De pratica* (Bibliothèque Nationale, Paris)

The remaining seven treatises are all to be attributed, directly or indirectly, to Guglielmo Ebreo (William the Jew), who was, in his own words, a 'most devoted disciple and fervent imitator' of Domenico in, presumably, their common occupation of choreographer–composer–theorist, and, though we are not certain in the case of Domenico, that of *ballerino* and dancing-master. The version of *De pratica seu arte tripudii* ('On the Practice or Art of Dancing') edited and translated here, may well have been the primary source not only for the six other treatises, but for three fragments as well as for two copies that are known to have existed but have since been lost. These are discussed below.

De pratica (as I shall henceforth refer to it), dedicated to Galeazzo Maria Sforza, then Count of Pavia, was completed on 11 October 1463 in Milan (see the colophon). The manuscript (Bibliothèque Nationale, fonds ital. 973) is still in its original green velvet binding[9] and is beautifully (and legibly) written on parchment in a humanistic hand. The scribe, who made remarkably few errors, was Pagano of Rho.[10] It is not known who illuminated the chapter initials (see Pl. 1), the borders of the first of the fifty-four folios,[11] and the dedicatory page illustrating the lineage and policies of the Sforzas with a series of emblems and mottoes (Pl. 2),[12] nor who painted the miniature depicting three dancers and

---

as a dance type, and a discussion of its musical characteristics, see the Glossary and Ch. 4. It is important, when evaluating Cornazano's affirmations, to keep in mind that—unlike Domenico and Guglielmo—he was neither choreographer nor composer, nor was he a 'professional' dancer or a dancing-master.

[9] The spine has raised bands and the outside edges of the leaves are gilded. Four holes on the front and back covers suggest that originally there probably were some sort of clasps. The velvet is faded and worn.

[10] Paganus Raudensis—Pagano from the town of Rho (near Milan)—is listed in Bradley's *Dictionary of Miniaturists, Illuminators, Calligraphers and Copyists* (London, 1887–9), as a copyist. A manuscript, in his hand, of *Terentii Poetae comici* is in the British Library. Four other manuscripts known to have been copied by him are in London, Milan, Florence, and the Vatican. In this last (Urb. lat. 460) he appears as 'librarian of Pietro Lalli, count of Montorio' (a town in the Sabine hills, near Rome). See E. Pellegrin, *La Bibliothèque des Visconti et des Sforza ducs de Milan au XVe siècle* (Paris, 1955), 340; and his *Supplement* (Florence and Paris, 1969), 40–1.

[11] The folios measure 255 × 165 mm. Chapter headings are red, and the large chapter initials are gilded and set against red, green, and blue backgrounds which are finely decorated in white.

[12] The emblems are as follows: (1) The gold flower, possibly a quince ([*mela*] *cotogna* in Italian), representing Cotognola, the birthplace of Muzio Attendolo, the first Sforza. (2) The ducal crown (emblem of the house of Visconti, the rulers of Milan and Pavia prior to the Sforzas) with two branches: the olive (or laurel) symbolizing peace, and the palm for victory and pre-eminence. (3) The shield, which displays the Sforza–Visconti arms: the imperial eagle and the snake with a babe in its fangs. The letters 'FS' (for Francesco Sforza, the first Sforza duke of Milan) appear on the sides of the shield. (4) The greyhound sitting under a pine tree alludes to 'the vigilant and fruitful peace established by Duke Francesco'. The symbolism of the celestial hand that takes off or puts on the dog's collar is not known but may well indicate the Duke's power to 'unleash the dogs of war'. (5) The little brush signifies the ridding of the state of invaders or anything foul; the motto *Merito et tempore* means 'deserving and in good time'. (6) The bridle bit with the motto *Ich verghes ni[ch]t* (I forget not) is a Sforza device favoured by Ludovico il Moro and the Montefeltro family. (7) Three linked rings, each with its small diamond, was a common device (also used by the Medici) and appears on numerous Sforza coins. Francesco Sforza presented the emblem to

a harpist, one of the rare representations of dance from this period (Pl. 3).[13] (It has been conjectured, though there is no evidence for this, that the male figure is none other than Guglielmo, and that the ladies—or perhaps all three —are singing as they dance.[14]) Of interest is the style of dress (note the long, chiffon-like handkerchief) and the manner in which the hands are joined.

De pratica was taken to France by Louis XII in 1499 when he carried off the bulk of the treasures from the magnificent Visconti–Sforza ducal library in Pavia to the royal residence at Blois.[15] In the following century the Royal Library was transferred to Fontainebleau (where, however, only Domenico's

various noble families in Milan as a sign of particular favour. (8) The scarf tied with a knot represents the 'veil with which Giangaleazzo [Visconti] was tied . . . before he was made duke in 1395 . . .'. (9) The mountain with three evergreens (perseverance) was used by Bianca Maria Visconti Sforza and her son Galeazzo Maria. The motto *Mit Zait* [*Zeit*] (literally 'with time') seems to have been common in Milan and Pavia. (10) The family colours, reproduced in various devices, were blue and dark red.

The citations above are from Guido Lopez, *Festa di nozze per Ludovico il Moro, nelle testimonianze di Tristano Calco, Giacomo Trotti ed altri* (Milan, 1976), 148 and Patrizia Castelli, 'La kermesse degli Sforza pesaresi', in *Mesura*, 31 n. 46. Other sources consulted include G. Bascapè, 'I sigilli dei Duchi di Milano', *ASL* 8 (1943); L. Beltrami, *Il castello di Milano sotto il dominio degli Sforza* (Milan, 1885); G. Bologna, *Milano e il suo stemma* (Milan, 1981); D. Sant'Ambrogio, 'Dell'impresa araldica dei tre anelli intrecciati concessa da Francesco Sforza a parecchie famiglie patrizie di Milano', *ASL* 18 (1891), 392–405; Pellegrin, *Supplement*.

[13] The miniature's artistic worth is indicated by its inclusion in the Catalogue (p. 154) of the exhibition *Dix siècles d'enluminure italienne (vi^e–xvie siècles)* (ed. F. Avril, Paris: Bibliothèque Nationale, 1984) where, together with the dedicatory page, it is attributed to the 'maître d'Ippolita'. This miniaturist used the same emblems to decorate other manuscripts formerly in the Sforza library in Pavia (figs. 133, 134, and 136 in the Catalogue). For the most complete collection, to date, of reproductions of 15th-c. Italian dance iconography, see *Mesura*, 92–111.

[14] The round mouths of the ladies give this impression. Chansons were occasionally used for dance-music. See, for example, Giovanni Ambrosio's letter (quoted in Ch. 2), which refers to Ippolita Sforza's composing two *balli* to French songs; Domenico's *ballo*, *Figlia Gulielmina* (in Pd), which is based on a French chanson; and the chansons used for *bassedanze* in the allegory performed in Urbino and in other *moresche* (see Ch. 3 and F. Alberto Gallo, 'La danza negli spettacoli conviviali del secondo quattrocento', in *Spettacoli conviviali dall'antichità classica alle corti italiane del '400* (Rome, 1982), 261–7). Chanson melodies were also used as tenors for *bassedanze* but, according to Bukofzer, these were extracted from their original sources and quite distorted in order to fit the purposes of the choreography ('A Polyphonic Basse Dance of the Renaissance', in *Studies in Medieval and Renaissance Music* (New York, 1950), 190–216). See also F. Crane, 'The Derivation of Some Fifteenth-Century Basse-Danse Tunes', *Acta musicologica*, 37 (1965), 179–88. At present there still is no documentation to the effect that ladies or courtiers sang while performing *bassedanze* or *balli*. See, however, Galeazzo Sforza's experience at Firenzuola in Ch. 3. (For a definition of the *ballo* as a dance type, and a discussion of its musical characteristics, see Glossary and Ch. 4.)

[15] G. Mazzatinti, *Inventario dei manoscritti italiani delle biblioteche di Francia* (Rome, 1886), i. The Pavia library, with its own librarian, was established in the 14th c., partly as a result of Petrarch's encouragement and personal donations. In 1459 it contained 951 volumes, which were attached to the library tables with silver chains! (Despite this precaution, a note written in 1453 reports that 'many books have been taken and are missing and some of the most beautiful are on loan to this or that person'; quoted by Mazzatinti, p. xv). Scholars from all over Europe visited the splendid collection of rare manuscripts, exquisitely copied and illuminated on parchment and bound in gold and silver brocade, velvet, damask, and satin. In an inventory made in 1469 of 'the books of the most Illustrious Lord Duke Galeazzo Maria' in the library of Pavia, *De pratica* is described as 'a little book of dances and songs [verses] in the vernacular'.

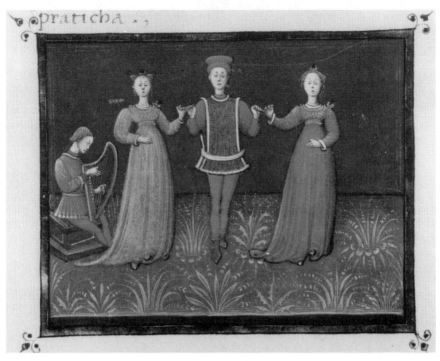

3. Miniature, *De pratica*, fo. 21ᵛ (Bibliothèque Nationale, Paris)

treatise appears in the 1544 catalogue[16]), and in 1666 the library was moved to
Paris, very near its present location. On the inside cover of *De pratica* there is
an inscription which reads: 'Ex Libris J. P. G. Chastre de Cangé. 1728.'.
Jean-Pierre Imbert Châtre de Cangé (d. 1756)—former mayor of Tours, War
Commissioner, first valet to the Duke of Orléans and later to the King—was
an amateur collector who owned a very rich library.[17] In his catalogue, printed
in 1733, *De pratica* is number 101. In the same year, for the sum of 40,000
livres, Cangé sold 170 manuscripts to the Bibliothèque du Roi. Presumably,
Guglielmo's treatise was amongst these, remaining then in the collection during the Revolution and after, when the royal library became the Bibliothèque
Nationale.[18]

---

[16] *De pratica* may have been misplaced, temporarily missing, on loan, or simply overlooked by
the cataloguer. See below, n. 18.

[17] Cangé's *cabinet*, probably located in his château in Touraine, contained military documents,
manuscripts, portraits, maps, and letters. See M. Prévost, *Inventaire sommaire des documents
manuscrits contenus dans la collection Châtre de Cangé* (Paris, 1910); and L. Delisle, *L'Inventaire des
manuscrits français de la Bibliothèque Nationale* (Paris, 1876), i.

[18] Guglielmo's treatise does not appear in Marsand's inventory of Italian manuscripts in the
Paris libraries, published in 1835 (*I manoscritti italiani della regia biblioteca parigina*, Paris), whereas

Guglielmo, on the title-page of *De pratica*, declares himself to be the author, but this point needs some clarification. When we compare the treatise's literary style with that of additions made to a later copy and with that of letters written or dictated by Guglielmo himself,[19] it becomes clear that someone other than Guglielmo is the author of the ornate and cultivated fifteenth-century prose. Who this person was—whether Pagano of Rho, who, like many scribes of the time, may also have been a scholar, or, possibly, Mario Filelfo, the author of *De pratica*'s final ode in praise of Guglielmo, or yet some other intermediary— is hardly likely to emerge.[20] Nor does it seem important, since this spokesman, ghost-writer, or collaborator is willing throughout the treatise to speak in the first person as Guglielmo, and no one other than Guglielmo has ever claimed authorship. The prose itself might well be taken for that of a Tuscan, according to F. Zambrini, who, in the preface to his edition of one of the copies of *De pratica*, declares the style and language good. He adds, however, perhaps out of a limited interest in the dance, that he finds the exposition 'tedious and boring'.[21]

Our version of *De pratica* opens with two dedicatory poems to Galeazzo Maria Sforza, then 19 years old and heir to the Duchy of Milan (see Pl. 4). The treatise proper begins with a sonnet (also present in the six other redactions) celebrating the art of the dance. A preface follows, in which Guglielmo extols the virtues of music, discusses its possible inventors, and then shows how dance was born from it. In a typically humanistic apology Guglielmo sets out to claim for dance the status enjoyed by music in fifteenth-century Italy, where

---

Domenico's manual and a later version of *De pratica* (by Giovanni Ambrosio) do. However, according to Gaston Raynaud, 'Inventaire des manuscrits italiens da la Bibliothèque Nationale qui ne figurent pas dans le catalogue de Marsand' in *Extrait du Cabinet Historique—année 1881*, ed. Picard and Champion (Paris, 1882), when Marsand began compiling his catalogue, the manuscripts in the Bibliothèque Nationale were not classified in any special or separate section, and it was not until 1860 that an Italian collection was established that included volumes overlooked by Marsand or acquired after 1838.

[19] See Ch. 2, nn. 19 and 37. The original of the first letter has unfortunately been lost, thus making it impossible to ascertain if it was written by Guglielmo himself.

[20] For Mario Filelfo, see below. On the role of the scribe and the preparation of manuscripts I found J. I. Whalley and V. C. Kaden, *The Universal Penman* (London, 1980) very helpful.

[21] F. Zambrini (ed.), *Trattato dell'arte del ballo di Guglielmo Ebreo pesarese* (Bologna, 1873; repr. Bologna, 1968). Marsand, on the other hand, writes (in his above-mentioned Inventory, 98–9) that the style and 'diction' betray 'the little skill of the writer in our language [Italian]'. One wonders what criteria Marsand used for drawing this rather drastic conclusion. The prose that Guglielmo used, together with his references to antiquity, had—in itself—to convince the reader that dance was a liberal art. So much of *De pratica*'s phraseology is of the kind found in Leon Battista Alberti's *On Painting* (both terminology and conceits) that the latter could almost have served as a model (see below, n. 22). However, as E. Winternitz points out in his analysis of Leonardo da Vinci's *Paragone* ('The Role of Music in the Comparison of the Arts', in *Leonardo da Vinci as a Musician* (New Haven, Conn., 1982)), 'Many notions were in the air' at the time, being disputed or echoed among courtiers and humanists. Some of these were 'rhetorical attempts to bolster the social status' of the artist and/or his art, though some notions did of course contain 'new and ingenious ideas'.

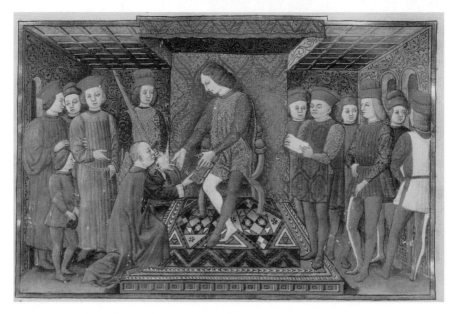

4. Duke Galeazzo Maria Sforza and members of his court, miniature
(Bibliothèque Nationale, Paris)

it was recognized as both art and science, just as Leon Battista Alberti before
him attempted to prove the worth of painting by basing it on mathematics
(though this was 'more appearance than reality').[22] Alberti and Guglielmo
were surely concerned to enlarge the scope of the *arti liberali* to embrace
painting on the one hand and the dance on the other. We may further speculate
that Guglielmo, by endeavouring to emulate the medieval and Renaissance
musicus (the philosopher of music who dealt only with the theory of his art),
was attempting to improve the standing of the dancing-master.

It is surely not by chance that after this theoretical introduction—which
proves the moral and ethical worth of the dance by citing classical philos-
ophers, pagan deities, and the God and heroes of the Old Testament—we
find a section dedicated to the fundamental principles of which the dance is
composed. For this was the format of most fifteenth-century treatises, whether
they dealt with rhetoric, painting, architecture, music, philosophy, or education.[23] And whoever drafted Guglielmo's work was clearly well aware of

[22] J. R. Spencer (ed. and tr.), *Leon Battista Alberti 'On Painting'* (2nd edn., New Haven, Conn.,
and London, 1966), 16 and 21.

[23] Besides Alberti's *On Painting*, see e.g. his treatise on architecture (completed in 1452); Filarete's *Architettura* (1464); Ghiberti's *Commentarii* (written after 1474); Gaffurio's *Theoricum opus*
(1480); Vergerio's *On Noble Behaviour* (c.1404); G. Manetti's *On the Dignity and Excellence of Man*

the conventions and specialized terminology. Indeed, as at the dawn of the Quattrocento the ideal of harmony dominated the humanists' universe, it is harmony—the source and sustenance of the dance—that dominates the introductory sonnet and Preface of *De pratica*.[24] Contemporary courtly literature provides themes for the dedicatory poems, as do heroes and heroines from antiquity, several of whom appear in a final ode. It is likely that these references were intended to give the dance a moral dignity, thus suggesting it as an appropriate pursuit for a prince. But it is the fundamental principles, rules, and exercises ('experiments') that give weight to Guglielmo's claim that dance is not only art but science. And these basic concepts—measure, memory, partitioning the ground (division of space), manner, air, movement —which Guglielmo, and Domenico before him, laid down and made intrinsic to the dance, are the same basic concepts found in other arts and sciences.[25]

In seven chapters, Guglielmo considers the fundamental principles of dancing. These include keeping in time to the music, remembering the sequence

(before 1459); Leonardo Bruni's treatise on a lady's education, *De studiis et literis* (c.1423–6). Patrizia Castelli discusses the relationship between the dance-treatises and Aristotelian and artistic theories in 'Il moto aristotelico e la "licita scientia": Guglielmo Ebreo e la speculazione sulla danza nel XV secolo', in *Mesura*, 35–57. See also M. Baxandall, *Painting and Experience in Fifteenth Century Italy* (Oxford, 1972), in particular 60, 77–8, A. Blunt, *Artistic Theory in Italy 1450–1600* (Oxford, 1940), and W. H. Woodward, *Vittorino da Feltre and Other Humanist Educators* (Cambridge, 1897).

[24] Guglielmo's emphasis on harmony, his defining dance as an expression of the emotions, and his references to gesture (see Sparti, 'Stile, espressione, e senso teatrale nelle danze italiane del '400', *La danza italiana*, 3 (1985), 46–7), suggest that, at some remove, Plato (e.g. in *The Laws*) may have been a source of inspiration.

[25] Manner, measure, and air (style) were, for example, important to the painter, as can be seen in the following poem describing the quality of Pisanello's work (Biblioteca Vaticana, Urb. 699; quoted in Castelli, 'Il moto aristotelico', 37 and Baxandall, *Painting and Experience*, 77). It is by the poet Angelo Galli, secretary and ambassador at the court of Urbino from 1432 to 1459, with whom Alessandro Sforza maintained a 'poetic correspondence' in 1456–7 (S. Eiche, 'Alessandro Sforza and Pesaro: A Study in Urbanism and Architectural Patronage', Ph.D. thesis (Princeton University, 1982), 127–8).

> Arte mesura aere et desegno
> Manera prospectiva et naturale
> gli ha data el celo per mirabil dono.

> Art, measure, style, and design [draughtsmanship],
> Manner, both perspective and natural,
> Has Heaven given him as admirable gifts.

Measure was also a fundamental principle in architecture and in music. References to movement can be found in Aristotle's *Ethics* and *Physics* as well as in the works of Alberti and in Leonardo da Vinci's treatise on painting. Guglielmo himself discusses not only body movement but the movements of the soul. Regarding the importance of memory in the Renaissance, see F. A. Yates, *The Art of Memory* (Chicago, 1966). The roots of the humanists' interest in the *ars reminiscendi* were probably Aristotelian and were echoed, among others, in Alberti's treatises on painting and architecture and, later, in the works of the Neoplatonist Marsilio Ficino. Lucian ('On the Dance', see above, n. 1) asserted that memory was the most important requisite for a dancer since he needed to know, by heart, and be able to give pantomimic representation to, all the best known events in history, mythology, and literature.

of the steps in a dance, spatial awareness, and ornamentation. While these precepts have counterparts in Domenico's and Cornazano's treatises, Guglielmo's descriptions supply significant particulars which help to clarify the concepts. Following the principles are exercises in which the aspiring dancer can acquire further skill and test his prowess in 'the aforesaid art'. The exercises, which deal with complex but fundamental relationships between the dance and its accompanying music, are unique to Guglielmo and give an idea both of his ingenuity as a dance-teacher and of the high level of achievement expected (theoretically at least!) of his pupils. The final chapters of Book I constitute another distinctive feature of *De pratica*: they give indications not only of how to compose dances and their music,[26] but they also offer advice on the comportment appropriate to young ladies who intend to take delight in the dance.

Book II consists of a Socratic dialogue between Guglielmo and his hypothetical disciples in which the 'master' defends the art of dancing and explains in more detail the reasons that make it indispensable to follow his precepts. (This same dialogue form, first used by Lucian in his defence of the dance, was to be used again, more than one hundred years after Guglielmo, by Thoinot Arbeau and Fabritio Caroso in their dance-manuals.[27]) The section ends with an autobiographical sketch in which Guglielmo comments on his thirty years of dance experience and cites the more important celebrations at which he had been present. He finishes by affirming that those who follow all the rules of his book 'will be loved, honoured, and revered'. The fine sonnet 'Il bel danzar' concludes this portion of *De pratica* devoted to *The Art* (or theory) *of the Dance*.

The Practice, or the practical part of the treatise, consists of descriptions of thirty-one dances (*bassedanze* and *balli*), the choreographies of which are important examples of early descriptive notation.[28] Of these thirty-one dances, fourteen were composed by Guglielmo, while the rest are his own accounts of dances by Domenico. (Domenico seems to have preferred the *ballo* as a dance form, while Guglielmo was more prolific as a composer of *bassedanze*.[29])

---

[26] Composition was also discussed in treatises on painting and architecture. (See e.g. Alberti's theory of composition, based on the humanists' concept of *compositio* in literature, in Baxandall, *Painting and Experience*, 135–7.) Filarete's work on architecture consists of a section on measure, one on techniques, and one on new creations. Another chapter in *De pratica* is devoted to the importance of measure as proportion, a basic tenet of Renaissance life and thought, used in mathematics, science, art, music, philosophy, and commerce.

[27] Thoinot Arbeau (pseud. for Jehan Tabourot), *Orchésographie* (Langres, 1589; Fac. repr. Langres, 1988; Geneva, 1972; copy with intro. by L. Fonta, Paris, 1888, repr. Bologna, 1969 (music and steps are misaligned); tr. M. S. Evans, new ed. J. Sutton, New York, 1967). Fabritio Caroso, *Nobiltà di dame* (Venice, 1600; repr. Bologna, 1970; tr. J. Sutton, 1986).

[28] While the 15th- and 16th-c. French *basses danses* are notated in step symbols or letters (see Crane, *Materials*), the Italian treatises of the same period use fully written out prose instructions for their choreographies.

[29] *De pratica* has 9 *bassedanze* and 5 *balli* by Guglielmo and 5 *bassedanze* and 12 *balli* by Domenico. (Domenico's own treatise contains 18 *balli* and only 5 *bassedanze* – two of which are versions of the same dance – while the last, a later addition, is probably not by Domenico.)

No explanation has yet been given for the interesting fact that five of the dances attributed to Domenico, including the famous *Rostiboli Gioioso*, are not present in Domenico's own treatise, but make their appearance here for the first time.[30]

The ode in praise of Guglielmo that concludes *De pratica* is by Giovanni Mario Filelfo (1426–80), a poet and humanist like his better-known father Francesco.[31] As a man of considerable standing—he delivered the oration at the lavish wedding festivities of Elisabetta Montefeltro and Roberto Malatesta (see Ch. 3)—he was certainly an excellent reference for a dancing-master. His own daughter, as we learn from the ode, had been taught by Guglielmo, but while this means that the two men were acquainted, it is not evidence for the authorship of the treatise's prose, although it does dispose one to hold Filelfo in mind as a candidate.

After the ode comes the scribe's dated inscription and then, still in Pagano's hand, the music for thirteen *balli*. These monophonic melodies, though spare, are (as I have had occasion to say elsewhere) 'a rare example of a type of secular instrumental music which was performed in the early Italian Renaissance— part of an important tradition of "unwritten" music'.[32] Together with Domenico's tunes, Cornazano's *bassadanza* tenors, and the melodies of four dances added to a later copy of *De pratica*, they form a unique collection of fifteenth-century dance-music.[33]

Within three years of the date of completion of *De pratica* (1463), Guglielmo

---

[30] For *Rostiboli Gioioso*, see the choreographic description and Ch. 2, n. 55, as well as references in Ch. 3. The other dances attributed to Domenico are *Reale*, *Phoebus*, *Flandesca*, and *Petit Rose*.

[31] In 1464, the same year that he was imprisoned for defiling Pope Pius II's tomb, Mario Filelfo (also known as Giovanni Mario Filelfo) composed a similar ode (*Canzon morale*) in 'adulation' of Federico Montefeltro. (C. H. Clough, 'Federigo da Montefeltro's Patronage of the Arts, 1468–1482', *Journal of the Warburg and Courtauld Institutes*, 36 (1973; repr. in *The Duchy of Urbino in the Renaissance*, London, 1981, 129–45)). In the last two years of his life, Mario was tutor to the sons of Federico Gonzaga, the Marquis of Mantua. (See Ch. 2 for further reference to Mario.) His father, Francesco, had been at the Visconti court in Pavia, at that of Lorenzo de' Medici, and then in Milan with Francesco Sforza who inspired his epic, the *Sphortias*. When Duke Francesco died, the funeral oration was delivered by the same Francesco Filelfo. According to Eiche, 'Alessandro Sforza', 127, 'In July 1470, when Alessandro [Sforza] was in Milan, Filelfo lamented to him about his sad financial state at the Milanese court, due to the circumstance of Galeazzo Maria having reduced by one-half the stipend he was used to receive from Francesco, and even this half not always forthcoming.' Francesco Filelfo had apparently also served Alessandro because 'In the same communication Filelfo alludes to a debt of two years ago which Alessandro had with him, amounting to 625 ducats.' Lorenzo de' Medici also received a letter from Filelfo complaining about discrepancies in the salary paid him by the Duke of Urbino for the years 1468 to 1472 (Clough).

[32] Sparti, 'The 15th-century *Balli* Tunes: A New Look', *Early Music*, 14 (1986), 346. See N. Pirrotta, 'The Oral and Written Traditions of Music', in *Music and Culture in Italy from the Middle Ages to the Baroque* (Cambridge, Mass., 1984), 72–9.

[33] Comparative transcriptions of the music from all four of the treatises have been published in O. Kinkeldey, 'Dance Tunes of the Fifteenth Century', in D. G. Hughes (ed.), *Instrumental Music: A Conference at Isham Memorial Library* (Cambridge, Mass., 1959). See also Marrocco, *Inventory*, for a transcription of the *ballo* tunes and *bassadanza* tenors.

converted to Catholicism and took the name of Giovanni Ambrosio.[34] Some time after 1471, and certainly before 1476, another redaction of *De pratica* was made in which the name 'Giohanne Ambrosio' was substituted consistently for that of Guglielmo Ebreo. This unsigned and undated manuscript (also in the Bibliothèque Nationale in Paris, fonds ital. 476) lacks the dedication and poems to Galeazzo Sforza, the miniature—although an appropriate space is provided for it—and Filelfo's ode.[35] It does, however, reproduce the earlier *De pratica* word for word, and, moreover, contains supplementary material of notable interest (included in the Appendices to this edition). The vocabulary and style of the additions have the flavour, in marked contrast to the rest of the treatise, of unadorned speech. It seems legitimate to suggest that Guglielmo, alias Giovanni Ambrosio, dictated the new material directly to copyists who, this time, rendered it literally or with a minimum of 'editing'.

Three new chapters are dedicated to the difference made by a man's dress to his style of dancing, and it is in discussing the appropriateness of capes and of long or short garments that Guglielmo/Giovanni Ambrosio incidentally reveals to us what cannot be found in so explicit a form in any other source, written or pictorial: the virtuosity and skill required of the fifteenth-century courtier–*ballerino*, who was expected to ornament his dancing with jumps, turns, and flourishes.[36]

[34] Given the weight of documentary evidence, most scholars today agree that Guglielmo Ebreo and Giovanni Ambrosio are the same person. See Ch. 2.

[35] The codex, containing 82 paper folios (including several lined and blank pages), measures 267 × 175 mm. It was written, probably over a period of time, in a hand similar to but less refined than Pagano's. There are no illuminations, and the only decorations appear at the end of some musical notations, where two notes (*longae*) are embellished with a design of other notes (see the facsimiles in App. II). Because these final *longae* are always notated on the middle line—whether musically appropriate or not—it seems likely that they were scribal ornamentations to mark the end of each tune (this was not at all uncommon in music manuscripts) rather than musical/choreographic indications of, for example, a final bow. Rubrics are in red, as are the many capital letters. On the back of the first folio, in a different but neat hand of, I believe, the same period, appears the beginning of a lauda(?):

O tu dolce singnore che nay creati   O thou, sweet lord, who hast created
Correnti fiumy de misericordia   Flowing streams of compassion,
I tuoy   Thy

The manuscript is bound in leather (now a dark red) on boards. The name *TRIPUDII* appears on its ridged spine, which is decorated with gold fleurs-de-lis. The front and back covers have a gold border and the emblem of the Royal Library of France (a crown with a chain and cross and three fleurs-de-lis encircled by a wreath). The table of contents in this version of *De pratica* (Pa) appears at the very beginning of the book. The composers of the dances are indicated here rather than after the title of each choreographic description, as in Pg.

[36] Flourishes (*fioretti*) were particular steps which were used to embellish late 16th-c. dances. Giovanni Ambrosio (see App. I) uses the verb *fioregiare* (to make or do flourishes), which is probably generic for ornamentation rather than an indication of a specific step. (Tinctoris, *Terminorum*, says that *contrapunctus diminutus* 'a quibusdam floridus nominatur', 'is called florid by some'.) Recently come to light are a *El gioioso fiorito* and *Tan geloso fiorito*, unique and ornamented versions of dances included in different redactions of *De pratica*; Q. Galli, 'Una danzografia in un protocollo notarile a Montefiascone nella seconda metà del XV secolo', *Arte e Accademia* (Viterbo: Accademia

A remarkable concept for its time is Ambrosio's unique exercise to discern the good dancer by his ability to shape his performance to the style and character of different instruments, each of which plays the same piece of music in turn.

This version of *De pratica* also contains the choreographic descriptions of a 'French' *bassadanza* and two 'French' *balli*, the first examples to appear in any Italian treatise. These are distinctively different from their Italian counterparts and, together with the Franco-Burgundian manuals of the period, help make a comparison of the two styles possible.[37] Three other *balli* and their music, composed by Giovanni Ambrosio himself, are also added (one being the popular *Rosina*[38]). Two of these have indications for a *riverenza* 'down to the ground', the first description of a bow in an Italian treatise. It is, moreover, this redaction alone that contains the music for the well-known [*Rostiboli*] *Gioioso*. Another significant characteristic is Giovanni Ambrosio's musical notation, which differs occasionally from Guglielmo's. There are some variations and the notation tends, on the whole, to be more precise. Whether this is because his scribe was more experienced in this sector than Pagano, or simply that Guglielmo/Giovanni Ambrosio himself made a corrected 'second edition', is not known.

Certainly, the most important feature of the Giovanni Ambrosio treatise is the eighteen-page Autobiography with which it ends. Written at different intervals, in at least two hands, it is the main source of information on Guglielmo's life and provides a particular picture of the role and activities of a dancing-master/court servant in the Italian Renaissance. While Giovanni Ambrosio is obviously fascinated by violent death, spectacular feats of tightrope-walkers and the like, and by the amount and variety of courses at banquets, he also describes public events such as princely weddings, ambassadorial receptions, entries, and visits of state. His inclusion of key names and places has made it possible to date and document these events. Also listed are expenditures for vestments, gifts, and particular festivities—some of this information admittedly from hearsay. The display of power through opulence required that expenditure—even that for small events—be noticed and talked about and, on many occasions, written down, and Giovanni Ambrosio's awestruck gossip shows effectively the success of the Renaissance policy of magnificence.[39]

di Belle Arti, 1989) 121–143. See Ch. 2, n. 55. Similarities between *fioreggiare* and *pavoneggiare* are discussed in Sparti, 'Style and Performance in the Social Dances of the Italian Renaissance: Ornamentation, Improvisation, Variation, and Virtuosity', in *Society of Dance History Scholars Proceedings* (1986), 31–52.

[37] Besides Michel Toulouze, *L'Art et instruction de bien dancer* (Paris, *c.*1488; fac. edn. London, 1936), see *Le Manuscrit dit des basses danses de la Bibliothèque de Bourgogne* (Brussels, Bibliothèque Royale, 9085). Fac., ed. Ernest Closson (Brussels, 1912; repr. Geneva, 1975).

[38] See Ch. 2, n. 55.

[39] F. Cruciani, *Teatro nel Rinascimento Roma 1450–1550* (Rome, 1983), 18–19. Leon Battista

A singular aspect of *De pratica* lies in the number of copies that were made of it both during Guglielmo's life and after his death. In addition to the 1463 redaction, here in translation, and to the Giovanni Ambrosio transcription already described, extant versions are to be found in the following libraries:[40]

Biblioteca Comunale of Siena[41] (S)

Biblioteca Estense of Modena[42] (M)

Biblioteca Nazionale Centrale of Florence[43] (FN)

New York Public Library[44] (NY)

Biblioteca Medicea Laurenziana of Florence[45] (FL)

Two other copies—both, interestingly enough, by Giovanni Ambrosio—are known to have existed in court libraries: one in the Sforza collection in Pesaro and the other in the Montefeltro library in Urbino.[46] These manuscripts, apparently lost after the looting by Cesare Borgia's troops in 1502, were undoubtedly a manifestation of Guglielmo's (Giovanni Ambrosio's) gratitude for the unfaltering support of his two lifelong patrons: Alessandro Sforza, lord of Pesaro, and Federico of Montefeltro, Duke of Urbino (see Ch. 2). According to a letter only recently brought to light, Giovanni Ambrosio had also prepared 'a work on dance' dedicated to Lorenzo de' Medici (presumably a copy of *De pratica*), which he intended to present in person in 1477.[47] (This will not have been the version now in the Biblioteca Nazionale in Florence since that copy is in Guglielmo's name.) The letter, written to the Magnificent by Alessandro Sforza's son, recommends Giovanni Ambrosio, and his treatise, most highly. It seems likely that this copy was an expression not only of

Alberti, in his treatise *Della Famiglia* (English edn., *The Family in Renaissance Florence*, by R. N. Watkins, Columbia, SC, 1969), confirms the positive influence of hearsay which, when concerned with expenditure, brings honour and fame to a family's house. Also see T. J. Tuohy, 'Studies in Domestic Expenditures at the Court of Ferrara (Artistic Patronage and Princely Magnificence)', Ph.D. thesis (Warburg Institute, 1982), and Ch. 3.

[40] For further information, bibliographic and other, on the treatises and their contents, see Gallo, 'Il "ballare lombardo" ', and Marrocco, *Inventory*, 2–3 and ch. II). On the lost copies, see Gallo, 'L'autobiografia artistica di Giovanni Ambrosio (Guglielmo Ebreo) da Pesaro', *Studi musicali*, 12 (1983), 195. For anyone interested in comparing the repertory and sequence, Gallo lists the complete contents of all (except N and Ven) the 15th-c. treatises.

[41] Codex L. V. 29. Ed. by C. Mazzi (incomplete), 'Una sconosciuta compilazione di un libro quattrocentistico di balli', in *La bibliofilia*, 16 (1914–15), 185–209.

[42] Codex Ital. 82. a. J. 94. Published by G. Messori Roncaglia, *Della virtute et arte del danzare* (Modena, 1885).

[43] Codex Magliabecchiano XIX. 88, published in Zambrini, *Trattato*.

[44] *MGZMB-Res. 72–254. Ed. A. Francalanci in *Basler Jahrbuch für historische Musikpraxis*, 14 (1990).

[45] Codex Antinori 13. See Beatrice Pescerelli, 'Una sconosciuta redazione del trattato di danza di Guglielmo Ebreo', *Rivista italiana di musicologia*, 9 (1974), 48–55.

[46] Gallo, 'L'autobiografia', 195. The Pesaro copy was registered in 1500 under 'Io. Ambrosio ballarino' (A. Vernarecci, 'La libreria di Giovanni Sforza signore di Pesaro', *Archivio Storico per le Marche e per l'Umbria*, 3 (1886), 518), and the Urbino manuscript appears in an inventory made after 1482 (C. Stornajolo, *Codices urbinates graeci Bibliothecae Vaticanae* (Rome, 1895), 138).

[47] Timothy J. McGee, 'Dancing Masters and the Medici Court in the 15th Century', *Studi musicali*, 17 (1988), 222–3'. See Ch. 2, nn. 50–1.

thanks to Lorenzo for previous favours but of Guglielmo's hopes of future employment in the service of the Medici.

The most impressive of all of the extant copies (the only one to be written on parchment) is the Siena manuscript.[48] Still in its original leather binding on wooden boards, it has illuminated initials and chapter-headings—some in gold, others in blue and red. The presence of a coat of arms (as yet unidentified), without, however, any dedication, suggests that this manuscript, rich both in dances and decoration, may have been commissioned for a princely library. The same hypothesis may indeed apply to the copies now in Modena and Florence (FN). These also have contemporary leather bindings; a few initials of the particularly beautiful Florentine manuscript are gilded, while the Modena rubrics are red.

Whereas all three of these copies were made by professional (anonymous) scribes, the manuscript in New York is an example of a personal copy belonging to a certain Giorgio, who may well have been a dancing-master.[49] It is written, for the most part, by a single hand (the script is a common one although somewhat illegible to a modern eye), perhaps by Giorgio himself. Giorgio's is the only one of the versions of *De pratica* to include dances from the Giovanni Ambrosio additions and to mention him—'Giovanambruogio, formerly a Jew'—along with Domenico and Guglielmo as one of the authors of the dances.

The Siena, Modena, and New York treatises reproduce all Guglielmo's theoretical chapters (Books I and II) and also include extracts from the introductory chapters of Domenico's own manual. Both the Siena and New York treatises contain numerous dances (many anonymous) that are not found in

---

[48] Besides the 1463 *De pratica* and the Siena copy, Cornazano's treatise is also parchment. All the other 15th-c. Italian dance-manuals are paper.

[49] The only indication for this, however, is the opening inscription: 'This is the copy of m.° [maestro] giorgio' (Master Giorgio). The inscription continues 'e del giudeo di ballare bassadanze e balletti, e questa e la tavola della conposizione del ballo e di bassadanze e baletti composti per messer domenicho da ferara e da m. giovanambruogio che fu ebre[?]'. The last letter is blotted, thus precluding the possibility of knowing if Giorgio wrote *ebreo* (Jew) or *ebrei* (Jews), and giving rise to speculations that Domenico too was originally Jewish; see W. Toscanini, 'Notizie e appunti sui maestri di ballo ebrei nel '400', *Il Vasari*, 18 (1960), 62–71. However, the verb (*fu* = was) is singular and indicates that only Giovanni Ambrosio was intended. The other enigma in this inscription is the phrase 'e del giudeo' (literally 'is of' or 'and of the Jew'). Marrocco, *Inventory*, reads it as Giorgio del Giudeo—'of the Jew'. However, Giorgio, at this time, was definitely not a Jew, for the above inscription begins with 'In the name of God and the Virgin Mary'. Besides, if Giorgio had been a Jew and converted—as Toscanini suggests—why did he not use of himself the expression 'che fu ebreo' (formerly a Jew) which he had used for Giovanni Ambrosio? It seems equally unlikely that Giorgio would have been called 'Giorgio e del Giudeo'; proper names followed by two family names joined by 'e del' still exist in Italy but are an indication of aristocratic lineage. A more plausible explanation is that the manuscript had two owners—or two authors: Giorgio, and the Jew. If, for example, the dancing-school run by Francesco, a Christian, and Giuseppe Ebreo, Guglielmo's brother, had a dance-book, might it not have been inscribed as being the property 'of Francesco and of the Jew'? (On the dancing-school, see Ch. 2.) Or, on the other hand, could it have been Giorgio's own copy of the Jew's (Guglielmo's) book?

any other copy, while the Modena 'edition' has fewer dances than any other redaction. (It is likely that the Siena treatise, or one similar, was the source for the abridged Modena copy.)

The copy of *De pratica* in the Medicea Laurenziana Library in Florence is still in its original tooled-leather binding and is dated 1510. It is written in a 'commercial cursive' hand and seems to be an almost identical copy (for personal or library use?) of the treatise in the Biblioteca Nazionale of Florence.[50] These two manuscripts present only the first part of *De pratica*'s precepts (Book I), and contain three additional *bassedanze*: two composed by Lorenzo de' Medici and one by Giuseppe Ebreo (Joseph the Jew), Guglielmo's brother.[51] Lorenzo's and Giuseppe's dances are also included in the Giorgio (NY) treatise, which was bought in Florence in 1932 and is considered to be of Tuscan origin.[52]

None of these copies of *De pratica* (S, M, FN, FL, NY) includes, as already noted, any dedication, and none contains any music; and while three refer to 'the miniature below' (and in two copies a space is provided), the illustration never reappears. None of the treatises is an exact replica of either the Guglielmo or the Giovanni Ambrosio *De pratica*, and only the Laurenziana manuscript (FL) is dated.

Besides the Giorgio codex, and possibly the Laurenziana 'edition', three fragments of Guglielmo's work are also probable examples of personal transcriptions. A two-leaf manuscript containing *De pratica*'s Preface and introductory chapters (bound up, very likely in the first half of the sixteenth century, with medical and pharmaceutical prescriptions) is now in the Biblioteca Nazionale in Florence.[53] Two other pages, which include the choreographies of four *balli* by Domenico and Guglielmo, were discovered in 1987 among various papers—these too apparently assembled haphazardly by later librarians—in the Biblioteca Marciana in Venice by A. William Smith, who has published the fragment (Ven) together with a critical study.[54]

---

[50] See Pescerelli, 'Una sconosciuta redazione', who points out that the date, while probable, is not absolutely certain, inasmuch as the third figure is unclear and may have been rewritten. After 'Here ends the book . . . and finished by me on the 6th day of December 1510[?]', the choreographies of a *bassadanza* and four *balli* (published in Pescerelli) are added in the same hand: *bassa di chastiglia, moza di biscaie, lipitier* [*Jupiter*?], *se no dormi dona alscioltta, mastri di t*[*r*]*o*[*n*]*boni*. (Note that a 16th-c. manuscript bound with the Giorgio [NY] codex and referred to as the 'Il Papa' manuscript contains 15 *balletti*, two of which are *Ippiter* and *l'Tromboni*.)

[51] On Giuseppe, see Ch. 2.

[52] According to Walter Toscanini, the paper in the Giorgio manuscript has a watermark (Briquet, i, no. 3387) similar to that found in use in Tuscany around 1450–60. (Letter to Dr I. Brainard, dated 16 Mar. 1962, in deposit at the New York Public Library's Dance Collection.)

[53] Codex palat. 1021. See P. L. Rambaldi and A. Saitta Revignas, *Biblioteca nazionale centrale di Firenze, I manoscritti palatini* (Rome, 1950), iii.16.

[54] It. II. 34 (= 4906), Libro di Sidrach, c. 105; see Smith, 'Una fonte sconosciuta'. The *balli* are *El gioioso* [*Rostiboli*], *Lioncelo, Berequa*[*r*]*do, Gracioxa*. Three lines are given to a description of the *saltarello* step, and two to *Moderna* (*bassadanza* in S).

Another small collection of eight choreographies, one of which is accompanied by a poem, can be found in the Biblioteca Jacobilli in Foligno.[55] Nothing is known of this manuscript's origin and no authorship is indicated for any of the dances. Two of the *bassedanze* are unique to the collection, whereas the remaining six appear in *De pratica*, where five are attributed to Guglielmo and only one to Domenico. The Foligno choreographies are written within lined margins in a neat cursive script with ornate initials by, it would seem, a single hand, probably on different occasions. Most significant is that after a number of blank pages, the codex contains household(?) accounts, apparently written in the same hand as the dances, with the dates 1445, 1461, and 1462. What is particularly perplexing, if these early dates are to be taken as an indication of when the dances were set down, is that some of the step and choreographic terminology is more similar to that found in the Siena and Giorgio manuscripts than to that used in the 1463 *De pratica*. Whereas it is difficult to establish a date for the Siena manuscript, it is obvious (because of its inclusion of Giovanni Ambrosio's name and his dances) that the Giorgio copy was made after Guglielmo's conversion (*c*.1466) and most probably after the Ambrosio treatise was terminated (*c*.1471—the last dateable entries of the Autobiography). Why there should be step descriptions peculiar only to the Siena, Modena, Foligno, and Giorgio manuscripts remains obscure, and the pronounced difference of dates, if exact, between Foligno and Giorgio, simply compounds the mystery.[56]

There are interesting and occasionally significant differences in how the dances are notated in the various copies of *De pratica*. (To date, no complete study has been made, although detailed comparative analyses of specific dances and steps have been undertaken.[57]) The most striking difference concerns the thoroughness and clarity of the choreographic descriptions. Domenico is by far the most precise annotator, whereas Guglielmo's renditions of both Domenico's and his own *balli* are inclined to be abridged, frequently omitting such information—vital to a correct reconstruction of a dance—as the *misura* and the number of step/music-units. (Giovanni Ambrosio is somewhat more explicit in the notation of his own *balli*.) Of all the redactions of *De pratica*, Giorgio's choreographic descriptions are the most detailed and complete, and

[55] Codex D. I. 42, published by D. M. Faloci Pulignani, *Otto bassedanze di M. Guglielmo da Pesaro e M. Domenico da Ferrara* (Foligno, 1887). One of the dances is described twice with only minor changes.

[56] Smith, 'Una fonte sconosciuta', poses similar questions regarding the Venice fragment.

[57] See, for example, A. Francalanci, 'La ricostruzione delle danze del '400 italiano attraverso un metodo di studio comparato delle fonti', *La danza italiana*, 3 (1985), 55–76 (Guglielmo's *Pellegrina*); A. W. Smith, 'Studies in 15th-Century Italian Dance: *Belriguardo in due*: A Critical Discussion', *Society of Dance History Scholars Proceedings* (1987), 86–105; Smith, 'Una fonte sconosciuta'; M. Lo Monaco and S. Vinciguerra, 'Il passo doppio in Guglielmo e Domenico. Problemi di mensurazione', in *Guglielmo*, 127–36; as well as L. Pleydell's contribution to *Guglielmo*. Peggy Dixon's paper at the Renaissance Dance Colloquium (Ghent, April 1985) was a comparative study of the *bassadanza Daphnes*.

Siena's the most condensed and vague. Most of the dance descriptions vary from treatise to treatise. Some, like those in the Tuscan (FN, FL, NY) and Foligno copies, have special, seemingly standardized endings; others have more subtle differences (compare the Pd, Pg, NY, and S versions of *Iove/ Jupiter*); and still others occasionally provide radical innovations (see Giorgio's ending of *Gelosia*).

In the past few years, research in Italy's libraries and archives has brought forth some extraordinary information regarding the dance treatises and their authors, making it pleasantly necessary—on different occasions—to rewrite these introductory chapters.[58] However, several questions regarding *De pratica* and its different versions remain unanswered. It is hoped that the present publication and translation, by stimulating and encouraging scholars to further study, will make a contribution towards their solution.

1. Was the 1463 *De pratica* commissioned? By whom? By the young Galeazzo Sforza himself? By his father, Duke Francesco, or his mother, Bianca Maria Visconti? Or was *De pratica*'s dedication to Galeazzo an attempt on Guglielmo's part to ingratiate himself with the future Duke of Milan? (Had he hopes of employment or payment—or both?[59]) If *De pratica* was not commissioned, who secured (and paid for) the services of the illuminator, of Pagano of Rho, and of whoever was responsible, if it was not he, for the urbane and relatively polished prose rendering?

2. Since none of the more beautiful extant copies of *De pratica* includes a dedication, is it possible that they were intended for particular libraries rather than as presentation copies for princely patrons? Who commissioned them?

3. Who made the copies? Were scribes attached to the Sforza library/court used, or were scribes (or dancing-masters) from other courts sent to Pavia to make copies? Was *De pratica* borrowed by other libraries or dancing-masters?[60]

---

[58] See the letters to Lorenzo de' Medici from the courts of Urbino and Pesaro—and from Giovanni Ambrosio himself—which shed light on Guglielmo's later years and show that Giuseppe Ebreo was Guglielmo's brother (McGee, 'Dancing Masters'); the documents from the Archives in Florence disclosed by A. Veronese which give the name, place of birth, and profession of Giuseppe's (hence Guglielmo's) father, as well as the contract establishing Giuseppe's dancing-school; the various letters referring to Giovanni Ambrosio found in the Archives of Milan and Pesaro. (For detailed accounts and complete references, see Ch. 2.) The Venice fragment, the Montefiascone *fiorito* dances (n. 36), and Domenico's dates according to salary-lists in the Este archives in Modena are other examples of recent findings.

[59] Pontremoli, 'Il ballare lombardo', 35, reports that two beautiful codices, containing Antonio Cornazano's description of the entertainments organized by Borso d'Este in Reggio Emilia in 1465 in honour of Ippolita Sforza's imminent marriage to the Duke of Calabria, were dedicated by Cornazano to Borso, who rewarded him with 60 ducats. (Ten years earlier, Cornazano's annual salary had been a mere 34 ducats; ibid., 33. For the value of the ducat, see Ch. 2 n. 41.)

[60] See n. 15. That works were consulted by many people and even lent out is confirmed in S. Eiche, 'Towards a Study of the "Famiglia" of the Sforza Court at Pesaro', *Renaissance and Reformation*, 9 (1985), 79–103, who cites the official responsibilities of the Duke of Urbino's

4. Since Domenico's and Guglielmo's treatises were evidently both in the Sforza library in Pavia, why were so many copies made of the Guglielmo manuscript and none of Domenico's (except for the excerpts from his theoretical preface included in the Siena, Modena, and New York copies)?

5. Where was the Giovanni Ambrosio copy located? If the hypothesis is correct that it ended up in Paris because it too had been in the Sforza library, then why do none of the *De pratica* copies, with the exception of the Giorgio manuscript, bear Giovanni Ambrosio's name or include his dances? If this were known it would help to establish a chronology for the treatises. Clearly the Giovanni Ambrosio manuscript was unavailable to the Siena and Florentine [FN] scribes because it was not in the 'right place' at the 'right time'.

6. Who added the choreographies, unknown elsewhere, to the Foligno and Siena manuscripts, and where did Giorgio get his new dances?

7. What criteria did Guglielmo use in determining which of Domenico's dances to include in *De pratica*? (Why, for example, did he choose *Mercantia* and not its counterpart *Sobria*?) And, while the first dances may well have been in honour of his patrons, with what *raison d'être* were the other choreographies assembled in *De pratica* and in the various redactions? What is the meaning, if any, of their sequence?[61]

8. Did Guglielmo know about the copies of *De pratica* (S, M, NY, FN) which were made during his lifetime?

9. Why do only the 1463 *De pratica* and the Giovanni Ambrosio redaction contain music?

10. As I have said above, the two lost Giovanni Ambrosio redactions of *De pratica* were probably Guglielmo's acknowledgement of the unfailing patronage of Alessandro Sforza and Federico of Montefeltro. The Pagano of Rho copy most certainly represented Guglielmo's hope of keeping the door to the Sforza court in Milan open and, at the same time, was an attempt to improve the status of both the dance and the dancing-master. What purpose, however, did the other dance-treatises serve? Judging by their condition today, they hardly seem, Giorgio's copy included, to have been consulted.[62] Does this mean that rather than working *aide-mémoires* for courtiers or dancing-masters, they were collectors' items for princely libraries, as well as repositories for the theory of the dance and catalogues of choreographies? Whom did Guglielmo envisage his readers to be? Considering the contents of Books I and II, it seems clear that he expected his work to reach more eyes and ears than just those of

---

librarian. Moreover, inventories were circulated so that court libraries might order copies of manuscripts for their own collections (Eiche, 'Alessandro Sforza').

[61] See n. 40. Is it significant that the *balli* tunes are notated in a completely different order from that of the choreographies (see below, 'The *Balli* Tunes'), and different again from the tunes as notated in the Giovanni Ambrosio redaction?

[62] This question, referred to me by Ingrid Brainard, was put to her—with a comment on the treatises' 'unused' condition—by John Ward.

Galeazzo Sforza. What was the significance to him of having his choreographies written down? Would they thus acquire the lustre of a work of art, shed on him honour and immortality, or gain for him—not copyright, certainly—the recognition of attribution?

Since *De pratica* may indeed be the primary source for all the other Guglielmo manuscripts, and because it is the only copy to have a dedication, miniature, date, and name of the scribe, and furthermore because it includes the music for the dances, it has been the obvious choice for transcription and translation (supplemented with the additional material from the Giovanni Ambrosio version). However, much of the contemporary theory and practice was taken for granted by Guglielmo—and his readers—and therefore either omitted by him or described in terms that are now obscure. Hence, for example, the scant musical notation, the almost total lack of descriptions of steps, and the often tantalizingly enigmatic introductory chapters. None the less, it is hoped that this edition will further the work, not only of specialists in early dance and music, but of scholars and others interested in the Italian Renaissance and in the contribution to it of the Jews.

2

Guglielmo's Life

THE main sources of information on Guglielmo's life are in his 'Conclusion' and in the autobiographical supplement at the end of the Giovanni Ambrosio redaction (App. III). Archival research—some very recent—has added several letters and other documents that have significantly supplemented our previous knowledge. Places where Guglielmo lived or worked are shown in Map 1.

Chronology of Salient Events in the Life of Guglielmo Ebreo/Giovanni Ambrosio

*c.*1420	Born in Pesaro, son of Moses of Sicily, dancing-master at the Pesaro court
1433	Begins his dancing-career
1437	*Marriage of Federico Montefeltro, Count of Urbino
1444	*Weddings in Ferrara; perhaps Guglielmo's first encounter with Domenico da Piacenza
1445	*Alessandro Sforza becomes Lord of Pesaro after his marriage to Costanza da Varano; Guglielmo probably enters his service
1450	*Francesco Sforza becomes Duke of Milan
1455	*Ippolita Sforza's betrothal to Alfonso of Aragon in Milan
1459	*Pope Pius II stops in Milan on his way to the Diet in Mantua
1460	Guglielmo prepares a *moresca* at the Sforza castle in Pavia
	*Federico of Montelfeltro's marriage to Battista Sforza in Urbino
	*Reception for King Louis XI's ambassadors in Milan
1463	Pagano of Rho completes the copy of *De pratica* dedicated to Galeazzo Maria Sforza
	*Marriage of Federico Gonzaga to Margaret of Bavaria in Mantua
1463–5	Guglielmo converts to Christianity and takes the name Giovanni Ambrosio; his godparents are the Duke and Duchess of Milan
1465	Guglielmo (now Giovanni Ambrosio) remarries, under the aegis of Alessandro Sforza; his wife is the daughter of a Christian citizen of Pesaro

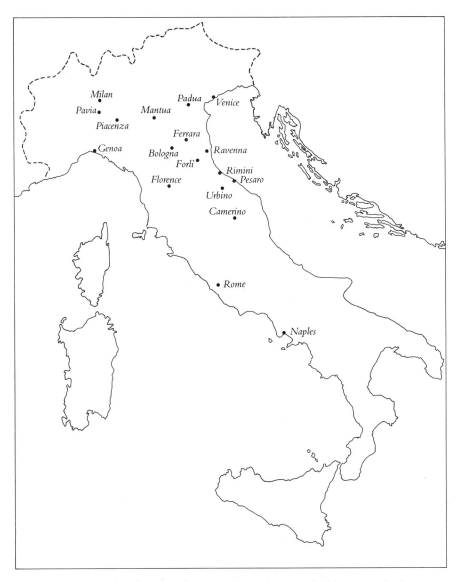

MAP I. Italy, showing the towns Guglielmo worked in and visited,
as well as those mentioned in the introductory chapters

	*Ippolita Sforza marries Alfonso of Aragon in Naples
1466	Death of Francesco Sforza, Duke of Milan
c.1466–7	Guglielmo in the service of the King of Naples for two years
1467	Guglielmo's brother Giuseppe (together with a Christian) opens a dancing-school in Florence
1468	*Wedding of Galeazzo Maria Sforza in Milan
1469	Guglielmo is knighted by the Emperor in Venice. He writes to Lorenzo de' Medici about his brother's conversion
	Galeazzo Sforza accuses Guglielmo of defaming an ambassador to his court and advises his own ambassador that he is not to be received
1469–71	Guglielmo is present at the courts of Pesaro and Urbino
1471	He prepares *moresche* for the betrothal of Elisabetta Montefeltro to Roberto Malatesta in Urbino
1473	Alessandro Sforza dies
c.1475–6	He and his son Pierpaolo are in the service of the Duke of Urbino
1477	He dedicates a treatise to Lorenzo de' Medici
1480	Costanzo Sforza (Alessandro's son) sends Guglielmo to the court of Milan with a letter of recommendation
1481	Guglielmo, referred to as the Duke of Urbino's dancing-master, dances with the 6-year-old Isabella d'Este in Ferrara
1482	Death of Federico of Montefeltro, Duke of Urbino
1483	Death of Costanzo Sforza
1484	Lorenzo de' Medici informs Camilla of Aragon, Costanzo Sforza's widow, that Florence cannot 'give alms' to Guglielmo as they have too many of their own poor

* Events attended by Guglielmo/Giovanni Ambrosio

Date and place of birth

In the 1463 version of *De pratica*, Guglielmo declares that he has been practising the art of the dance for thirty years. If we assume that he began his dancing career between the ages of twelve and sixteen, then he was probably born about 1420. (The year of his death is unknown, but it cannot have been before 1484.) Guglielmo and his brother Giuseppe were the sons of Moses of Sicily, probably the same Moses who was—for a time at least—dancing-master at the court of Pesaro,[1] and Pesaro, it would seem, was also their birthplace.[2]

Early Years: Patronage of Alessandro Sforza of Pesaro and his wife Costanza da Varano of Camerino

Alessandro Sforza became Lord of Pesaro in 1445 through his marriage to Costanza da Varano of Camerino, and it is probable that shortly thereafter Guglielmo entered his service.[3] Of the preceding twelve years of his career, all that is thus far known is that he attended the wedding of Federico of Montefeltro, Count of Urbino, in 1437, but we do not know in what capacity or in whose retinue.[4] For the present we can merely speculate that during those early years he began practising his art in Pesaro, where his father had taught, and in the neighbouring Marches of Camerino and Urbino.[5]

[1] Moyse (referred to also as 'of Pesaro' and as Musetto) is described in a letter written by Camilla Sforza del Drago, wife of the Lord of Pesaro, as being 'a fine person and he teaches dancing to the children of my lord'. The letter, dated 30 Aug. 1429, is cited in A. Veronese, 'Una societas ebraico-cristiana in *docendo tripudiare ac cantare* nella Firenze del Quattrocento', in *Guglielmo*, 51–8, and published in A. A. Bernardy, 'Les Juifs dans la république de San Marin du XIVe au XVIIe siècles', *Revue des études juives*, 48 (1904), 241–64. On his brother Giuseppe, see below. To date I have been unable to identify any Camilla Sforza del Drago, wife to a lord of Pesaro.

[2] The designation 'of Pesaro' after Guglielmo's name indicates that Pesaro was either where he was born or the place he considered his home. Since Guglielmo's mentor Domenico was known as both Domenico of Piacenza (his birthplace) and Domenico of Ferrara (the court he served), it is conceivable that Guglielmo was not born in Pesaro but considered himself a citizen of that city after he entered Alessandro Sforza's service. According to V. Colorni, the name 'Guglielmo' corresponded, in 15th-c. Italy, to the Hebrew name 'Biniamin' (Benjamin), and this was because of a kind of homophonic resemblance. While the Italian Jews used their Hebrew or biblical names —or those Italian/Latin names that had already been assimilated—for written documents within their community, outside it was common practice to use established Latin/Italian equivalents, except in the case of the best-known biblical names. (The first study of the equivalent Latin/Italian and Hebrew or 'Hebrew-ized' names was made at the end of the 17th c.) See V. Colorni, 'La corrispondenza fra nomi ebraici e nomi locali nella prassi dell'ebraismo italiano', in his *Judaica Minora—Saggi sulla storia dell'ebraismo italiano . . .* (Milan, 1983), 660–825, particularly 672, and 716–17 for examples of Italian Jews known as Guglielmo/Benjamin.

[3] The title of Lord of Pesaro was ceded to Alessandro by Costanza's grandfather Galeazzo Malatesta when he sold the March to Alessandro's brother, Francesco Sforza (see Eiche, 'Famiglia', 80). Alessandro and Costanza were betrothed on 8 Dec. 1444 in the Varano castle of Sentino (near Camerino) and princely guests and numerous entourages from all over Italy were in attendance; see A. A. Bittarelli, *Camerino* (Camerino, 1985). The March or Duchy of Camerino (*c.*1300–1545) was extensive, but prior to the dual reign of Costanza's brother Rodolfo and his cousin Cesare— which began in Dec. 1443—it had passed through a tumultuous period. Up until this time court life, if any, will have been so unsettled as to make it unlikely that a professional dancing-master would have found employment.

[4] For the date of this event, as well as for the dating of the other festivities mentioned in Giovanni Ambrosio's Autobiography (App. III), see Gallo, 'L'autobiografia'. The numbers in square brackets that appear in this chapter are also from Gallo and correspond to entries in the Autobiography.

[5] In the mid-15th c. the Marches of Pesaro, Urbino, Camerino, and Rimini were ruled respectively by the Sforza, Montefeltro, Varano, and Malatesta families.

Both Alessandro and Costanza were well-educated and cultured princes,[6] and while Renaissance Pesaro has been largely neglected by historians, an inventory of their library includes—among more than twenty-two paintings —works by Mantegna, Perugino, and van der Weyden, thus suggesting a most civilized court.[7] The relationship between the dancing-master and his patron, honoured with the presentation of a copy of *De pratica*—now unfortunately lost—lasted until Alessandro's death in 1473.[8]

Guglielmo was present at Alessandro's and Costanza's betrothal in 1444 [2],[9] but even earlier in the same year he had been taken to Ferrara by Costanza's brother, Rodolfo da Varano, to attend Rodolfo's own marriage to Niccolò d'Este's daughter Camilla [1].[10] (See Pl. 5.[11]) During the festivities—which lasted a month—Leonello d'Este's wedding to Maria of Aragon was also celebrated. It is not known if Domenico da Piacenza had anything to do with the 'great balls' that took place,[12] and if so, if this was Guglielmo's first meeting with him.

[6] Alessandro, whose father was then in the service of the Marquis of Ferrara, was educated there together with his brother Francesco and the Este children; Annibale degli Abati-Olivieri Giordani, *Memorie di Alessandro Sforza signore di Pesaro* (Pesaro, 1785). (The Marquis, Niccolò III, presented Palazzo Schifanoia to Alessandro, who, however, sold it some time before 1458; Eiche, 'Alessandro Sforza'.) Costanza is said to have been a poetess (Bittarelli, *Camerino*), and at the age of 14 she recited verses in Latin in the presence of Bianca Maria Visconti Sforza.

[7] Vernarecci, 'La libreria di Giovanni Sforza', 518. See also Eiche, 'Famiglia', who cites Vespasiano da Bisticci's biography of Alessandro Sforza: '[A] most learned [and] well paid man' was 'in charge of this library'. For further information on art and culture at the court of Pesaro before and during Alessandro Sforza's signory, see Eiche, 'Alessandro Sforza'.

[8] See Ch. 1 n. 46 for information regarding this copy. Three years after Alessandro's death Guglielmo/Giovanni Ambrosio sent a letter to Lorenzo de' Medici (see n. 37 below), signing it 'Giohane Ambroxio Alixandresscho' (of the household of Alessandro [Sforza]).

[9] I have been unable to discover when the marriage itself took place, but it seems to have followed close upon the betrothal celebrations.

[10] Guglielmo, or Alessandro Sforza, apparently remained in contact with the Varano family even after the deaths of Costanza (1447) and Rodolfo (1464), for in 1471 Guglielmo was present at the wedding of Rodolfo's daughter [29].

[11] This painting (53.5 × 83.5 cm.), now in the Musées Royaux in Brussels (cat. no. 515, inv. no. 2407), is generally agreed to be from the workshop of Rogier van der Weyden and to have belonged to the Sforza library in Pesaro. Because of the device in the right corner, critics are now agreed that the donor (whose head has been retouched) is Alessandro Sforza. In the Museum's catalogue the other figures are identified as Costanza da Varano and her brother Rodolfo. However, art historians elsewhere claim that because of the probable date of the painting (*c*.1460), it cannot be Costanza who is represented. Germano Mulazzani ('Observations on the Sforza Triptych in the Brussels Museum', *The Burlington Magazine*, 113 (1971), 252–3) and J. Mesnil (*L'Art au Nord et au Sud des Alpes à l'époque de la Renaissance* (Brussels and Paris, 1911), 32–9) suggest that Alessandro's and Costanza's daughter and son, Battista and Costanzo, are portrayed. A third hypothesis, sustained by Josée Mambour, is that the female figure is Alessandro's second wife, Sveva of Montefeltro. Mambour, too, is of the opinion that the young man is Costanzo (because of the resemblance to Costanzo's portrait on medals), and notes that his tabard recalls the coat of arms of the Varano family ('Sveva de Montefeltre est-elle la donatrice représentée sur le triptyque Sforza?', *Musées Royales Beaux-Arts*, 17 (1968), 99–110).

[12] It is unfortunate that in English 'great balls' conjures up 19th-c. Assembly Rooms. The Italian is 'gran balli'. 'Balls' is used here and in the following chapter to mean entertainments dedicated to dancing.

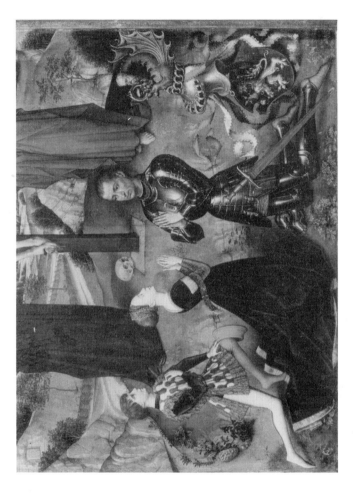

5. Rogier van der Weyden (workshop), *The 'Sforza' Triptych* (detail)
(Musées Royaux des Beaux-Arts, Brussels)

Domenico da Piacenza/da Ferrara

In his Autobiography, Guglielmo/Giovanni Ambrosio[13] mentions his esteemed mentor, Domenico, on only two occasions. One is a wedding celebration in Forlì in 1462, which indeed seems to have had as its only attraction for him the fact that Domenico and he were there together [9]. On that occasion no specific reference is made to dancing, whereas at the lavish celebrations for the betrothal of the 10-year-old Ippolita Sforza to the Duke of Calabria in Milan in 1455, Guglielmo and Domenico apparently performed in and collaborated on the choreography and direction of *moresche* (dance entertainments in costume), as well as composing *balli* for, and organizing, the general dancing [11].[14]

Francesco Sforza: Duke of Milan 1450–1466

The close relationship that existed between Alessandro Sforza and his brother Francesco (who assured to himself the position of first Sforza Duke of Milan through his military defence of that city and his marriage to Bianca Maria Visconti, the last Visconti heir to the Duchy) explains the numerous occasions mentioned in the Autobiography in which Alessandro, together with Guglielmo, was at Francesco's side.[15] One of the earliest autobiographical entries by Guglielmo/Giovanni Ambrosio is the account of a visit that Francesco— not yet Duke—and his wife Bianca Maria (see Pls. 6–7) paid to Alessandro and Costanza in Pesaro in 1447 [3].[16]

It has been generally assumed that Guglielmo was, for a time, in the service of the Sforzas in Milan.[17] According to his Autobiography, however, at almost every one of the festivities that was held in Milan between the years 1450 and

[13] The Autobiography is written in Giovanni Ambrosio's name, that is, the name Guglielmo took on his conversion. For the sake of clarity, however, I have preferred in this chapter to use the name Guglielmo throughout—even after his conversion, although when quoting from the Autobiography I shall often put both names. I have modernized and standardized the various spellings of Giovanni Ambrosio's name (Zuan Ambrosio, Giovanni ambruogio, Giohane Ambroxio, govananbruozio, Joanni Ambroxo, Giohambrosio, etc.) to avoid confusion.

[14] That dancing was a part of the festivities in Forlì is confirmed in a contemporary chronicle (Castelli, 'Il moto aristotelico', n. 57). For a discussion of *moresche*, see Ch. 3. Guglielmo/Giovanni Ambrosio states here, and on other occasions in his Autobiography, that he was present at the festivity to 'fare moresche e molti altri balli', which translates literally as 'to make' or 'do' *moresche*. Not only is the verb ambiguous (Guglielmo may have performed *or* choreographed them, or both), but even *balli* (see Glossary) may refer to a specific dance type, or to dances in general.

[15] Prior to Alessandro's marriage, Francesco had already made him a governor in the Marches (Litta). On many occasions Alessandro fought alongside Francesco in his military campaigns.

[16] This is confirmed by Abati-Olivieri Giordani, *Memorie*, who mentions other visits prior to this one. The first took place in 1445 when Costanza was pregnant. The following year Francesco came alone, once during the winter and again when Battista was born.

[17] See, among others, Gallo, 'L'autobiografia', 193; M. Padovan, 'La danza alla corte degli Sforza', in the catalogue of the exhibition *Leonardo e gli spettacoli del suo tempo* (Milan, 1983), 77; Bianchi, 'Tre maestri di danza alla corte di Francesco Sforza', *ASL* 89 (1962), 290–9; Toscanini, 'Notizie', 70. Marrocco, *Inventory*, 13, assumes that Galeazzo Sforza was Guglielmo's patron.

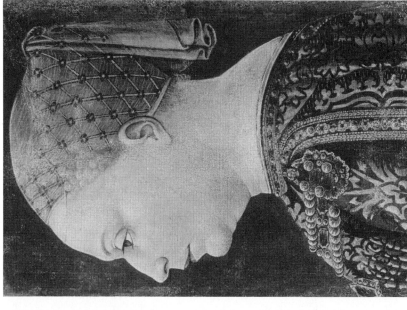

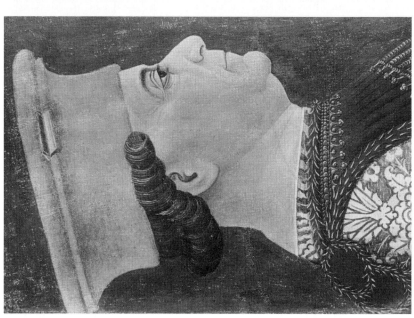

6–7. Bonifacio Bembo (attributed to), *Francesco Sforza and Bianca Maria Sforza* (Brera, Milan)

1466 (Francesco's reign as Duke), Guglielmo was there present in the company of Alessandro Sforza or of Alessandro's son Costanzo. This is the case when Francesco made his entry into Milan in 1450 [10]; at Ippolita Sforza's betrothal in 1455 [11]; at various receptions in 1459 connected with the visit of Pope Pius II, who was on his way to the Diet in Mantua [13] [16] [12?]; and at the celebration of Francesco's becoming lord of Genoa in 1464 [15].

There are two entries (dated 1460 in Gallo, 'L'autobiografia') in which Guglielmo describes being at Francesco Sforza's court, and no mention is made of Alessandro. This, however, does not necessarily mean that Alessandro was not present nor—were that even the case—that Guglielmo was no longer in his service. The first is an account of an entertainment in Pavia given by Francesco and Bianca Maria (almost certainly at the Sforza castle), at which Guglielmo was asked to 'fare' (prepare and/or perform) a *moresca* [26]. The other describes an important reception in Milan in which Francesco honoured the ambassador of King Louis XI of France. A great deal of dancing took place, but who organized it is not specified [27].[18]

Positive evidence supporting the theory that Guglielmo remained in Alessandro's service throughout Francesco's reign is contained in the letter, dated 15 July 1466, which Guglielmo sent from Naples to Bianca Maria Sforza: 'I believe that your Excellency must know that I am with his Majesty the King [Ferdinand I of Naples, Ferrante] *inasmuch as he sent to his Lordship Messer Alessandro [Sforza] that I was to come and teach* Madonna Lionora, his daughter, and Madonna Beatrice the Lombard [style] of dancing'. Guglielmo adds that the King of Naples has not allowed him leave to go to Milan but that he and Madonna Lionora (Eleonora, presumably still betrothed to Bianca Maria's son Sforza Maria) 'cannot wait for that day to come'.[19]

---

[18] It is worth noting that Antonio Cornazano was in the service of Francesco Sforza from 1455 to 1465, and although—according to his own account (V)—he did teach Ippolita Sforza dancing, he was not a professional dancing-master. (Whether Cornazano was Ippolita's only teacher, how much he taught her, and under what circumstances, is not known.) Furthermore, despite his being present at Ippolita's betrothal—and presumably at other festivities that Guglielmo also attended—the latter never mentions him.

[19] As of 1986 there is no longer any trace of this letter which was transcribed and published in E. Motta, 'Musici alla corte degli Sforza', *ASL* 4 (1887), 61–3, where it is listed as being in Potenze sovrane: Ippolita Sforza in the State Archives of Milan. The fact that Guglielmo had to inform Bianca Maria that he was in Naples because the King had sent to Pesaro for him to teach *his* (Ferrante's) daughters casts serious doubts on the assumption (see for example, Pontremoli and La Rocca, *Il ballare lombardo*, 53, and M. Padovan, 'Guglielmo Ebreo da Pesaro e i maestri del XV secolo', in *Mesura*, 77) that Bianca Maria's daughter Ippolita brought Guglielmo with her from Milan to Naples at the time of her wedding in 1465. The betrothal—or marriage— of (E)Leonora of Aragon to Sforza Maria was arranged earlier that year, just before Francesco's death. Four years later (1472) it was rescinded when the new duke, Galeazzo Maria, decided to make a more important alliance with Naples: that is, the marriage of his own son Giangaleazzo to Isabella, daughter of the Duke of Calabria and granddaughter of the King of Naples. The King, for his part, had arranged for Eleonora to marry Ercole d'Este, Duke of Ferrara. (Caterina Santoro, 'Nozze Sforzesche del Quattrocento', in *Città di Milano*, 70 (1953), 95.)

Naples: c.1465–c.1467

Six days later one of Bianca Maria's emissaries in Naples sent her another letter which included, among other things, a description of a banquet and dancing at which 'the palm was given to Lady Beatrice, the King's daughter, and her partner was our Giovanni Ambrosio, formerly a Jew, who, I understand, has been her teacher'.[20] It is not surprising that Guglielmo—while continuing in Alessandro Sforza's service—passed two years [17] (presumably 1465–7) at the court of Naples, inasmuch as Alessandro, an important ally of the King of Naples, had been given an official position at that court, and he and his son Costanzo spent long periods there between 1462 and 1466.[21] Moreover, it was common practice in fifteenth-century Italy to send a member of one's retinue to another court to teach the young princes or to help organize special festivities,[22] and it is quite possible that prior to Guglielmo's stay in Naples he also served Francesco and Bianca Maria Sforza on special occasions or for brief periods.

Guglielmo's letter to Bianca Maria suggests that he was seeking her help to enable him to return to Milan. However, Francesco Sforza's death earlier that year and the investiture of his son Galeazzo as Duke of Milan will have curtailed her powers of patronage. Guglielmo had dedicated *De pratica* to Galeazzo three years earlier. He may well have been disappointed that his gift had borne no fruit, for at Galeazzo's wedding in 1468 he limits himself to a terse account of what appears to be his last participation at a Sforza function in Milan, the high point for him being the presence of Count Federico of Urbino (who was

---

[20] '. . . tute ballavano bene. Ma l'honore fu dato a madama Beatrice figlia regale et con Ley balava il nostro Johan ambrosio che fu Judeo, quale secondo ho inteso e stato il magistro suo.' The letter, dated 21 July 1466, also reports on the warmth and affection shown to Ippolita Sforza (Bianca Maria's daughter) by both her husband and the King of Naples and describes a tournament at which Ippolita and 'Elionora' were the judges (Milan, State Archives, Sforzesco, Potenze estere, c. 215).

[21] Alessandro had helped the Aragons to drive the Angevins out of Naples, and so grateful was King Ferdinand I that in 1462 he gave Alessandro the Duchy of Sora and made him his deputy-general and the *Gran Conestabile* of the Realm. Alessandro spent more than a year in the Kingdom of Naples and returned there again in 1464. Two years later he sent his son Costanzo, to whom the King had promised his niece Camilla in marriage, to represent him in Naples. (Abati-Olivieri Giordani, *Memorie*; Eiche, 'Alessandro Sforza'.)

[22] In 1480 Bona of Savoy, the widow of Galeazzo Sforza, allowed the dancing-master Lorenzo Lavagnolo—in her retinue since the preceding year—to return briefly to his former patrons, Federico and Margaret Gonzaga of Mantua, who requested his services prior to the marriage of their daughter (Chiara) (Motta, 'Musici', 63–4). Back in the Gonzagas' service (at least in 1483), Lavagnolo was sent by them to Ferrara in 1485 to teach the sisters Isabella, Beatrice, and Lucretia d'Este. The following year the Bentivoglio family arranged for him to go to Bologna in December to prepare the festivities for Lucretia d'Este's marriage to Annibale Bentivoglio in January. In April 1488, after having spent some time with Elisabetta Gonzaga in Urbino (following her marriage to Guidobaldo of Montefeltro in February of that year), Lavagnolo returned to Mantua. (A. Luzio and R. Renier, *Mantova e Urbino: Isabella d'Este ed Elisabetta Gonzaga* (Turin and Rome, 1893; repr. Bologna, 1976), 6 n. 1, 41–3). Also see the description of Roberto Malatesta's wedding, in which the engineers came from Florence, the musicians from Ferrara, and the cooks from Bologna (below), and n. 59.

later to become his patron) [19]. His desire, however, to make the 'Milan connection' must have been very strong, and Guglielmo was to make at least two more attempts to this end before he died.

Guglielmo's conversion and marriage

Guglielmo's letter to Bianca Maria has another, quite different, importance. It begins 'Yhesus' and ends 'lo vostro figliolo [your son; godson] Giovanni Ambrosio da Pesaro'. The date of Guglielmo's conversion is not known, but one year before this letter—in May 1465—Alessandro Sforza had written to his brother Francesco informing him that he had arranged for 'our Giovanni Ambrosio . . . who is Christian to marry again'. (All that is known of this second wife is that she was the daughter of Pier Paolo di Berardi, 'a good citizen of Pesaro'.) Guglielmo's conversion, therefore, took place between 11 October 1463 (the date on which *De pratica* was terminated) and 5 May 1465, the date on which di Berardi himself wrote to Francesco Sforza thanking him for consenting to the marriage.[23] It is probable that Guglielmo, who took the name Ambrosio, after the patron saint of Milan, was baptized in that city, and that Bianca Maria Sforza and Duke Francesco were his godparents.[24]

There have been various conjectures regarding the motives for Guglielmo's conversion, including the suggestion that he had been the victim of anti-Semitism. This seems improbable, however, because, despite isolated episodes, fomented for the most part by fanatics of the Franciscan order, Jews in fifteenth-century Italy had citizenship and their everyday relations with Christians were cordial.[25] Many popes and princes, including the Estes, the Gonzagas, Lorenzo de' Medici, and Francesco Sforza, are known to have treated Jews with consideration.[26] Moreover, when Jews began to escape from

[23] Padovan, 'Guglielmo Ebreo' (78 and 82), publishes facsimiles and partial transcriptions of both letters. The originals are in the State Archives of Milan, Sforzesco, Potenze estere, Marca 147.

[24] Presumably Guglielmo's conversion resulted in his becoming an *all[i]evo* ('foster child or servant of one's bringing up', Florio) of Francesco Sforza (see below, Costanzo Sforza's letter to Bona of Savoy), as well as the Duke's 'most faithful servant, retainer, and slave' (di Berardi's letter; see n. 23), and explains the Milanese emissary's reference to him as '*our* Giovanni Ambrosio'. This does not prove, however, that Francesco's patronage of Guglielmo was either exclusive or more than honorary, inasmuch as Guglielmo, soon after di Berardi's letter, was sent to Naples *by Alessandro*, and the letter to his godmother, Francesco's wife, expressing his desire to return to Milan, went unheeded.

[25] See, for example, L. Poliakov, *I banchieri ebrei e la Santa Sede del XIII al XVII secolo* (tr. from the French; Rome, 1974), 144–5, etc.; A. Milano, *Biblioteca historica italo-giudaica* (Florence, 1954). Pontremoli affirms: 'Although conditions were far better than in the preceding century, there were still episodes of anti-Semitism', and cites A. Antoniazzi Villa, 'Fonti notarili per la storia degli Ebrei nei domini sforzeschi', in *Libri e documenti*, 3 (1981), 1–10.

[26] According to Milano, *Biblioteca*, 156 and 158, 'Under Pope Eugene IV various Roman Jews preferred to move to Mantua under the tranquil marquisate of Gianfrancesco Gonzaga, just as under Nicholas V others turned to the equally welcoming one of Leonello d'Este.' When Pope Pius II (1458–64) asked the Jews for an annual contribution of 5% of their property, 'The Duke of Milan informed him that his Jews were unable to meet the new tax or any other . . .'.

the persecution rampant in Spain, it was the independent Kingdom of Naples and other Italian states that granted them asylum, and this a whole generation after Guglielmo's conversion.[27] In fact, it was not until Naples fell under the direct control of Aragon, in the early sixteenth century, that the Jews were expelled from that part of southern Italy.

On the other hand, it is conceivable that Guglielmo was urged to convert by his patron Alessandro Sforza, in whom 'A marked turn towards piety and a certain sobriety can be noted in his private affairs from the early 1460s on'.[28] He founded 'charitable and pious institutions' and 'gave himself into the care of . . . the Franciscans'. His 'intense religious fervour' and 'newly-found spirituality' extended also to his relationship with his mistress . . . He spared no pains in entreating her to pursue, as he himself was doing, a more pious mode of living'.

Another hypothesis is that Guglielmo changed his name and religion when his reputation was already made and he was at the peak of his career because he had high hopes regarding further advantages that might accrue from Bianca Maria Sforza's and Duke Francesco's guardianship, and, like other artists after him, he aspired to the recognition and honour of knighthood, to attain which it was almost always requisite to be a Christian.[29] If it was in this hope that he converted he was not disappointed, for early in 1469 he was indeed knighted in Venice by none other than Frederick III, the Holy Roman Emperor himself, during a magnificent visit of state [20].[30] The title conferred was Knight of the Golden Spur.[31]

[27] Cecil Roth, *History of the Jews* (New York, 1961).

[28] Eiche, 'Alessandro Sforza', 91–3.

[29] According to Walter Toscanini, who first made a connection between Guglielmo's conversion and his knighthood, it was advantageous—and not unusual—to convert under the patronage of some noble person. (Correspondence, 1965, New York Public Library, Dance Collection.) It is interesting to note the following commentary in the 1985 Caravaggio exhibition in Naples: 'Probably attracted by the desire—common to many of his fellow artists—to receive the title of Knight of the Order of Malta, Caravaggio moved to that island.' Joyce Mollow, whose paper 'Interaction of the 15th Century Jewry with the Italian Renaissance' (in *Guglielmo*) mentions the knighthood bestowed on the rabbi and physician Messer Judah Leon by the Holy Roman Emperor Frederick III, informed me that this took place *without* a conversion. And Alessandra Veronese has confirmed to me in a letter that '*in most cases*' conversion was necessary prior to knighthood. There were, however, a few exceptions, which apparently provoked a certain amount of protest, since it was contrary to contemporary practices. M. Inglehearn also addresses the question of knighthood and Italian Jews, but is of the opinion that Guglielmo and Giovanni Ambrosio were two different people ('A Little-Known Fifteenth-Century Italian Dance Treatise', *Music Review*, 42 (1981), 174–81). As late as 1966, Dante Bianchi, in a letter to Walter Toscanini, draws similar conclusions regarding Domenico of Ferrara and Domenico of Piacenza. (See also his 'Tre maestri di danza'.)

[30] In December 1468, sixteen years after his coronation journey, Frederick III returned to Italy on a pilgrimage (Eiche, 'Alessandro Sforza', 230–4). He stopped in Pesaro on his way to and from Rome. 'Throughout his journey the Emperor sold titles and honours at considerable profit to himself. This disreputable practice was standard procedure . . .' (as can be seen by another reference in Eiche: 'On the return north from his coronation trip in 1452 Frederick created Borso d'Este Duke of Modena and Reggio for an annual census of a staggering 4,000 *fiorini d'oro*'

A few months later, at the end of July, Galeazzo Maria Sforza, now Duke of Milan, was sent a recommendation on Guglielmo's behalf together with a request to receive him—the occasion being the forthcoming wedding festivities of the Duke's sister—from the Count of Urbino (Federico of Montefeltro) through Galeazzo's ambassador at that court. The young Duke's reply, written the following October, is shocking, particularly in the light of the mutual esteem which had existed between his father, Francesco Sforza, and Guglielmo, and of the recent knighthood probably procured for Guglielmo (as a favour to a devoted member of the household) by Alessandro Sforza. 'Give no hearing to that Ambrosio, alias Jew, who has said certain things against Camillo, but treat him for what he is.' (It has been suggested that 'Camillo' refers to Camillo Borzi, the ambassador of Urbino at the court of Milan.[32]) For the present it is impossible to know if this statement is an example of Galeazzo's general arrogance (he was considered a cruel, corrupt, and greedy ruler[33]), his contempt for dancing-masters, for Jews, or for Guglielmo in particular, or whether, on the other hand, it tells us something, albeit enigmatically, about Guglielmo's personality.

Giuseppe Ebreo of Pesaro

In May 1467 a contract was signed in Florence between Guglielmo's brother Giuseppe ('Joseph the Jew of Pesaro, dancing-master') and a Christian named Francesco ('dancing- and music-teacher') in which a 'society' was established where men and women could learn dancing, singing, and instrumental

(412 n. 25)). However, during this second journey, the Emperor was so impressed with the great honour paid him by Alessandro, that he gave him permission to use his coat of arms (the imperial eagle), and he granted a great many privileges to all his household, cost free (231). It may help to date Guglielmo's knighthood if we consider that Messer Leon (n. 29) was knighted that same year—on 21 Feb.—in Pordenone, 93 km. north-east of Venice, and on 13 Apr. Guglielmo (back in Urbino) wrote to Lorenzo de' Medici saying he had just returned from Venice where he had been knighted (McGee, 'Dancing Masters', Doc. II).

[31] The title 'Equitis Aurati' follows Giovanni Ambrosio's name in the library listing of the lost Urbino manuscript (Ch. 1, n. 46). Domenico was also 'cavaliere aurato' (see V, fo. 29ᵛ; Motta, *Nozze principesche*; Gallo, 'L'autobiografia', 193 and 195). That this was a distinguished order can be seen in the list of courtiers and household staff at the court of Duke Federico of Urbino discussed below, where in third place, after the princes and counts, come five 'Cavalieri a Speron d'Oro'. At the time only the Emperor or the Pope could confer this honour. The Order of the Golden Spur, which dates from the 14th c., still exists in Italy, although it has undergone many changes and the cross itself has been modified. (G. Bascapé, *Gli ordini cavallareschi in Italia nella storia e nel diritto* (Milan, 1972).)

[32] I wish to thank Maurizio Padovan for this information as well as for having sent me the copies he made of the two letters he discovered in the State Archives of Milan (Sforzesco, Potenze Estere, Marca, c. 147).

[33] See, for example, Litta, and V. Ilardi, 'The Assassination of Galeazzo Maria Sforza and the Reaction of Italian Diplomacy', in L. Martines (ed.), *Violence and Civil Disobedience in Italian Cities: 1200–1500* (Berkeley, Calif., 1972), 72–103.

music.[34] The agreement, drawn up by Leonardo da Vinci's father (the notary Piero di Antonio da Vinci), was to last one year and stipulated that all expenses, including rent, were to be equally shared.

Two years later we find Giuseppe in the employ of the 20-year-old Lorenzo de' Medici. (When and how this appointment came about is not known.) On 13 April 1469 his patron was sent two almost identical letters: one from Guglielmo/Giovanni Ambrosio, who had just returned from Venice where he had been knighted by the Emperor, the other from the Duke of Urbino.[35] The subject is Giuseppe's conversion, which had not taken place the year before in Milan at the time of Galeazzo Maria Sforza's wedding (according to a plan, Guglielmo claims, made by the brothers), because the plague in that city had prevented the attendance of the Florentine contingent. Guglielmo/ Giovanni Ambrosio is so concerned that Giuseppe be baptized that he suggests to the Magnificent that he himself come to Florence, adding that if Giuseppe 'should obstinately refuse to carry this out [that is, to become a Christian], I would not wish to have anything to do or share with him'.

Whether Giuseppe did convert is not known. His name, with the appellation 'the Jew', appears in the three Tuscan copies of *De pratica* as the composer of the *bassadanza Partita crudele*.[36] (Two *bassedanze* by Lorenzo de' Medici, *Lauro* and *Venus*, are in the same treatises.) The last extant reference to Giuseppe appears in another letter which Giovanni Ambrosio sent to Lorenzo seven years later, in 1476, in which he begs the Magnificent, in a rather obscure phrase, 'to remember my brother with regard to the office [appointment].[37]

Guglielmo's career: 1444–71

In the almost thirty-year span of his recorded career, Guglielmo's attention is to occasions where he danced and to court festivities he attended. In 1459 he

---

[34] Published and discussed in Veronese, 'Una societas', who gives the location of the original contract, in Latin, as the State Archives, Florence, Notarile Antecosimiano, P. 350 (1465–7), fo. 276ᵛ.

[35] Published in Italian with an English translation and a commentary in McGee, 'Dancing Masters'. The originals are in the State Archives, Florence: MAP (Mediceo avanti il Principato), Filza XX, no. 477 and Filza XXIII, no. 241. The second letter is also published in S. Cerboni Bairdi *et al.* (eds.), *Federico di Montefeltro: Lo Stato* (Rome, 1986), 480–1.

[36] NY, FL, FN. A version of *Partita crudele* (anonymous) also appears in S.

[37] Published and translated into English in McGee, 'Dancing Masters'. The letter, written 29 May 1476, is in the State Archives, Florence, MAP, Filza XXXIII, no. 414. (I have examined the handwriting of both this letter and the one Guglielmo sent to Lorenzo seven years earlier. It seems to me that the letters are in different hands and that they are the work of professional scribes.) McGee reports (210 n. 18) that none of the Medici household records from this period has survived nor are any dancing-masters listed in the pay records of the civic government during the years of the Republic. He suggests that Giuseppe may have been employed privately by the Medici family, and adds that tracing him 'is further complicated by the possibility that he may have converted to Christianity and, like his brother, changed his name . . . .'.

was in Padua at a wedding at which the entire Council of Venice was present [18]. He visited Bologna three times for wedding celebrations, the first taking place in 1454 when Alessandro Sforza's daughter Ginevra married into the influential Bentivoglio family [6], [7], [14].[38] He attended the marriage of Federico Gonzaga to Margaret of Bavaria that was held in Mantua in 1463 [22]. In 1469 and 1471 he was in Pesaro again at two entertainments (both included dancing) given by Alessandro Sforza: one at the port [28] and the other an eighteen-course banquet—with 'sets of masques'—for Shrovetide [24].

Guglielmo was in Ravenna in 1448 when Francesco Sforza celebrated his victory over the Venetians at Caravaggio, though he had come not to dance but to buy grain. This fact suggests that the relationship between Guglielmo and Alessandro may have been more than the simple one of court dancing-master and patron. On this occasion, at least, Guglielmo is a trusted retainer engaged in a special mission [4].[39]

Alessandro Sforza died in 1473, and nothing is known of Guglielmo's whereabouts until 1476. It was heretofore supposed that in this interim Guglielmo returned to Naples, inasmuch as his Autobiography (which, however, is not in chronological order) ends with descriptions of three events which took place in Naples (Gallo 'Autobiografia'). But at least one of these events happened 'many years ago'; while the first, an entertainment with which the King of Naples did honour to the ambassador of the Duke of Burgundy (Charles the Bold), is described as having 'French balli performed by the Duchess [of Calabria, Ippolita Sforza] and by Lady [E]Leonora [of Aragon]'.[40] Clearly, this entry must be dated before Eleonora left Naples in 1473, on her way to her wedding with Ercole d'Este in Ferrara (Ch. 3, n. 30).

Guglielmo also noted that during the entertainment 'Don Federico', the 22-year-old son of the King of Naples (whose sisters—including Eleonora—Guglielmo had taught to dance), performed with his brother Alfonso, Duke of Calabria, 'a mummery of masques, dressed in the French fashion'. In the late autumn of 1474, the same Don Federico arrived in Urbino on his way to Burgundy. Duke Federico of Montefeltro received him grandly and among the entertainments in his honour there was a spectacular allegory with moresche

---

[38] Guglielmo's bassadanza Genevra was probably composed for her, perhaps even for the occasion of her marriage. It is the third choreography in De pratica, the first being Domenico's Reale, which may have been composed in honour of Francesco Sforza, while the second is Guglielmo's Alexandresca, almost certainly in honour of Alessandro Sforza.

[39] According to Eiche, 'Alessandro Sforza', 46, 'The significance of grain in the economic life of the Marches is evinced by the establishment of a market square devoted solely to the trade in cereals.'

[40] See App. III [30]. Gallo ('Autobiografia') has documented a visit of the Duke of Burgundy's ambassador in 1474, and Pontremoli and La Rocca, Il ballare lombardo, have noted another one in 1475 (50). I am presuming, but have so far not been able to confirm, that an ambassador from Burgundy also came to the Kingdom in 1466, the year that we know for certain that Guglielmo was in Naples.

(see Ch. 3). We do not know who arranged the dancing or whether Guglielmo was asked—by either the Duke of Urbino or the King of Naples—to
participate in any of the festivities, or if he was included in the entourage that
accompanied the young Aragonese prince on his long journey.

And although we know that Guglielmo had arranged some of the dance
entertainments for Elisabetta Montefeltro's engagement to Roberto Malatesta
in Urbino in 1471 [23], neither his name, nor that of any other dancing-master,
appears in the documents for the actual wedding, which took place in Rimini
four years later. (The festivities, which included jousts and mock battles, lasted
eight days, and cost 35,000 ducats.[41] Duke Federico, the bride's father, was in
attendance, and Mario Filelfo and Pietro Bono were among the guests.[42])

We also remain in ignorance about the name of the person responsible for
the dancing and spectacles performed at the marriage of Alessandro Sforza's
son Costanzo to Camilla of Aragon (Pesaro, May 1475, see Ch. 3); but let us
hope that Guglielmo's faithful service to both families gave him some part
in them.

Federico of Montefeltro, Duke of Urbino

Presumably, sometime after Alessandro Sforza's death (1473), Guglielmo
entered the service of Federico of Montefeltro in Urbino. It is from here that
he wrote to Lorenzo de' Medici in May 1476, signing the letter 'Your faithful
servant Giovanni Ambrosio Alessandresco, in the retinue of the Duke of
Urbino'.[43] And in 1481 another letter informs us that the 6-year-old Isabella
d'Este 'danced twice with that Ambrosio, formerly a Jew, and [who] is with
the most illustrious lord Duke of Urbino as his dancing-master'.[44] Guglielmo,
who clearly admired Federico, had continued to have contact with him ever
since Federico's first marriage in 1437. Federico alone is mentioned among the
guests both at Alessandro Sforza's wedding in 1444 [2] and at that of Galeazzo
Sforza in 1468 [19].

[41] From a paper by Daniel Bornstein, 'The Wedding Feast of Roberto de' Malatesta and Isabetta
da Montefeltro: Etiquette and Power', delivered at the 19th International Congress of Medieval
Studies, May 1984, Kalamazoo, Michigan. Most of the documents consulted for the paper were
from the Civic Library in Rimini. The value of 35,000 ducats can be grasped if it is compared
with the average yearly earnings of a labourer, which was about 48 ducats (see McGee, 'Dancing
Masters', 216 n. 30. See also Ch. 1, n. 59).

[42] Pietro Bono, who appears in Castiglione's *The Book of the Courtier*, was a singer and the
most celebrated lutenist of the Italian Renaissance. He spent most of his life at the Este court in
Ferrara and was in the retinue sent to Naples to accompany Ercole d'Este's bride, Eleonora of
Aragon, to Ferrara. Filelfo gave the wedding oration for which he received '50 ducats and some
cloth' (Clough, see Ch. 1, n. 31).

[43] For my interpretation of 'Alessandresco', see above, n. 8. McGee, 'Dancing Masters', on the
other hand (208), suggests that Guglielmo refers 'to himself as "an Alexandrine", probably an
identification with Alexandria, Egypt, his ancestral origin (or possibly his place of birth)'.

[44] An excerpt from this letter, written by a certain Guido di Bagno and sent from Ferrara on
24 Jan. 1481, was first published in A. Luzio, *I precettori di Isabella d'Este* (Ancona, 1887), 12.

Guglielmo's two patrons were doubly connected. Alessandro had made a political second marriage in 1448, taking to wife Federico's half-sister Sveva Colonna of Montefeltro [5].[45] In 1460 the two families became even more closely tied when Alessandro's daughter Battista married Federico himself in Urbino [8] (see Pls. 8 and 9). In the same year Guglielmo, who had attended these weddings, was at the reception that Federico gave for Alfonso of Avalos [25]. It was Carnival and there was dancing and *moresche*, but it is not clear what part, if any, Guglielmo had in their organization or performance. In 1471, however, for the betrothal celebrations in Urbino of Federico's daughter Elisabetta to Roberto Malatesta, Lord of Rimini, he arranged a suite of *moresche* [23].

Federico was proclaimed Duke of Urbino in 1474. Some time earlier that same year he was in Naples where he was invested as a Knight of the Ermine. We do not know if Guglielmo attended either of these events. The copy of *De pratica* which Guglielmo/Giovanni Ambrosio dedicated to Federico was donated after he became Duke,[46] and was, no doubt, Guglielmo's tribute to a staunch patron and a noble prince, whose qualities and glorious palace were later to be admired and praised by Castiglione in the opening pages of *The Book of the Courtier*.

Guglielmo and his son are listed as dancing-masters and 'ballarini' ('Maestro Giovanni Ambrosio' and 'maestro Pierpaulo suo figluolo') in a record of the courtiers and retinue attached to Duke Federico's court.[47] The document is uncompromising about the position of the dancing-master, even at a court as humanistically inclined as that of Urbino. After the princes (Orsini, Colonna, Farnese, etc.) come the counts, then five 'Knights of the Golden Spur', and various gentlemen and counsellors. These are followed by the Duke's masters of grammar, logic, and philosophy (one of whom is Mario Filelfo); the Duke's secretaries and ambassadors; his chancellors; stewards; chamberlains; the carvers, squires, and readers for his table; his library scribes; his pages; his architects and engineers; singers of the chapel and choirboys; lackeys . . . and kitchen stewards; weavers and upholsterers; miniaturists; fencing-masters to the pages; and finally—though not quite at the end—our dancing-masters.[48]

---

[45] In the Siena redaction of *De pratica*, Guglielmo's *ballo Colonnese* bears the dedication, 'Composed for Madonna Sveva of the Colonna family'. She may appear in the Sforza Triptych; see above, n. 11.

[46] The copy, which has not survived, bore a dedication to Federico as Prince and Duke (Gallo, 'L'autobiografia', 195).

[47] The document is in the Biblioteca Vaticana, cod. Urb. 1204, according to G. Zannoni, who reprints it in his 'I due libri della Mariados di Giovan Mario Filelfo', in *Rendiconti della Reale Accademia dei Lincei*, ser. 4, iii (1894), 666–71. It is without any date, but was set down at the beginning of the 16th c. by an old courtier called Susech, after the death of Federico's son Guidobaldo. (Mentioned as being at Guidobaldo's court are the various personages in *The Book of the Courtier*, including the 'Venetian Pie[t]ro Bembo' and Castiglione himself.)

[48] The list concludes with four captains employed in peace and war; three health officers; organists; old servants (including Guidobaldo's wet-nurse) and retired gentlemen; the warden of

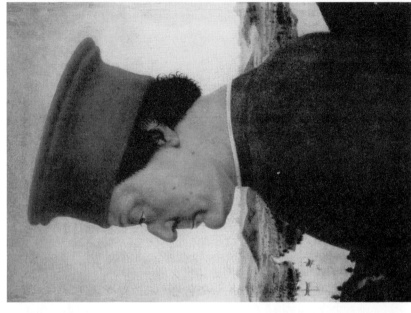

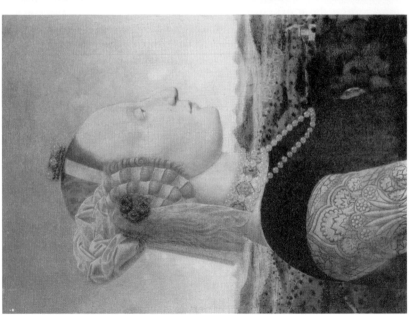

8–9. Piero della Francesca, *Battista Sforza and Federico of Montefeltro* (Uffizi, Florence)

One may well ask where in all of this—not necessarily rigorous—hierarchy is Giovanni Ambrosio, created Knight of the Golden Spur by the Emperor himself in 1469.

Nothing is known of Guglielmo's son, who may have been named after his maternal grandfather. If he is the same Pierpaolo described by Castiglione in *The Book of the Courtier*, it would seem that he did not inherit his father's talents:

We can truthfully say that true art is what does not seem to be art . . . So you see that to reveal intense application and skill robs everything of grace. Who is there among you who doesn't laugh when our Pierpaolo dances in that way of his, with those little jumps and with his legs stretched on tiptoes, keeping his head motionless, as if he were made of wood, and all so laboured that he seems to be counting every step? Who is so blind that he doesn't see in this the clumsiness of affectation?[49]

Lorenzo de' Medici

As mentioned above, in 1469 Guglielmo wrote to Lorenzo de' Medici concerning his brother's conversion, suggesting that if he were invited to Florence, he and Giuseppe would arrange 'pleasant and novel' entertainments. When, or if, Guglielmo and the Magnificent ever met is not at all clear. According to a letter sent to Florence in 1476, Guglielmo, while still in the retinue of the Duke of Urbino, was also serving Lorenzo. He writes, for example, that because of illness he has been unable 'to carry out my duty toward your magnificence', that 'I cannot offer you anything else except to be a devoted ambassador for your magnificence always', and that 'I shall always want you to choose me for your servant'. He thanks Lorenzo 'a thousand times over' for his 'most worthy gift' and announces his arrival in Florence a month before Carnival (1477) 'so that we can prepare things that are most excellent and that have never been done in Florence'.

One wonders if Guglielmo did in fact participate in the Carnival festivities that winter, for Costanzo Sforza writes a letter to Lorenzo the following June (1477) informing him that 'Messer Giovanni Ambrosio, master of dancing', whom he recommends most highly, 'is coming first to visit your magnificence

the keys; the pantry servant; the armourer; and the bailiffs in charge of hemp, straw, and provender. McGee, 'Dancing Masters', 213, has recently found a similar document (also undated) in the Biblioteca Universitaria in Urbino (*Manoscritti comunale*, Busta 118, fos. 14 ff.) in which 'M[aestr]o Ambrogio' and 'M[aestr]o Pietro Paulo suo figlio', again listed as dancing-masters and 'ballarini', are numbers 183 and 184 on a list of 203 members of Duke Federico's 'famiglia' (household).

[49] Castiglione, *The Book of the Courtier*, tr. G. Bull (Harmondsworth, 1967; repr. 1976), 67–8. The events described in the book take place in 1507. McGee, 'Dancing Masters', 213, confirms that 'no record could be found in the archives of Urbino providing any other details of the life of Pietro Paulo'. Another possible interpretation of Pierpaolo's 'gracelessness' is that he was dancing in an outmoded style—that of his father.

and secondly to give you a work on dance that he composed and dedicated to you'. He begs Lorenzo to accept his recommendation since he knows Giovanni Ambrosio 'to be the affectionate servant of your magnificence'.[50] Did Guglielmo in fact present himself at the Medici court, and did Lorenzo receive such a copy of *De pratica* dedicated to him by Guglielmo as Giovanni Ambrosio?[51] At all events, the relationship between the dancing-master and the Magnificent was such as to justify an appeal to Lorenzo by Camilla of Aragon, the widow of Alessandro Sforza's son Costanzo, to which the Medici prince replied on 21 April 1484, 'excusing us for not being able to offer any charity to M[esse]r Giovanni Ambrosio because of the multitude of poor here [in Florence]'.[52]

Guglielmo's last years

This touching letter is, to date, the last news we have of Guglielmo, and one would like to think that although he had outlived his patrons—Alessandro Sforza having died in 1473, Duke Federico of Urbino in 1482, and Alessandro's son Costanzo in 1483—that 'Lady Camilla' continued to look after the faithful old servant of the house of Sforza. Three years earlier, the report of him dancing with the young Isabella d'Este in Ferrara indicates that he was well and still in the service of the Duke of Urbino.[53] The preceding year, 1480, Guglielmo seems to have made one more attempt to obtain a position at the Sforza court in Milan. On 1 August Costanzo Sforza wrote to Galeazzo Sforza's widow Bona and her son, the 11-year-old Duke of Milan, Giangaleazzo:[54]

Messer Giovanni Ambrosio, the bearer of this letter, godson of the late lord, Duke Francesco of happy memory, and of the lord my father and old servant of [our] house, more gifted in the art of dancing than anyone in Italy, and having understood that your Excellency is now ready to take up such accomplishments, it behoves me to set out how great his accomplishments are in this field. And since I know him [to be] the

---

[50] Published and translated into English in McGee, 'Dancing Masters'. The letter is dated 1 June 1477 and is in the State Archives, Florence, MAP, Filza XXXV, no. 483.

[51] Where is this copy? (The two Florentine redactions of *De pratica*, without dedications, are in Guglielmo's name, not Giovanni Ambrosio's.) Is it listed in any inventory of the Medici library? Is there an extant list of expenditures for the Carnival festivities of 1477 and if so, is Giovanni Ambrosio's name on it?

[52] Published and translated into English in McGee, 'Dancing Masters', 213. Whereas McGee has translated *elemosina* ('alms' according to Florio) as 'pension', I prefer 'charity'. State Archives, Florence, MAP, Filza LXIII, p. 287. The letter itself is lost; the citation is from an annotation in a register of Lorenzo's letters.

[53] See above and n. 44.

[54] This letter, in a most beautiful hand, and the reply (most probably a chancellery minute) are in the State Archives, Milan, Sforzesco, Potenze estere, Marca 150. Published and translated into English in Sparti, 'Questions Concerning the Life and Works of Guglielmo Ebreo', in *Guglielmo*, 42–3, 46–7; transcriptions and photographic reprints in Padovan, 'Guglielmo Ebreo', 78–9, 83.

foremost in this art and that he can truly be called the master, and that he taught all the gentlemen and the children of gentlemen and ladies who were in Italy during his lifetime; and [because I know] him to have the best method and manner of teaching of anyone in the world, I had the idea of trusting him to you and recommending him to your excellencies, and I assure [you] again that for teaching this sort of accomplishment, no one can be found in Italy who is the equal of him, as you will be able to see for yourselves.

The reply, dated Milan, 10 September, is signed 'Duces' and is addressed to Costanzo, 'Our beloved illustrious kinsman':

We received the jars that your lordship sent us with Messer Giovanni Ambrosio, the bearer of this, and we saw them gladly and received them most gratefully both because they are very beautiful and because of the love of your lordship, who we know sent them out of the goodness of his heart, as well as out of respect for Messer Giovanni Ambrosio who brought them, a most well-mannered and virtuous person. We saw him gladly and took pleasure in his accomplishments and it seems as if he deserves every commendation. And we therefore send him back so that your lordship and the illustrious lady your wife may take pleasure from his dancing and his other accomplishments and we recommend him to your lordship as a favour.

Guglielmo's heritage

After Guglielmo's death the popularity of at least one of his dances lived on into the sixteenth century and earned particular distinction. Around 1530, the humanist Giangiorgio Trissino cited what is almost certainly Giovanni Ambrosio's dance [*Voltati in ça*] *Rosina* together with what we presume to be Domenico's [*Rostiboli*] *Gioioso* and his *Leoncello* 'as examples . . . of the highest artistic production, of the same standard as Jannequin for music, Leonardo da Vinci for painting, and Homer, Dante, and Petrarch for poetry'.[55]

During his lifetime Guglielmo achieved a certain level of eminence as a dancing-master, attested not only by his knighthood and Filelfo's ode, but by the letters of Costanzo Sforza and Federico of Montefeltro. They considered

---

[55] Cited in Gallo, 'Il "ballare lombardo"', 82. *Rosina* was a well-known *frottola* which seems to have also been a dance-tune. According to K. Jeppesen, *Balli antichi veneziani/Old Venetian Dances* (Copenhagen, 1962), 'The . . . song is to be found in the later part of the 15th c. and lives on, with various texts, until the end of the following century, perhaps even longer.' (See App. II.) The name keeps cropping up—as does that of the *Gioioso* [*Rostiboli*?]—as a favourite, but it is difficult to know if or when the references are to those dances composed by Giovanni Ambrosio and Domenico. Both dances are mentioned as late as *c.*1540 in a letter written by the Venetian actor–playwright, Andrea Calmo (see *Le lettere di Messer Andrea Calmo*, ed. V. Rossi (Turin, 1888), 232). They appear again in *La Bilora* (*c.*1525), the comedy by Angelo Beolco (Ruzante), where old Andronico, racked by love for the young Bilora, says: 'I tell you that my legs are still so good that I have the spirit to dance four *tempi* of the *Gioioso* and can even perform it scrambled; and *Rosina* as well—done complete with flourishes—which would be no small feat.' (See D. Heartz, 'A 15th-Century Ballo: *Rôti Bouilli Joyeux*', in J. La Rue (ed.), *Aspects of Medieval and Renaissance Music, A Birthday Offering to Gustave Reese* (New York, 1966), 359–75 at 374.)

him 'more gifted in the art of dancing than anyone in Italy'; 'the foremost
in this art', one who could 'truly be called the master'; 'exceptional in his
profession'.[56] Alessandro Sforza described him as 'persevering in good and
honest living' characterized by 'good works and conduct' (see above). Yet
he suffered bitter experiences and disappointment. *De pratica* contains two
indicative and rather scathing passages in which he gives vent to his contempt
for both the general public and for some of his colleagues. Regarding the first
group, Guglielmo claims that the 'multitude of the spectators' judge dancing
subjectively—according to their pleasure and instinct rather than according to
reason or any understanding or knowledge of the art'.[57] In the Conclusion of
the theoretical part of his treatise, Guglielmo affirms that even after thirty
years' experience at various courts he still does not know all there is to know
about the art of dancing, whereas he has met others who call themselves
masters who 'hardly know their right foot from their left, and they believe
themselves to be truly expert in three days'.

Dancing as such, though an integral part of most entertainments and festivities, did not rank among the leading pursuits at Renaissance courts, and some
princes seem to have managed without any permanent dancing-masters at all.
Indeed, as I have already said, it is likely that *De pratica* was, in part at least,
an attempt to gain recognition for the dance. That Guglielmo himself felt the
need of recognition can, perhaps, be inferred from the condescension and
vehemence with which he speaks of 'mechanicals' and 'plebeians' (Preface and
Rejoinder I), not an unusual indication that one's own status may have been,
until recently, altogether too similar.[58] In effect, Guglielmo's social position,
as revealed in the list of Duke Federico's household, his futile attempts to
improve it through conversion and knighthood, as well as the fruitless dedication of *De pratica* to Galeazzo Sforza, can be summed up in the contemptuous
remark made by the same Galeazzo, to 'treat him for what he is'. Guglielmo's
unheeded requests to the King of Naples and to Bianca Maria Sforza to be
allowed to go to Milan, the humiliating experience of his being sent to the
young Duke of Milan—Giangaleazzo—and his mother simply to be packed
back to Pesaro, as well as Lorenzo de' Medici's refusal to 'give alms' for the
support of his last years, represent the more sombre sides of Guglielmo's
professional life.[59] These, together with the splendid festivities in which he

---

[56] Federico writes 'singulare . . . nel suo mestiere', which I have translated as 'exceptional'
rather than McGee's 'excellent'.

[57] See Rule II.

[58] It is also possible that Guglielmo may once again be emulating the humanists, for whom
scorn, disdain, and 'contempt for the multitude, the vulgar herd' (i.e. Alberti's 'the lazy and
cowardly plebeians') were common attitudes, virtue being equated with nobility, moral worth
with social rank (L. Martines, *Power and Imagination* (Baltimore, Md., 1979; repr. 1988), 212–15).

[59] In 15th-c. Italy, painting—like dancing—was not considered a liberal art and the worth of
a court painter was often measured by how much his work increased his patron's stature. Indeed,
it is interesting to note the parallels that exist between the career of Guglielmo Ebreo, dancing-

did take part, help to make more complete the picture of the art of the dance in Italy, of the fifteenth-century dancing-masters, and of the enigmatic Guglielmo/Giovanni Ambrosio himself.

master, and that of a painter such as Andrea Mantegna. When the Pope demanded that Mantegna work for him for two years, he was sent to Rome—against his will—by his patrons, the Gonzagas of Mantua. Mantegna too was knighted and his patrons also gave one of his sons a position at court. (Tuohy, 'Studies', and K. Simon, *A Renaissance Tapestry: The Gonzaga of Mantua* (NY, 1988).)

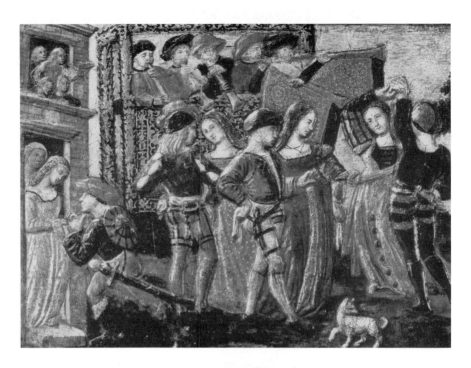

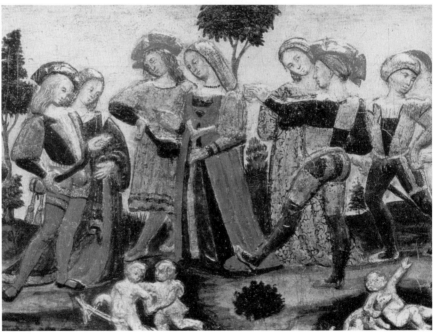

10. Details from a wedding *cassone* (Hermitage, St Petersburg)

3

Dancing in Fifteenth-Century Italian Society

IN his Autobiography, Giovanni Ambrosio (Guglielmo Ebreo) offers a pano-
rama of princely and public festivities which, because of the prestige of the
participants, or because of some spectacular happening, particularly impressed
him. Thus, on the one hand we have his accounts of receptions given in
honour of emissaries of the King of France and the Duke of Burgundy, as
well as of the visit to Venice by the Emperor, Frederick III, and on the
other, his reports of violence and last-minute reprieves, of fireworks, tightrope
walkers, and conjurers. Guglielmo tells of banquets with as many as twenty
courses, where peacocks wandered about the tables and the platters were made
of gold. On one occasion he ate so much he was ill for a week! Jousts are also
recorded, as is a remarkable hunt that was held in Naples. At many of these
magnificent fêtes 'si fece un gran dançare'—there was a great deal of dancing.

Just how this dancing for hundreds of people was arranged is not known.
What we can glean from available documentation, several examples of which
are presented in this chapter, is that there were three distinct sorts of dancing
at a festivity: the dances performed by the host and his or her princely guests,

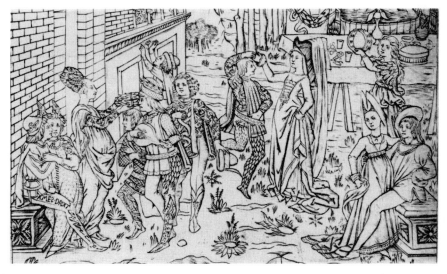

11. Detail from the engraving (anon., *c.*1460) *The Planet Venus*
(British Museum, London)

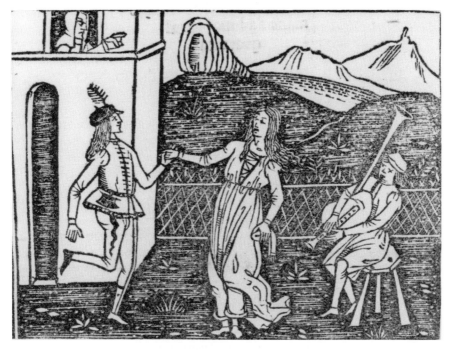

12. Woodcut (anon., early sixteenth century) (Biblioteca Marciana, Venice)

often accompanied by one or two young ladies at court; the general dancing for all, during which couples and trios danced *saltarello* and *piva* (for examples see Pls. 10–12) and specific *balli* in vogue at the time; the *moresche*—mimed and costumed interludes—danced for the entertainment of the assembled company.[1] Occasionally there would be a special exhibition by a particularly talented young girl performing with a dancing-master.[2]

In April 1459, Pope Pius II stopped in Florence on his way to the Diet in Mantua. Count Galeazzo Sforza (the future recipient of *De pratica*), then a youth of fifteen, had been sent by his father Francesco, Duke of Milan, to pay homage to the Pope. This state visit (Galeazzo was accompanied by 500 men, all Cosimo de' Medici's guests) is immortalized in Benozzo Gozzoli's frescoes in the chapel of Florence's Medici Riccardi palace (see Pls. 13–14). Galeazzo Maria is next to Sigismondo Malatesta, lord of Rimini, in the mounted procession following the Wise Men. Lorenzo de' Medici, 11 years old at the time, is glorified as one of the Magi. The city organized grand festivities, which

---

[1] See Glossary for a discussion of these dance types.
[2] See below, n. 17.

included a sumptuous banquet, jousts in Piazza Santa Croce, a combat with savage beasts in front of Palazzo della Signoria, and a great ball held in the Mercato Nuovo.[3] The dancing began with a *saltarello*, to the accompaniment of shawms and sackbuts, during which 'every squire' chose a partner, some promenading around, some skipping, others changing hands. Then two charming girls, bowing deeply, asked Galeazzo to join the dancing. When their dance had finished, the young count himself invited two ladies to dance, after which one of his courtiers—Tiberto Brandolino[4]—followed suit, and then other gentlemen as well. The dancing having lasted an hour ('love had tied more than one knot'), refreshments were served—special wines and sweetmeats—and then everyone 'danced the *saltarello* for a long time'. Following this, favourite dances were requested, including the *Chirintana* (a popular dance for 'as many as will'[5]), *Leoncello*, and *Bel Riguardo*.[6]

[3] The most complete account of the dancing appears in an anonymous manuscript in Florence, Biblioteca Nazionale, Magl. VII, 1121, fos. 66ᵛ–69ᵛ, and published with a few omissions—indicated by ellipsis points—in V. Rossi (ed.), *Un Ballo a Firenze nel 1459* (Milan, 1885). (Another anonymous description, which includes details of Cosimo de' Medici's hospitality—Magl. XXV, 24, is published by G. M. Tartini (ed.), 'Ricordi di Firenze 1459' in *Rerum italicarum scriptores*, ed. L. A. Muratori, 27, pt. 1 (repr. Città di Castello, 1907), 1–38.) See also Galeazzo Maria's own report of the festivity in his letter to his father written in Florence on 30 Apr. 1459 (State Archives, Milan, Potenze Sovrane, Galeazzo Maria Sforza, cited in R. Magnani, *Relazioni private fra la corte sforzesca di Milano e casa Medici 1450–1500* (Milan, 1910), xxi–xxii, doc. 28, and in Pontremoli and La Rocca, *Il ballare lombardo*, 160–1; 167–71). The Mercato Nuovo is now Piazza della Repubblica. For the term 'ball', see Ch. 2 n. 12.

[4] Tiberto Brandolino was a condottiere who fought at the side of Sforza Sforza (II) (the recipient of Cornazano's treatise) and the Angevins against the Aragons in Naples. In 1458 Guglielmo/Giovanni Ambrosio was present at Tiberto's second marriage and at that of his son who married into the influential Bentivoglio family of Bologna. (See Autobiography, [14].)

[5] A *Chirintana* (*Chiaranzana*, *Giranzana*, *Chirentana*, etc.) is found in the Siena redaction of *De pratica* (fos. 66ᵛ–67ʳ), where—like all the *balli* in this codex—it is attributed to Domenico. (C. Mazzi cites a possible etymology from Crusca in a note on p. 202 of his edition of S.) The description of the choreography is extremely cursory, but it does bear a resemblance to the long and detailed anonymous version that appears in F. Caroso, *Il ballarino* (Venice, 1581; repr. New York, 1967). The *Chiaranzana* was a dance that seems to have enjoyed a long popularity in rural and urban areas as well as in courtly circles. It appears as early as 1415 in a sonnet ('they danced to the music of the *chiarentana*', M. Padovan, 'Da Dante a Leonardo: la danza italiana attraverso le fonti storiche', *La danza italiana*, 3 (1985), 26 n. 35). We find it again in a chronicle describing pre-nuptial festivities in Rome under Pope Leo (1513–21); as the *Grand Bal* with which Marie de' Medici and Henry IV opened the dancing at their wedding in Lyons in 1600; and in Goldoni's play, *Scuola di ballo* (1759), where it is mentioned as being sung. (References in A. G. Bragaglia, *Danze popolari italiane* (Rome, 1950).)

[6] The chronicle reads: 'missero amendue gli arrosti in danza [they put both the roasts into dance]/ con *laura, communia e carbonata,/ lioncel, bel riguardo e la speranza/ l'angiola bella e la danza del re*'. It has been suggested (Heartz, 'A 15th-Century Ballo', 360) that the roasts, together with the grilled meats (*carbonata*), referred to the *ballo Rostiboli* (*rôti bouilli*—roasted and boiled). On the other hand, as is pointed out in Padovan, 'Da Dante a Leonardo', the *carbonata* is mentioned in the *ballo Principessa* (S) where it clearly indicates a specific dance. *Communia* (*comino* or cumin seed?) does not have any known dance concordance, while *Laura* (laurel, if written with a final 'o') is the name of a dance composed by Lorenzo de' Medici. McGee, 'Dancing Masters', maintains (213 n. 25), that because Lorenzo was only 11 years old at the time and is never mentioned in the poem/chronicle, 'it is highly unlikely' that his dance was intended. *Leoncello* and *Belriguardo* are

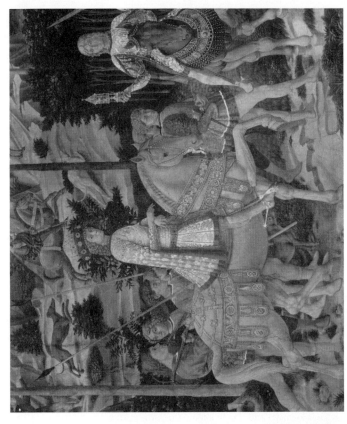

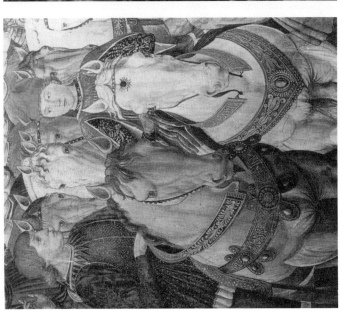

13–14. Benozzo Gozzoli, Details from *Procession of the Magi*: (*13*) Galeazzo Maria Sforza (on the right) and his uncle Sigismondo Malatesta; (*14*) Lorenzo de' Medici (Palazzo Medici Riccardi, Florence)

The anonymous description of this festivity is in verse and is not as detailed and precise as one would wish. Did the *saltarello* have a particular choreography? How many couples (or trios) performed it simultaneously?[7] While the text seems to imply that no one else danced when Galeazzo himself was dancing ('as he passed all stood up'), was this also the case when the other important courtiers danced with their partners? Were the *balli* and *bassedanze* performed by more than one set of dancers at a time? Was there a prescribed order to the ball in terms of what dances were performed, and by whom?[8]

In another festival poem, written about 1454, Gaugello Gaugelli describes the dancing that took place in Pergola, a small medieval town situated amid rolling hills not far from Pesaro.[9] First we are presented with a list of the instruments that played at the fête. Aside from the ever-present shawms and sackbuts, there were *organetti* (portative organs) and 'sweet-sounding' strings: harps, lutes, viols, dulcimers, *cit[h]are*, and a psaltrey. As to the dancing itself, 'You will see these lovely ladies dance—two by two with the other damsels —*bassadanza* and *Lioncello*, some the *piva*, some the *saltarello*, others *Rostiboli* . . . and others *Gelosia* . . .'. Once again we cannot tell from the poetic rendering if several couples performed particular dances at the same time or if one couple danced alone followed by the next in turn.

On 13 January 1490, Ludovico il Moro, unofficial ruler of the Duchy of Milan, organized an entertainment at the Sforza castle to celebrate the marriage between his nephew Giangaleazzo Sforza, the 21-year-old Duke of Milan, and Isabella of Aragon.[10] One hundred of the richest and most beautiful ladies of

balli by Domenico (included in *De pratica*) which enjoyed particular popularity. *La speranza* may well have been Guglielmo's *Spero*; and S includes a *ballo* called *Angiola* and another entitled *danza di Re*.

On fo. 67[r] of this account (the section quoted above appears on fol. 69[r]), Galeazzo's dancing is described: 'Ballato quella danza peregrina . . .'; 'having danced that *danza peregrina*, the ladies led him back to his place'. Some historians have interpreted this to mean that Guglielmo's *bassadanza Pellegrina* was danced. It seems to me, however, that *peregrina* (*pellegrina*) is used here—as it is in various places in *De pratica* and on fo. 68[v] of the chronicle where the guests are described as 'singnori e gente peregrine'—as a descriptive adjective, meaning rare and lovely, and not as the name of a dance.

[7] The description suggests a certain amount of choreographic freedom inasmuch as, in the midst of the *saltarello*, dancers would 'drop out'—presumably as they tired—while others joined in.

[8] We learn from Galeazzo's letter to his father (see above, n. 3) that after all his men had danced (one after the other?), four damsels simultaneously invited two of the Duke of Burgundy's ambassadors to dance.

[9] Published in Heartz, 'A 15th-Century Ballo', 372–3, where its location is given as Biblioteca Vaticana, Urb. 692. According to Heartz, the occasion was a celebration by 'the petty bourgeois'.

[10] The marriage had, in fact, taken place one year before, but the festivities had been interrupted owing to the death of Ippolita Sforza, the bride's mother. The chronicle is published in E. Solmi, 'La Festa del Paradiso di Leonardo da Vinci e Bernardo Bellincione', *ASL* 1 (1904), 75–89, who gives its location as cod. ital. a. J. 421 in the Biblioteca Estense of Modena and attributes it to Giacomo Trotto (see below, n. 14). Included are detailed descriptions of the hall decorations, seating arrangements, and the dancers' attire, as well as the protocol and unfolding of the festivity. Stella Mary Pearce's 'The Paradise of Ludovico il Moro', in James Laver (ed.), *Memorable Balls* (London, 1954), is a general, not always precise, description—in English—based on Solmi.

the city were present.[11] The evening began with Isabella dancing two dances in the company of three of her ladies-in-waiting. Next came performances by dancers from Spain, Poland, Hungary, Germany, and France, each group —characteristically clad—sent by their sovereigns to honour the bride and groom.[12] Eight maskers then danced 'a la piva' and did 'many sorts of capers, leg shakes, and jumps'.[13] At Isabella's invitation, some of her ladies danced Neapolitan and Spanish dances. Following this, the Spaniards were requested to dance with their ladies, after which the French company performed a dance, which Isabella liked so much that she asked them to repeat it. The culmination of the evening, the dancing having already lasted about four and a half hours, was the spectacular theatrical production of 'Paradise' (*Festa del Paradiso*), directed by Leonardo da Vinci.

Ludovico il Moro's own marriage to Beatrice d'Este (Isabella d'Este's sister) was celebrated one year later. It was followed immediately by two other weddings which further strengthened the Sforza–Este alliance: that of Anna Sforza (Giangaleazzo's sister) to Alfonso d'Este (brother to Beatrice and Isabella) and Ercole d'Este, Sigismondo's son, to Angela Sforza, daughter of Carlo Sforza. On 24 January a great ball was held. It was opened by the Duchess of Milan—Isabella of Aragon—dancing with a lady-in-waiting. Then came the turn of Beatrice and Isabella d'Este, who were followed by Anna Sforza and her sister Bianca Maria (who was to become the wife of the future Emperor, Maximilian).[14] There was a delightful entertainment provided by couples wearing colourful costumes (French, Spanish, Hungarian, Turkish, Egyptian), whose 'gestures and improvised movements were most pleasing'.[15] The dancing, which had begun about 1.30 p.m., continued until dark, when some of the guests performed *Maura*, 'receiving due praise for their outstand-

[11] It was a custom in Renaissance Italy to invite a group of one or two hundred beautiful damsels and ladies—adorned in magnificent dresses and jewels—to ornament important festivities. This was done in Florence at the ball in Mercato Nuovo (see above) and in Siena for Ippolita Sforza's visit in 1465 (Gallo, 'La danza', 262). Other examples are in Giovanni Ambrosio's Autobiography [24, 27, 28, 29] and in Pontremoli and La Rocca, *Il ballare lombardo*, 176.
[12] The groups were composed of four maskers from Poland, eight from Germany, four couples (men and women) from France and Spain, and about six couples from Hungary.
[13] Solmi, 'La Festa', 86: 'cavriole, scambiti et salti'. According to Florio, *scambietti* were 'wrigglings', while *sgambettate* meant 'gambols, shakes'.
[14] This was the order according to Giacomo Trotto, the Duke of Ferrara's ambassador at the Sforza court in Milan (letter dated 24 Jan. 1491 and published in Pontremoli and La Rocca, *Il ballare lombardo*, 235–7). (For Domenico's relations with the Trotto family, see Ch. 1. Solmi, 'La Festa', 82, notes an ode by Cornazano praising Trotto.) Somewhat different is the account by Tristano Calco, the Milanese historian, who states that 'the queens' (Isabella of Aragon and Beatrice d'Este) opened the dancing, taking as their partners two newly dubbed knights (Pontremoli and La Rocca, *Il ballare lombardo*, 158).
[15] '. . . nec minùs gesticulis & incondito motu placebant . . .', from Trotto's official record of 'The Nuptials of the Milanese Princes and the Este Princes', reprinted in Latin with an Italian translation in Lopez, *Festa di nozze*, 121, 124, 126.

ing ability and agility'.[16] The very next day the marriage between Ercole d'Este and Angela Sforza was celebrated and dancing followed the ceremony. After an entertainment in costume, the guests admired the extraordinary grace, agility, and beauty of 'a Tuscan girl, accompanied by a [dancing-] master, who performed with all sorts of turns and twistings of her body'.[17]

An ambassadorial report of the 1502 New Year/Carnival festivities of Pope Alexander Borgia's court in Rome gives us another account of dancing-as-spectacle intermingled with more casual domestic dancing.[18] The guests were seated on benches and on the floor while a *moresca* was performed on a low stage. An excellent dancer, dressed as a woman, led forth a group of nine men masquerading as animals. (One of them was no less a personage than the Pope's son, the infamous Cesare Borgia.) All wore masks and magnificent brocades. Each of the nine dancers then took hold of a silk streamer which was hanging from a tree, and to the music of shawms, and under the direction of a youth who sat on top of the tree reciting verses, they danced round the tree intertwining the ribbons. When the performance ended, at the Pope's bidding, his daughter Lucretia danced with one of her Spanish ladies-in-waiting, after which the maskers danced one couple at a time.

Moresche, 'theatre-dance' pieces performed for the amusement of an audience, were very popular in fifteenth-century Italy. Because they often broke up lengthy—and occasionally tedious—banquets and plays, they were also referred to as *intermezzi (tramezzi)*.[19] *Moresche*, maskers, 'liveries', and 'mummeries of masques' are mentioned frequently in chronicles describing private and public entertainments, as well as in the Guglielmo/Giovanni Ambrosio Autobiography. Towards the end of the century, these musical, mimed, and

---

[16] Ibid. 121 and 126. This dance may have been in honour of Ludovico Sforza, who was popularly known as the Moro (Moor or mulberry). His given name, according to Lopez (17–18), was Ludovico Mauro, and although his second name was changed to Maria for 'a grace received', Moro persisted because of his dark colouring.

[17] Ibid. 123: '. . . subijt Tusca Puella, Magistro comitata: quae, saltu flexuquè corporis multifariàm rotata, omnes humanae agilitatis venustatisquè numeros non modò referre decenter, sed supergredi etiam admirantibus visa est'. The girl, one may suppose, was the daughter or pupil of the dancing-master with whom she performed. Another instance of a young girl performing at a courtly entertainment is mentioned by Gallo, 'La danza', on p. 265: during the festivities for the wedding of Annibale Bentivoglio (son of the lord of Bologna) to Lucretia d'Este, which took place in Bologna in 1487, a 6-year-old Florentine girl, accompanied by a man, danced to pipes and tabor with such incredible grace, agility, virtuosity, and musicality that she caused a veritable sensation.

[18] See F. Gregorovius, *Lucrezia Borgia* (Italian edn., Bologna, 1968), 184, as well as 341–2, where the original letter—written by El Prete on 2 Jan.—is published as Document 35, and where the source is given as the Gonzaga Archives, Mantua. The dancing was preceded by a pastoral play and an allegorical poem recited in Latin. Costumes are described as well as room and stage decorations.

[19] N. Pirrotta, *Music and Theatre from Poliziano to Monteverdi*, tr. K. Eales (Cambridge, 1982), has some excellent references to and descriptions of 15th-c. *intermedi* and *moresche*. See his chapter, 'Classical Theatre, *intermedi* and *frottola* . . .', 37–75. Further research will undoubtedly result in the discovery of still more material.

danced interludes became more important than some of the staged tragedies themselves. Performed, for the most part, in costume, they made use of distinctive headgear, masks, scenery, and special effects—fire in particular. They portrayed allegorical, heroic, exotic, and pastoral scenes. Mock skirmishes were common, the Fool a popular character, and the grotesque was frequently represented by doddering old men and fantastic monsters. Depending upon the occasion, the *moresche* were danced by courtiers, 'squires', *ballerini*, or dancing-masters.[20] The extant descriptions unfortunately make little mention of the music involved and provide no detailed choreography, thus making it difficult to know if the step vocabulary differed—and in what way—from that of Guglielmo's and Domenico's dances.[21] Songs—and special singers—were occasionally used to accompany the dancing,[22] and several references are made to *tamburini* (pipe- and tabor-players) who helped 'to keep the measure'.[23] There is no doubt that with the *moresca*, the seeds for the sixteenth-century *intermedio*—and the future theatrical ballet—were already sown.

Dancing also played an important part in spectacles to celebrate state visits, such as that made to Urbino in 1474 by Federico of Aragon.[24] A morality in

[20] According to Castiglione, *Book of the Courtier*, a courtier could demonstrate his skill in dancing by performing a *moresca* in public—but only if properly masked (p. 118), and, as we have seen, Cesare Borgia himself took part in *moresche*. (See also [30] of Autobiography, where Guglielmo/Giovanni Ambrosio notes how the two sons of the King of Naples, Federico and Alfonso, danced in a 'mummery of masques dressed in the French fashion'.) *Scudieri* (squires, i.e. future knights or courtiers, the sons of gentlemen or the attendants of noblemen) are mentioned as participating in 'social' dancing (*saltarello* and *piva*) at the ball in Florence in 1459 and at a private Carnival party in Piacenza (*Proverbi di messer Antonio Cornazano in facetie*, 1865; repr. Bologna, 1968, and below); and an account of Costanzo Sforza's wedding includes an impressive entertainment performed by 180 squires (see below as well as T. De Marinis, *Le nozze di Costanzo Sforza e Camilla d'Aragona celebrate a Pesaro nel 1475* (Florence, 1946), 45–6). A dancing-master was also referred to as a *ballarino*, as Giovanni Ambrosio is in the record of courtiers and staff attached to the Urbino court (Ch. 2 nn. 47–8).

[21] However, on two occasions, at least, a *bassadanza*—presumably with its characteristic steps —was danced as part of a spectacle. Wolfgang Osthoff describes one, performed by 'nymphs' and 'queens', that took place during an entertainment presented in Urbino in 1474 (*Theatergesang und darstellende Musik in der italienischen Renaissance*, 2 vols. (Tutzing, 1969), i. 33–8 ii. 34–7). For the wedding festivities of Annibale Bentivoglio and Lucretia d'Este in 1487 a similar sort of *bassadanza*—nymphs dancing in a ring—was performed to instrumental accompaniment (Gallo, 'La danza', 266).

[22] Gallo, 'La danza', cites a *moresca* performed in Siena in 1465 in honour of Ippolita Sforza in which twelve dancers and 'a nun' danced to a well-known *ballata* 'Oramai che fora son'. (See A. W. Atlas, *Music at the Aragonese Court of Naples* (Cambridge, 1985), 220–1, for the music and text. The version in E. Southern, 'A Prima Ballerina of the Fifteenth Century', in A. D. Shapiro (ed.), *Music and Context: Essays for John M. Ward* (Cambridge, Mass., 1985), is imprecise.) At the festivities in Bologna in 1487 some of the dancing was accompanied by a group of six singers. Their performance included a 'caccia' (hunting song), to which Diana and her nymphs danced.

[23] *Tamburini* can also mean drummers. For other references to the music in *moresche* see Pirrotta, *Music and Theatre*, and Osthoff, *Theatergesang*, i. 33–6.

[24] A. Saviotti, 'Una rappresentazione allegorica in Urbino nel 1474', *Atti e memorie della R. Accademia Petrarca di Scienze, Lettere ed Arti in Arezzo*, 1 (1920), 13–14 and 18–26. (The source given is Cod. Palat. 286 in Florence, Biblioteca Nazionale.) For other descriptions see Osthoff,

praise of Chastity (but incuding Cleopatra leading various 'lascivious women of antiquity') culminated in a *bassadanza* performed around Chastity by six 'queens', followed by twelve 'nymphs' who danced in a ring around them, all to the music of two well-known chansons.[25]

Other favourite themes for *moresche*, besides Chastity, were the Planets and the activities of country folk.[26] Alessandro Sforza's son Costanzo married Camilla of Aragon in Pesaro in May 1475. In the intervals between the various orations, refreshments, and presentation of gifts there was dancing for all, as well as magnificent scenes with maskers who made 'praiseworthy jumps and movements'.[27] Especially notable was the spectacle given by the Jewish community of Pesaro. Not only was a dance of the Seven Planets performed, but there was a lively *moresca* in which 'country folk' hoed and mowed with imitation gold and silver implements, sowing the ground with flowers from golden baskets.[28] During the banquet 'the shawms played a slow and gentle *piva*' and 180 of Costanzo's young squires 'entered the hall dancing gracefully', bearing on their heads or in large baskets on their shoulders all kinds of gold and coloured castles, animals, and flowers made of marzipan. In order for all of them to fit into the hall and be seen, they danced 'freely in the space like a snake in the form of an S . . . and dancing the *piva* they all, at certain parts [of the music], knelt at the same time in a bow'.[29] The sweetmeats were

Theatergesang, i. 33–6 and Gallo, 'La danza', 263–5. It should be noted that the grandiose musical and choreographic spectacle that is reported to have taken place in Tortona in 1489 as part of the banquet offered to Giangaleazzo Sforza and Isabella of Aragon by the nobleman Bergonzio Botta, and which continues to be referred to in Italian books and articles on the history of dance and theatre (including Saviotti), is based on an 18th-c. Italian re-write (largely invented) of the original Latin chronicle. The actual presentation had neither dancing nor music. See Eugenia Casini-Ropa, 'Il banchetto di Bergonzio Botta . . . Quando la storiografia si sostuisce alla storia', in *Spettacoli conviviali dall'antichità classica alle corti italiane del '400* (Rome, 1982), 291–306.

[25] *J'ay pris amour* and *Gent de cors*. (For transcriptions see Osthoff, *Theatergesang*, ii. 34–7.)

[26] The *Festa del Paradiso*, directed and staged by Leonardo da Vinci, included the Seven Planets, each of which spoke in praise of the Duchess Isabella (Solmi, 'La Festa', 87–8). During the 1499 Carnival and again, three years later, at the festivities for the marriage of Lucretia Borgia and Alfonso d'Este, Ferrara witnessed *moresche* representing the labours of the fields. See, among others, Pirrotta, *Music and Theatre*, 50; Gregorovius, *Lucrezia Borgia*, 214; William Gilbert, *Lucrezia Borgia* (London, 1869); B. Zambotto, *Diario ferrarese* (Rerum italicarum scriptores, xxiv); M. Sanuto, *Diarii*, ed. F. Stefani *et al.* (Venice, 1879–1903), iv. 225–30.

[27] De Marinis, *Le nozze*, 34, 37. This edition comprises a reprint of the 1475 printed account as well as the reproduction of 32 miniatures included in a 1480 manuscript version (Biblioteca Vaticana, Urb. 899), depicting scenes from the festivities. The same text was published in 1870 in Florence by Marco Tabarrini with the title *Descrizione del convito e delle feste fatte in Pesaro per le nozze di Costanzo Sforza e di Camilla d'Aragona . . .* See also E. Povoledo, 'From Poliziano's *Orfeo* to the *Orphei tragoedia*', pp. 286–7 in Pirrotta, *Music and Theatre*.

[28] De Marinis, *Le nozze*, 38.

[29] Eiche, 'Alessandro Sforza' (especially 176–8) has a detailed description of the hall and of the particular arrangements made for this occasion. For example, at the 'head' was a platform (exact dimensions given) which was the place of honour for the wedding couple and their most illustrious guests; at the 'foot' of the hall was the entrance. Also included are the locations of: the windows (which provided natural illumination); the musicians' gallery; a ladies' balcony; the fireplace; the raised sideboard—nearly touching the ceiling—with its display of silver plate; an organ; and

presented to the newly-weds, to the ladies and gentlemen, and then strewn throughout the hall, after which all the squires took up the dance again with joy and grace. Then Costanzo and Camilla rose to dance, after which almost every lord, gentleman, doctor, and cavalier took a partner 'and performed a long and grand dance'.

The dancing that took place on state occasions and at official Carnival celebrations had a specific function and was not mere diversion. The allegorical themes and symbolism of the *moresca* flattered and idealized the prince, his image reinforced through the highlighting of his virtues, values, and power.[30] Dancing also played its part in the lavish entertainments that included magnificent banquets, orations, jousts, and plays, and gave the Renaissance prince an opportunity to show largesse towards his subjects (and thus hinder or dilute any discontent), and served to impress political allies and rivals as well.[31] Protocol during these entertainments and balls demanded a hierarchy in the seating arrangements, which was often respected in the order of the dancing. No amount of expense was spared. Whether the dancing was held out of doors or in the great halls of palaces,[32] tiered platforms were often erected along one side for the princes and their guests. Opposite might be a dais for the band of players, while the host's gold and silver plate—displayed on appropriate sideboards, as was the custom—was often raised on yet another platform, in good view of all.[33] Bright velvets, brocades, and cloth of gold and silver hung everywhere and draped the platforms. Festoons of garlands and boughs added

benches and tiers of seats for guests. The hall was decorated with festoons and tapestries and a blue cloth sky on which mirrors and gold and silver rays represented the stars and planets.

[30] The quintessential allegorical 'representation' is probably the banquet organized in Rome in 1473 by Cardinal Riario for Eleonora of Aragon, on her way to Ferrara for her marriage to Ercole d'Este. The event ended with a magnificent *ballo* centring on Hercules, the groom's namesake. After dancing with other heroes and nymphs, Hercules engages in battle and—in a grand finale —defeats the Centaurs. (See, among others, Cruciani, *Teatro*, 151–64.) For further examples of dances or mimed allegories, see Pontremoli and La Rocca, *Il ballare lombardo*, 205–17.

[31] Besides Giovanni Ambrosio's Autobiography, this is attested to in chronicles and in innumerable ambassadorial reports and letters, many of which are referred to in this chapter.

[32] See, for example, the splendid state rooms in the ducal palaces of Urbino and Mantua, as well as those in Ferrara—in the palace of Ludovico il Moro and the Este summer residence, 'Schifanoia' (Shun Boredom—see Ch. 2 n. 6). The great halls, also used for banquets, plays, and receptions, were on the *piano nobile* (the first storey), and although the floors were almost always stone or terracotta, they were laid over wooden beams, which gave them a definite spring. None the less, even when covered with carpets, the floors would have been cold and hard to the foot, particularly since the more refined courtier, and his lady, wore no shoes indoors, the fashion being to attach protective soles to the hose. (Sumptuary laws in Florence in 1464 prohibited this luxury to nurse- and housemaids; E. Polidori Calamandrei, *Le vesti delle donne fiorentine nel quattrocento* (Rome, 1973), 94–8.) It was not usual for these halls to possess a musicians' gallery.

[33] Tuohy, 'Studies' (ch. 4) explains that the element of display was a particular reflection of princely magnificence. The most important work—and the least practical—would have been exhibited. Little plate has survived inasmuch as, in times of need, the objects would not only have been pawned, but melted down, or minted.

further decoration and torches provided illumination. On special occasions, a cloth sky was suspended above the entire scene.[34]

It was not, however, dancing as such that contributed to this conspicuous display of wealth as power, an essential part of the quattrocento policy of 'magnificence'.[35] Indeed, the chroniclers of great weddings and receptions, while occasionally mentioning the names of illustrious personages who participated in the dancing, took little or no notice of the dancing (or dance music) itself, describing instead—and thus carefully recording their value—the clothes and jewels of all those present.[36] The success of the *moresche*, attested to in diaries and reports written by secretaries and ambassadors attached to host and foreign courts, was undoubtedly owing to their combining the spectacular, the sublime, and the expensive.[37]

Dancing is also ignored—and at times explicitly condemned—in the approximately thirteen treatises on education written in Italy in the fifteenth century.[38] The humanist curriculum was directed at educating princes as well as upper- and upper-middle-class males—and some females. It was based on moral and religious studies, intellectual training, and physical development, and aimed at producing moderate, ethical, self-sacrificing, and, above all, civic-minded statesmen, soldiers, and citizens. The only two humanists not to have excluded dancing left it, none the less, in a very ambiguous position. At his Estense school in Ferrara, Guarino admitted dancing as one of the possible outdoor activities, together with ball games, hunting, walking, and riding.[39] And Vittorino da Feltre warned that dancing, like choral singing and instrumental music, should have a place in the curriculum in circumscribed situations only, that is, where it was certain not to lead either to indolence or to sensual excitement.[40]

[34] See, for example, De Marinis, *Le nozze*, Solmi, 'La Festa', Gregorovius, *Lucrezia Borgia* (208–9), Luzio, *Mantova* (19), Rossi, *Un ballo*, Lopez, *Festa*, and Benedetto Capilupo's letter (16 Feb. 1488) reprinted in Padovan, 'Da Dante' (30–1), as well as above, n. 29.

[35] See Tuohy, 'Studies'. Also see the chapters 'The Princely Courts' and 'Art: An Alliance With Power' in Martines, *Power and Imagination*.

[36] See, for example, Gregorovius (above, n. 18), the description of the festivities culminating in the *Festa del Paradiso* (above, n. 10), and n. 11.

[37] See, among others, Burchard (papal master of ceremonies) and El Prete (Isabella d'Este's ambassador) in Gregorovius, *Lucrezia Borgia*; Sanuto (*Diarii*); Giacomo Trotti (Este ambassador to the Sforza court) and Tristano Calco (historian at Sforza court) in Lopez, *Festa*, as well as B. Zambotto (above, n. 26).

[38] See Woodward, *Vittorino da Feltre*, 180–1, for a complete list and approximate dates. The most well-known authors are Vergerio, Leonardo Bruni, Francesco Barbaro, Aeneas Piccolomini (Pope Pius II), Guarino of Verona, Maffeo Vegio, Jacopo Porcia, and Gianozzo Manetti. (See Ch. 1 n. 23.)

[39] Besides Woodward, see Eleanor B. English's 1978 UCLA thesis, 'Physical Education Principles of Selected Italian Humanists . . .', as well as the chapter 'Humanism: A Program for Ruling Classes', in Martines, *Power and Imagination*. Paul Grendler's *Schooling in Renaissance Italy: Literacy and Learning 1300–1600* (Baltimore, Md., 1989) has an interesting chapter called 'Girls and Working-Class Boys in School'.

[40] See English (n. 39) and Woodward, 241.

Little is known of the dancing which took place outside the courts. The setting of one of Cornazano's *Proverbs in Jest* is a private Carnival party in the city of Piacenza. After dinner a squire and a provincial lass, the hero and heroine of this risqué ballad, take part in the dancing, together with a great crowd of people. The music seems to have been supplied by a single player (if we can trust Cornazano's poetic rendering), and the only dances mentioned are the *saltarello* and *piva*.[41]

An interesting document dated 1517 provides what may prove to be a precious insight into urban dancing.[42] It is the work of Johannes Cochlaeus, a German pedagogue and music theorist, who, one may conjecture, personally observed some dancing when visiting Bologna. Responding to a request made to him by the daughters of a leading citizen of Nuremberg, he set down and sent off to Germany his own description of the choreographies of eight Italian dances—seven of which had appeared 30–50 years earlier in one or more of the redactions of *De pratica*.[43] The value of this document (N) is a measure of our scant knowledge. We would need to know far more to determine how and when Guglielmo's and Domenico's dances began to pass from the courts and noble 'ballrooms' into lesser households, and to discover where else dancing took place (in the main square? at the universities?). We know that Guglielmo's brother, Giuseppe, had a dancing-school in Florence (see Ch. 2). Where else were there schools? Who ran them and who were the teachers? What dances were taught and how were they learned? Who attended? What was the role of the Jews in the dancing profession?[44]

[41] Cornazano, *Proverbi*, Proverb 15, 95–100. I wish to thank Peggy Dixon for first bringing this ballad to my attention. For another example of what may be bourgeois dancing, see the description above of the festivity that took place in the town of Pergola.

[42] Described in detail in I. Brainard, 'The Art of Courtly Dancing in Transition: Nürnberg, Germ. Nat. Mus. MS. 8842, a Hitherto Unknown German Source', in Edelgard E. DuBruck and Karl Heinz Göller (eds.), *Crossroads of Medieval Civilization: The City of Regensburg and its Intellectual Milieu* (Medieval and Renaissance Monograph Series, 5; 1984), 61–79. Ingrid Wetzel's transcription of the German text and her Italian translation are published in *Guglielmo*, 321–43, together with photographic reproductions of the original manuscript.

[43] The eight dances are (in the original spelling) *der spanier* (a dance with only 'double' steps, perhaps to the *bassadanza* tenor *la Spagna*); *Rostibin* (*Rostiboli gioioso*, Pg etc.); *angelosa* (NY and S); *L[']amorosa* (Pa, NY, S); *leoncell[o]*, *bellregwerd* (*Belriguardo*), *mercasan* (*Marchesana*)—all three by Domenico and included in *De pratica*; and *vite de Colej* (*Vita de Colino*, NY).

Some of the choreographies included in the various versions of *De pratica* were 'hits' for almost one hundred years (see Trissino's remark in Ch. 2). Despite Cornazano's statement that several of Domenico's dances 'are either too old or too well known' to include in his treatise (V, fos. 29ᵛ, 30ʳ), the fact that these same dances were being performed in Bologna in 1517, and that almost all the ones he dismisses are reported in one or more of the redactions of *De pratica* (Pg, Pa, NY, FN, FL, S, all of which are considered to have been completed after 1455, the date of Cornazano's own treatise), testify to their lasting popularity.

[44] Bonnie Blackburn has kindly pointed out to me a most interesting document from Venice, dated 7 Jan. 1444/5, and summarized in the catalogue of the *Mostra documentaria: Vivaldi e l'ambiente musicale veneziano* (Venice, 1978), 16: 'For good reasons, the Council of Ten orders that the teachers of music, singing, and dance close their schools, attended by the young and the very young, no later than the 24th hour [in this case, sunset].' Unfortunately, the undocumented claims

The dances described by Guglielmo and Domenico are certainly not the only ones that were danced at the time. In no treatise, for example, is there a reference to a circle dance, although we can see one being performed by three courtiers and their ladies in a miniature preserved in the Bible of Borso d'Este, Duke of Ferrara (Pl. 15).[45] Moreover, when Galeazzo Maria Sforza arrived in Firenzuola, on his way to Florence (April 1459), he and his courtiers were invited to a private home where, after supper, they took part in round dances with a group of girls who sang as they danced. The dancing was so merry and the singing so beautiful that Galeazzo and his courtiers enjoyed themselves immensely, 'particularly those who have never [before] seen this kind of sport'.[46] Round dances are shown in Pl. 16, from the second edition (1562) of *Canzone a ballo* ('Songs to dance to'), a collection of poems by Lorenzo de' Medici, Angelo Poliziano, and others.[47]

The dancing that took place in the private apartments—generally the ladies' chambers—of princely palaces may well have included some of the dances from *De pratica*. Isabella d'Este, the Duchess of Mantua, received from her informant in Rome the following report (written on 29 December 1501) concerning her future sister-in-law, Lucretia Borgia.

That evening I went to her room and her Ladyship was sitting next to the bed; and in the corner of the room were about twenty Roman ladies dressed in the Roman fashion . . . Then there were her ladies-in-waiting, ten in all. The dancing was begun by a gentleman of Valencia with a lady-in-waiting by the name of Nicola. Then My Lady danced elegantly and with particular grace with Don Ferrante . . . A lady-in-waiting from Valencia, Catalina, danced well; another was seductive.[48]

of Cecil Roth (*The Jews in the Renaissance* (1959; repr. New York, 1965), 276) that Jews ran dancing-schools in Venice (closed by the authorities in 1443), and that Jewish women who taught music and dancing to ladies in Parma were expelled from the city in 1466, have not as yet been confirmed.

[45] The artist is Taddeo Crivelli (*c.*1425–before 1479), who painted the miniature—representing the court of Solomon—between 1455 and 1461. The Bible (probably 15th-c. Italy's most expensive book; Tuohy, 'Studies') is in Modena, Biblioteca Estense, MS V. G. 12, i (fo. 280ᵛ). Round *bassedanze* were performed in *moresche* (see above, n. 21).

[46] From a letter to Galeazzo's mother, dated 15 Apr. 1459 (State Archives, Milan, cited in Magnani, *Relazioni private*, and in Pontremoli and La Rocca, *Il ballare lombardo*, 160–1). See above n. 3. (Firenzuola, then called Fiorenzuola, is 50 km. north of Florence.)

[47] According to a handwritten entry in the British Library copy, this same engraving is from a first edition, dated 1533. It is almost certainly based on a much more rudimentary woodcut that appears on the title-page of Lorenzo de' Medici's *Ballate e Rispetti*, probably printed at the end of the 15th c. (and included in the 1915 Florentine reprint of the 1533 edn. of *Canzone a ballo*). Besides the gentleman and the two kneeling girls, the woodcut shows only six ladies. They do not seem to be singing, and are dancing round a column topped with the Medici device of six balls. Yet another version of the engraving exists in the 1568 edition of the *Canzone*, also in the British Library. Technically the most refined of the three, it shows the twelve girls—in typical 15th-c. dress—dancing out of doors, in front of a *palazzo* that displays the Medici device. The three foreground figures are reversed.

[48] Gregorovius, *Lucrezia Borgia*, 179, 181. See also Bianca Maria Sforza's description of the evenings spent in Innsbruck, just before her wedding to the Emperor Maximilian, when there

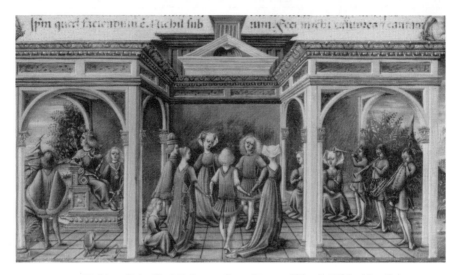

15. Taddeo Crivelli, Miniature from Borso d'Este's Bible (detail)
(Biblioteca Estense, Modena)

16. Frontispiece (anon.), *Canzone a ballo* (1562)

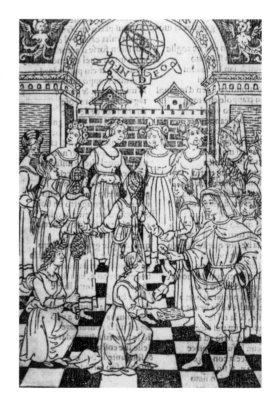

This informal 'after-dinner dancing', in contrast to that organized for state occasions, seems to have been engaged in primarily as a pleasant, cultivated pastime. It followed a tradition—first reported by Boccaccio in 1353[49]—which continued into the sixteenth century, as Castiglione's description of an evening at the palace in Urbino testifies:

'Since the hour is late . . . let the short time that is left be spent on some less ambitious entertainment.' As everyone agreed with this, the Duchess called on Madonna Margherita and Madonna Costanza Fregosa to dance. And then immediately Barletta, a delightful musician and an excellent dancer . . . began to play, and the two ladies, taking each other by the hand, danced first a bassa [danza] and then a roegarze, extremely gracefully, and to everyone's satisfaction.[50]

The distinction that exists today between theatrical and social dancing cannot be applied to the fifteenth century. Courtiers were the performers whether they danced the traditional, improvisatory saltarello and piva or donned costumes and danced, before an audience, the choreographed, spectacular moresche. If one of Guglielmo's bassedanze or one of Domenico's balli was danced by princesses during a great festivity, its purpose—in that context—would have been to impress the onlookers; if it was danced by the same ladies in their rooms at night, its intention would have been to delight the performers themselves; if it was danced during a moresca, it will have taken on another— possibly allegorical—significance. For the creators, Guglielmo and Domenico, each one of the dances was a unique composition and work of art.[51]

was dancing both 'in public [festivities] and privately in our room'. Prior to this, she and her aunt Beatrice d'Este—occasionally in Spanish dress and accompanied by their ladies-in-waiting— would spend their evenings in her mother's rooms in the castle in Milan, dancing until one in the morning (Beatrice's husband Ludovico il Moro having retired at nine). Pontremoli and La Rocca, Il ballare lombardo, 154.

[49] See e.g. the endings of each of the ten days of The Decameron.

[50] Castiglione, Book of the Courtier, 104. Nothing is known regarding the roegarze.

[51] Most of the dances included in De pratica, more particularly the balli, were explicitly designed for men and ladies dancing together. The chronicles, however, present us with another picture. While it appears that men and ladies did indeed dance the saltarello and piva in couples and trios, we do occasionally find groups of girls dancing together. As for the bassedanze and balli themselves, they seem to have been performed primarily by ladies, whether at public festivities or in private chambers. The moresche, on the other hand, seem to be dominated by squires, princes, and ballerini, while solo performances were the speciality of young girls.

4

The Music in *De pratica*: Transcribing the *Balli* Tunes[1]

DANCE without music was inconceivable for Guglielmo, who devoted ten out of his sixteen introductory chapters to musical problems. Like Domenico before him, he composed not only the choreographies of his *balli* but the music as well. The spare monophonic dance-tunes notated in *De pratica* are undoubtedly merely skeletal outlines, and when performed would have been elaborated and accompanied by one or two other voices.[2] A dancing-master's knowledge of musical notation may not have been extensive, dance-music at the time being performed and passed on as part of Italy's rich oral tradition, and in the recording of the melodic lines (as with the choreographies themselves), many formulae were taken for granted.[3] In transcribing the *balli* tunes in modern notation—with barlines, time signatures, and particular note-values —my primary consideration has been to match the choreographies and their music.[4] While specific observations are noted in the commentary following each transcription, some basic musical and choreographic conventions used in the treatises will be discussed in this chapter.

[1] The conclusions in this chapter, many of which have already been discussed in Sparti, '15th-century *Balli* Tunes', are based on a study of Pg, Pa, Pd, and V. Several new ideas have been introduced, thanks to the generosity and expertise of Véronique Daniels. See Glossary for step descriptions as well as for musical and choreographic terms left in Italian.

[2] The iconography of the period shows that the instruments used most frequently to accompany dancing in 15th-c. Italy were the so-called 'high' instruments—shawms, bombards, or chalumeaux (all part of the same double-reed family), and sackbuts. Most often depicted in a trio, performing on a dais, they are also present in groups of two, four, or five. Examples of solo string-players (and occasionally a duo) are also plentiful, these 'low' instruments—primarily lute and harp—appearing on the same level as the dancers. Both groups of instruments are portrayed playing in as well as out of doors. See Pls. 3, 10, 11, 12, and 15. Whereas on certain occasions a pipe and tabor accompanied the dances, there is no evidence that other percussion instruments were used. See M. Mingardi, 'Gli strumenti musicali nella danza del XIV e XV secolo', in *Mesura*, 113–55, and below, n. 35. R. Mullaley ('The Polyphonic Theory of the Bassa Danza and the Ballo', *Music Review*, 41 (1980), 1–10) and most recently William Tuck ('Man and Woman— Flute and Drum', *Proceedings of the European Association of Dance Historians*, Leuven, Belgium, 1990), argue for a monophonic—rather than polyphonic—interpretation of the dance tunes.

[3] See Ch. 1 n. 32.

[4] Besides Kinkeldey's and Marrocco's transcriptions of the *balli* tunes and Cornazano's tenors, Mary Criswick has transcribed the music in V (in M. Inglehearn and P. Forsyth, *The Book on the Art of Dancing. Antonio Cornazano* (London, 1981), four *balli* tunes have been transcribed and the dances reconstructed in I. Brainard, *The Art of Courtly Dancing in the Early Renaissance* (West Newton, Mass., 1981), and Domenico's tunes have been reproduced in Wilson, *Domenico of Piacenza*.

Step durations and tempi

In their treatises, Domenico and Cornazano give the duration of almost every step, so that one *doppio*, one *ripresa*, a *riverenza*, a *meza volta*, two *sempii*, two *continenze*, and two *movimenti* all last one *tempo* (a *volta tonda* lasts two *tempi*).[5] A *tempo*—or *tempus*—is a time-unit which is the mensuration of the *brevis* and, in this context, the equivalent of a modern musical bar. These theoretical step durations seem to apply primarily to *bassadanza misura*, inasmuch as in *piva* and *quadernaria* a *volta tonda* is occasionally performed with only one *doppio* (one *tempo*), and a *ripresa* is done in half the time of a *doppio*.[6] A *tempo* can also indicate a step-unit, so that 'four *tempi* of *saltarello*' means not only four bars of *saltarello* music but four *saltarello* steps.[7] Each *tempo* usually lasts the length of a *doppio* or its equivalent in step and music.[8]

The four misure

A *ballo* is composed of different *misure* that vary in metre and tempo. *Bassadanza* is the slowest, *quadernaria* follows, then *saltarello*, and finally *piva*. Domenico stresses that each *misura* increases in speed by one-sixth: the *quadernaria* one-sixth faster than the *bassadanza*, the *saltarello* two-sixths (a third) faster, the *piva* three-sixths or twice as fast.[9] What emerges, theoretically at least, is a ratio of 6 : 5 : 4 : 3. However, Domenico and Cornazano also dedicate several pages to explaining how each of the four *misure* can be danced not

---

[5] V, fo. 9ᵛ; Pd, fo. 2ᵛ. See also S, fos. 30ʳ⁻ᵛ. (It is more than probable that Domenico's statement that the *meza volta* lasts a half-*tempo* is an error.)

[6] For *volta tonda* with one *doppio* in *quadernaria* or *piva* see Pg's *Gelosia, Legiadra, Petit Rose, Petit Riense, Marchesana,* and (?)*Voltati in ça Rosina.* For examples of a *ripresa* half the length of a *doppio*, see the finale of *Petit Riense* (*piva*), the *saltarello* in *piva* fashion in *Ingrata*, and *Tesara* (Pd, fo. 24ᵛ, *piva*).

[7] According to Domenico (fo. 6ʳ), a *saltarello* step is a *doppio* and hop (*salteto*). Cornazano confirms that *saltarello doppii* are performed with a rise, although his explanation is somewhat obscure (fo. 5ᵛ).

[8] In *Ingrata*, however, Guglielmo has nine patterns or bars of *saltarello* music for 'six *tempi*', that is, six *quadernaria* step-units 'in *piva* fashion': three *doppii* (in this case, six bars of music), three *riprese* (three bars of music). And it is not clear if in his chapter on Manner the term *tempo* refers to the time-unit of a *sempio* step: '[W]hen in the art of the dance someone does a *sempio* or a *doppio* he should . . . for the entire duration of the measured *tempo* turn his body . . . .'.

[9] Pd, fos. 3ʳ⁻ᵛ, 4ᵛ, and Wilson, *Domenico of Piacenza*, 11, 13. 'La prima la quale e piu larga de le altre se chiama per nome Bassedanza de mazor imperfecto: La 2ᵃ mexura se chiama quadernaria de menore imperfecto: la quale per distantia de tempo e piu strecta de la bassadanza uno sesto. La 3ᵃ mexura se chiama per nome Saltarello de mazor perfecto voi dire passo brebant e questa mexura per distantia de tempo e piu strecta de la quadernaria uno altro sesto che vene ad essere uno terzo piu strecta de la bassadanza: La 4ᵃ et ultima mexura se chiama per lo vulgo piva de menore perfecto. Questa calla del Saltarello per distantia de temp[o] uno sesto. Siche adonque questa mexura ultima dicta piva vene ad essere piu strecta de la bassadanza tri sesti che contene la mitade.' Cornazano, who begins his scale of *misure* with the *piva*, does not specify any particular proportion between the *misure*, but he does confirm that one *tempo* of *bassadanza* can be danced with two *tempi* of *piva* and each *misura* will thus 'have its [correct] order' (fo. 13ʳ). On the proportional relationships between the *misure* Guglielmo is silent, although S (fos. 30ᵛ–31ʳ) reproduces most of Domenico's scale of *misure* word for word, albeit with errors.

only in its 'natural order' but according to 'intellectual artistry', by doing one dance type in another *misura* (for example, dancing *saltarello doppii* steps to *bassadanza* music).[10] This artistic dialectic, which creates quite different relationships between the *misure*, together with Domenico's table of *misure* (Pd, fo. 4ᵛ), and the unusual—and perhaps purely notional—ratio of 6 : 5 : 4 : 3, have provoked a rethinking of Domenico's proportions and given rise to new interpretations.[11]

Theoretical mensurations of the four misure

Each *misura* has, in addition to its own tempo (relatively proportioned with the others), a particular metre. In the dance-treatises, however, the concept of mensuration would seem to be fraught with discrepancies, since theoretical principles, mensural signs, and notation often contradict each other. Domenico ascribes the four prolations to the four *misure*, and he and Guglielmo agree only on the mensuration of *quadernaria*.[12] Cornazano has his own scale of mensurations, which again seems to contrast with his statement that every

[10] Pd, fos. 5ʳ–7ʳ; V, fos. 11ᵛ–13ʳ. On fo. 5ʳ of Pd (Wilson, 14), Domenico states, for example, that the *bassadanza* '. . . se po danzare per modi cinque, de li cinque dui hanno suo ordine per motto de compartitione de tempo [*bassadanza* and *piva*]. li altri tre per acidentia lo intelecto li po spartirli e danzarli [*quadernaria*, one slow *saltarello* step to one *tempo* of *bassadanza*, two fast *saltarello* steps to one *tempo*]: Ma piu difficille sono quisti altri tri motti che li dicti dui . . .'. In the choreographies themselves, the following *misure* are performed 'out of their natural order': *quadernaria* and *saltarello* in *bassadanza misura*; *saltarello* and *piva* in *quadernaria misura*; *quadernaria* in *saltarello* and *piva misure*. *Piva* is also danced to *bassadanza misura*, but it is 'within the system', being twice as fast.

[11] I am thinking here, for example, of Véronique Daniels with Eugen Dombois and their 'Die Temporelationen im Ballo des Quattrocento: Spekulative Dialoge um den labyrintische Rätselkanon De la arte di ballare et danzare des Domenico da Piacenza', *Basler Jahrbuch für historische Musikpraxis*, 14 (1990). For Daniels, who spoke on the same theme at the NEMA Conference ('The Marriage of Music and Dance') in London, 1991, the *piva* is twice as fast as the *quadernaria* (as suggested by Cornazano; see below and n. 13). She also proposes a constant *semibrevis* between the *misure*, which results in a ratio of 6 : 4 : 3 : 2. Maurizio Mingardi, on the other hand, has expressed to me his belief that Domenico's proportions are formal hints for the stylistic perform-ance of the four *misure*. Yet another hypothesis for 'Domenico's comparison of one *misura* to the next' is formulated by A. William Smith, who sees the proportions as 'schematic, rather than related to actual tempi (in the modern sense)'. Smith speculates that 'Domenico's references to sixths and thirds are based on his diagram containing six spaces. The chart establishes a relativity which Cornazano makes concrete, perhaps absolute, in a diagram where the relationship of the sizes of the rungs on the ladder have proportions related in sixths.' Furthermore, 'Guglielmo avoids reference to the relationship of *misure* in terms of sixths very likely because it was not actually practiced by musicians.' John Caldwell, in his 'Early Keyboard Tablatures and Medieval Dance Theory', in *Atti del XIV Congresso della Società Internazionale di Musicologia. Trasmissione e recezione delle forme di cultura musicale*, ed. A. Pompilio, D. Restani, L. Bianconi, F. A. Gallo, iii (Turin, 1990), 681–6, states that 'the tempo-relationships of neither strict mensural theory nor dance can have been observed in practice. The dance theory of the period points to a loosening of convention and a more pragmatic approach that can also be found in various form of keyboard tablature.'

[12] Pd, fo. 3ʳ⁻ᵛ. See below, Book I n. 13. In the list of mensurations in Pg (see 'Aliud experi-mentum [V]' in this edn.), the names of the four *misure* are omitted. They are specified, however, in S (fo. 30ᵛ) and M (fo. 19ʳ).

note (*semibrevis*) of his tenors should get three beats in its 'natural' form (*saltarello*); six or twelve in *bassadanza*; four if played in *quaternaria*; and four also in *piva* which, though faster, 'is born' from the *quaternaria*.[13] See Table 1.

TABLE 1. *Mensurations according to the dance theorists*

	Domenico	Guglielmo	Cornazano
bassadanza:	mazor imperfecto	perfetto magiore	perfecto magiore in ragione di canto
quadernaria:	menore imperfecto	quaternario [imperfetto minore][a]	quattro per tre di perfecto magiore[b]
saltarello:	mazor perfecto	perfetto minore	perfecto magiore
piva:	menore perfecto	imperfetto minore	perfecto minore

[a] Specified in S, fo. 30[v].   [b] Corrected in MS from *dimperfecto*.

According to fifteenth-century theory, *perfecto* (or *imperfecto*) usually indicated the *tempus*, and major/minor indicated the prolation. (See Guglielmo's and Cornazano's mensurations.) However, Domenico, and other fifteenth-century theorists, invert word order and meaning: *mazor imperfecto* = *tempus perfectum, prolatio minor*. See Table 2.

TABLE 2. *The mensurations according to Domenico*

mazor imperfecto (perfetto minore) = tempus perfectum, prolatio minor:

menor imperfecto (imperfetto minore) = tempus imperfectum, prolatio minor:

mazor perfecto (perfetto magiore) = tempus perfectum, prolatio maior:

menor perfecto (imperfetto magiore) = tempus imperfectum, prolatio maior:

[13] Cornazano's scale of *misure* is on fo. 11[r] of V and is reprinted in Sparti, '15th-century *Balli* Tunes', and in Inglehearn and Forsyth, *Book on the Art of Dancing*. His explanation of the tenor note-values is on fo. 30[v]: '. . . ogni tenore si puo fare a quatro mesure. Delle quali a bon sonatori la prima e il suo naturale a tre botte per nota. et questa a gli Taliani si dança in saltarello. Siconda in quaternaria mettendo quatro botte per nota, e questa in dançare e piu usata da Todeschi. Terça la cacciata che e misura di piva; alcuni la chiamano figliola de la quaternaria, perche per nota van pur tante botte, ma si dan piu preste della mitate. ['. . . some call it the daughter of the *quaternaria* because for [each] note there are the same number of beats, but they go twice as fast.'] Quarta e la Bassadança, misura imperiale, dove ogni nota si radoppia et le tre vagliono sei, et le sei dodeci.'

Mensural signs

When used, the mensural signs in the notations of Domenico, Guglielmo, Giovanni Ambrosio, and Cornazano simply compound the inconsistencies, rather than clarify the situation. In the four *balli* tunes composed by Guglielmo (*Colonnese*, *Gratioso*, *Legiadra*, and *Spero*), and in the three added to the Giovanni Ambrosio copy (*Petit Vriens*, *Amoroso*, [*Rostiboli*] *Gioioso*), almost no signs are used. (In the Giovanni Ambrosio version of *Spero*, however, there are signs for each of the *misure*, with the exception of the final *piva*.) Domenico uses more signs in his *balli* tunes than Guglielmo does for either his own *balli* or for those versions of Domenico's tunes that he includes in *De pratica*. Guglielmo (or Pagano, his scribe for the 1463 copy) seems to have had less interest in notation and mensural signs and, in general, to have been less precise than Guglielmo/Giovanni Ambrosio and his scribe. Cornazano, on the other hand, tends, in his treatise, to reproduce faithfully Domenico's notation and the mensural signs. Some of Domenico's *balli*, presumably the earlier ones like *Leoncello* and *Belriguardo* (also included in *De pratica*), have only the *bassadanza* sections signed, whereas complex *balli* like *Jupiter* (*Iove*), *Verçepe*, and *Sobria* have every section marked.

₵ (6/4, 6/8) is the symbol that appears most frequently. It is used by both Domenico and Guglielmo to indicate eleven *bassadanza* sections and by Domenico for five *saltarelli*. (The Giovanni Ambrosio treatise has it in *Gratioso* for both German *saltarello* in *quadernaria misura* and for *bassadanza*.)

⊙ (9/4, 9/8) is used three times by Guglielmo, in his versions of Domenico's *balli*, for *bassadanza* sections which, however, are marked ₵ in Domenico's and Giovanni Ambrosio's treatises.[14] It is also used once by Domenico—and his three 'followers'—and again by Guglielmo and Giovanni Ambrosio, as a sign of a change of *misura* from *saltarello* (₵) to *bassadanza*.[15]

○ (3/4) is the symbol Domenico (and Cornazano after him) uses for *saltarello* sections in three *balli*, and for *bassadanza* in one other.[16] (Whether signed ○ or ₵, the notation of the *saltarello* sections in the various *balli* tunes is basically the same.) It is also the sign used in the Giovanni Ambrosio copy for the final part of [*Rostiboli*] *Gioioso*, which is probably *quadernaria* in *piva misura*. Moreover, it indicates German *saltarello* (*saltarello* in *quadernaria*) in all the versions of *Jupiter/Iove*.

₵ (2/4) appears in eight *balli* as the symbol for *quadernaria* sections and in three

---

[14] *Iove* (first *bassadanza*), *Mercantia*, and *Presoniera*. The version of *Presoniera* in Pa, however, has the sign ○.

[15] *Jupiter* (Pd, V), *Iove* (Pg, Pa), and *Spero*.

[16] The *bassadanza* section is in *Marchesana* and the symbol is repeated in the Pg and Pa versions. It is the only sign used by Domenico in this *ballo*. The Giovanni Ambrosio copy, however, has a ₵ for the opening *saltarello* in *quadernaria*, as well as for the final section. Moreover, it has *breves* instead of Domenico's repeated *semibreves* in the *bassadanza*.

balli for those in *piva* (one of which, *Tesara* in Pd, would seem to be in 6/8: ♩ = ♩. : ♩ ♪ ♩ ♪ .[17]

It seems clear that both Domenico and Guglielmo occasionally use 'inappropriate' (as we see it) symbols to indicate a change of *misura* or tempo when the mensuration (metre) itself, and/or the notation, does not change, for example, when a *saltarello* section follows a *bassadanza* section (6/4 to 6/8), or a *piva* (♩ = ♩. : ♩ ♪ ♩ ♪ ; ♩ ♪ ♪ ♩) follows a *saltarello* (♩ = ♩. : ♩ ♩ ♪ ♩).

Metres implicit in the balli tunes

After barring the *balli* tunes according to the number of *tempi* stipulated in the choreographies, it is possible to determine which metre is being used simply by observing the notation. What emerges is:

bassadanza, whether notated in two or six *semibreves* per *tempo* (probably an instrumental indication), is always in 6/4;

quadernaria is in duple time and must always be barred in 4/4;[18]

saltarello is always in 6/8 except for two *balli* that have *saltarello* sections which appear to go back and forth between a 3/4 and 6/8 metre.[19] These can, however, be transcribed throughout in 6/8;

piva seems to be notated like a 6/8 *saltarello*, or like a fast *quadernaria* (see below).

In conclusion, the four *misure* are written in only *two* mensurations (and in only one *tempus*—*imperfectum*). An explanation sometimes given for the inconsistencies and apparent inaccuracies in mensuration is the inexperience of the authors of the dance-treatises in dealing with written music. But it has also been argued, by Véronique Daniels, that Domenico, at least, knew more than this supposition would credit him with. Furthermore, the scheme of the four *misure*, together with Domenico's particular proportion of tempi, may well have been an attempt to reflect, theoretically at least, the complete system of *tempus*, *prolatio*, and *proportio* found in music at this time and, by this means, to raise the dance to a status not only enjoyed by music but by the other arts

---

[17] See below on the transcription of the *piva*.

[18] If the proportional relationship 6 : 5 between *bassadanza misura* (in 6/4) and *quadernaria* (one-sixth faster in 4/4)— ♩ ♩ ♩ ♩ ♩ ♩ to ♩ ♩ ♩ ♩ —is taken literally, then the crotchet of the *quadernaria* will be somewhat longer in duration than that of the *bassadanza*. In other hypotheses—based on different proportions—the crotchet remains invariable in all the *misure*. (See n. 11.)

[19] See the notations of *Sobria* (Pd) and *Pizocara* (Pd, Pg). The blackened notes in *Pizocara* seem to confirm the change of metre between 3/4 and 6/8, inasmuch as blackening (or coloration) produces a shift in accent, referred to today as 'courante patterns'. (Sparti, '15th-century *Balli* Tunes', 356 n. 27; W. Apel, *The Notation of Polyphonic Music 900–1600* (Cambridge, Mass., 1953), 126–7.)

and sciences that embodied doctrines of number and proportion. A system (*misura*) whereby the dance was proportioned and measured by all four of the mensurations then used in secular music would bring it in line, hypothetically, with the humanistic ideals of the Renaissance. In their attempt to have dance considered a true *arte liberale*, Domenico and Guglielmo composed a complex theory, and it is just possible—and would not have been uncommon at the time—that their system of four mensurations was more of an abstract speculation than a working formula.[20] Indeed, according to Eugen Dombois,[21] the system may have been designed by Domenico to be purposely and artfully enigmatic, stimulating the clever reader—then as now—to search for hidden keys to different levels of meaning. One wonders, however, if even Guglielmo and Cornazano were able to unravel the master's riddle. It is also conceivable that the dance-theorists used the principle of the four prolations and tried to relate them to the four *misure* not in terms of music at all but in terms of dance, in much the same way as they based their aesthetic theory on a terpsichorean interpretation of humanistic conceits. Even were this the case, it would, unfortunately, not explain the contradictions amongst them. John Caldwell claims that the reason for the 'anomalies in the mensural nomenclature attached to the steps by the theorists' is that 'the mensural theory from which the four *misure* were drawn' was 'only half-understood' (the 6 : 5 : 4 : 3 ratio being 'a schematic rationalization' of the same 'half-understood' mensural theory).[22]

Proportional changes of tempo

There are specific indications, besides different mensural signs, that Domenico and Guglielmo—in the Giovanni Ambrosio *De pratica*— tried to notate *misura* relationships and changes of tempo. There are instances of proportion signs (three in Pd and one in Pa, all noted in the commentary on the musical transcriptions[23]) which imply a proportional change in tempo from *saltarello* to *piva*, or from *bassadanza* sections to *piva* or *saltarello* (*misure* that in these examples are all similarly notated and therefore suggest the same mensuration). The symbol that appears in *Voltati in ça Rosina* when the *ballo* changes from *quadernaria* to *piva* (no change in notation) indicates that the *steps* are to go twice as fast, thus requiring a different barring and metre. Although the proportion signs used (C3, ₵3, 3, ₵, ₵) do not always correspond to their contemporary or modern meaning, their main intention seems to have been

---

[20] This is certainly the case with the abstruse proportions listed by Tinctoris (*Proportionale musices*, *c.*1472) and Gaffurio (*Practica musicae*, Milan, 1496). As mentioned in Ch. 1, Alberti's basing painting on mathematics to prove its worth has been called 'more appearance than reality'.

[21] See above, n. 11.

[22] 'Early Keyboard Tablatures', 683.

[23] The notations of *Ingrata*, *Jupiter/Iove*, and *Pizocara* are also included in Pg, without, however, any proportion signs. [*Rostiboli*] *Gioioso* is the Giovanni Ambrosio *ballo* tune.

to denote a proportional change of tempo.[24] Moreover, in two *balli* in the Giovanni Ambrosio *De pratica*, notes with different time-values are actually used. In the notation of *Spero*, and similarly in *Presoniera*, one *tempo* of *bassadanza* is indicated by two *breves* (▫ ▫) and one *tempo* of *saltarello* by two *semibreves* (◦ ◦ or ◦ ♩ ◦ ♩). In the earlier 1463 version of *Spero* Guglielmo used the same note-values for both the *bassadanza* and *saltarello* sections, a convention he maintained in all the other *balli* tunes in that treatise.[25]

Transcriptions of different misure: the relative tempi and scales of reduction

Proportion signs were used instead of writing passages in the next smallest note-values (as was done in the Giovanni Ambrosio versions of *Spero* and *Presoniera*). With this in mind, I have used different note-values in transcribing the four *misure* in order to bring out their increasing speeds: see Table 3.

TABLE 3. *Transcriptions of the four* misure

misura	transcription	metre
bassadanza	◦ = ♩. [a]	6/4
quadernaria	◦ = ♩ [b]	4/4
saltarello	◦ = ♪.	6/8
piva	◦ = ♪ (♩.)	2/4 (6/8)

[a] In mensural notation a *semibrevis* ◦ can either be duple ♩ or triple ♩., depending on the mensuration of the piece. In *Colonnese*, *Legiadra*, and [*Rostiboli*] *Gioioso*, where there are six—rather than two—*semibreves* per *tempo*, ◦ has been transcribed as a crotchet, but in the *saltarello* as a minim.
[b] In order to match the notation and choreography, some *quadernaria* sections have also been transcribed ◦ = ♪ , and, particularly in the case of German *saltarello* (*saltarello* in *quadernaria misura*), as ♬ = ♪.

Transcription of piva

There is a lack of uniformity in the notation of the *piva*: its prolation (the subdivision of the *semibrevis*) is sometimes minor and sometimes major. This

[24] See, for example, Apel, *Notation*, 190: '[P]roportional signs . . . represent the tempo marks, nay the metronomic marks, of the 15th and 16th centuries'. Domenico's signs (C3 , 3, ₵ 3) do, in fact, correspond in all three *balli* to a diminution sign or *sesquialtera* and suggest not only a proportionate increase in tempo, but a barring of *piva* in 2/4 with triplets.
[25] There seems to have been a kind of evolution in Guglielmo/Giovanni Ambrosio's notation which led up to this differentiation in Pa between *bassadanza* and *saltarello*. Guglielmo (Pg) began by notating his own *balli* tunes (e.g., *Spero*) in the same manner as Domenico before him. Then he seems to have experimented with new techniques in *Gratioso*, after which he changed the notation of the *bassadanza* and *saltarello* sections in his last *balli* to six repeated *semibreves* for each *tempo*.

occurs when an identical *piva* melody appears in different *balli* as well as when it appears in the same *ballo* transcribed in different treatises, so that the same *tempo* of *piva* is notated ♩ ♩ ♩ ♩ or ♩. ♩♩. ♩ or ♩♩♩♩ or 𝅝 ♩ 𝅝 ♩.[26] Cornazano's claim that the *piva* is '[the] daughter' of the *quadernaria*[27] would seem to suggest that all *piva* sections can be transcribed in 2/4, even if they look different in structure. When the notation intimates a 6/8 character, the 2/4 metre can be kept by using triplets. It is probable that because of the quickness of the *piva misura* there was not a strict difference in the performance of the various notations, the rhythmical disparities indicating, quite possibly, a kind of 'inequality' or 'ambivalence'.[28] Furthermore, by using a transcription in 2/4, rather than 6/8, the *saltarello* and *piva* are clearly differentiated, and a faster tempo is implied.

Transcription of German saltarello and German piva

What Guglielmo refers to in his *balli* as 'German *saltarello*' is, for the most part, the equivalent of Domenico's *saltarello in quadernaria*, that is, *saltarello* steps (*doppii* with hops) danced to music in *quadernaria misura*. A very popular variation of the *quadernaria*, it appears in half of Guglielmo's and Domenico's choreographies. In transcribing *saltarello in quadernaria* (and also *piva in quadernaria*), particular care should be taken to use the appropriate reduction and barring so that the music matches the *tempi* indicated.

The term 'German *saltarello*' also appears in two *bassedanze* in *De pratica*, where it presumably means a specific *quadernaria* step performed to *bassadanza* music.[29]

In yet another context German *saltarello* seems to mean *quadernaria doppii* performed to *saltarello* music. Guglielmo's *ballo Spero*, for instance, begins with four *doppii* 'in German' [*saltarello?*],[30] and in order to fit the choreography to the music (eight patterns or bars of what appears to be *saltarello misura* in 6/8), one *quadernaria* (four-beat) *doppio* is done to two bars of *saltarello* music.[31] Similar examples of what appear to be *quadernaria* steps to *piva* music are found

[26] See *Presoniera* and *Gelosia*. Compare the endings of *Spero*, *Gratioso*, *Legiadra*, and *Colonnese*.

[27] See above, n. 13.

[28] *Inégal* means the unequal performance of equally notated notes. An analogy can be found in the technical notion of 'ambivalence' in regional dance-music, past and present.

[29] In Guglielmo's *bassedanze Principessa* and *Caterva*, the choreography specifies not only *saltarello* steps (performed to the *bassadanza* music), but German *saltarello* as well. Clearly, German *saltarello* —as *saltarello doppii* danced to *quadernaria* music—does not apply here. Presumably Guglielmo intended a specific step (to be done to the *bassadanza* music), such as Domenico's *quadernaria* step —a *doppio* followed by a *frapamento*—or Cornazano's *quaternaria* or German *saltarello* step, two *sempii* and a *ripresetta* (a little *ripresa*). (Pd, fo. 6ᵛ; V, fo. 5ᵛ.)

[30] Specified only in NY, where the choreography calls for 'four *tempi* of German *saltarello*'. See below, *Balli*, n. 113.

[31] See the musical transcription and commentary on *Presoniera*, n. 2, alternative version, and *Spero*, I.

in the finales of *Spero*, *Legiadra*, *Colonnese*, *Gratioso*, and [*Rostiboli*] *Gioioso* and are barred accordingly.

Doppii *on or upon the same foot*

The *contrapasso* (literally 'counter-step') does not appear in any of Guglielmo's or Domenico's choreographies in Pg, Pa, or Pd, although it is present in later versions of the dances in V, S, NY, and FN. According to Cornazano (V, fo. 10ᵛ) and the Siena treatise (fo. 30ᵛ), three *contrapassi* ('on one foot', S) were performed in two *tempi* (bars of music). What is significant for the transcription of the *balli* in *De pratica* is that the equivalent type of performance applies to what Guglielmo and Domenico both refer to as 'three *doppii* per foot', that is, sequences of *doppii*, each *doppio* beginning 'on [with, upon] the same foot', rather than with the usual alternating of left and right feet.[32]

Introductory saltarelli

The *saltarello* was to begin, like the *bassadanza*, with the dancer initiating a preparatory movement—together with the soprano player—on the up-beat, his first step coinciding with the entrance of the tenor on the down-beat.[33] Two of Guglielmo's and six of Domenico's *balli* begin with an introductory *saltarello*.[34] With only one exception, Domenico's *Tesara*, all these *saltarelli* have an extra *tempo* of music, which may well have served as a brief introduction, providing, moreover, the necessary half-*tempo* of music for the initial *movimento*.

While many of Guglielmo's and Domenico's intentions still elude us, there are encouraging attempts (some included in this chapter) to unravel and to solve what, only a few years ago, were considered to be erroneous assertions, confused theorizings, or unfathomable mysteries of dance theorists.[35]

---

[32] See Lo Monaco and Vinciguerra, 'Il passo doppio'.

[33] Pd, fos. 3ʳ–4ᵛ.

[34] The *balli* in *De pratica* with introductory *saltarelli* are *Ingrata*, *Belriguardo*, *Colonnese*, *Legiadra*, *Mercantia*. (See also *Verçepe*, *Sobria*, and *Tesara* in Pd.)

[35] On a practical level, too, musicians specializing in early music have begun to make valid advances in the performance of 15th-c. Italian dance-music, improvising melodic lines around *bassadanza* tenors and *balli* tunes with the appropriate techniques and instrumentarium (for example, the Basle-based Ferrara Ensemble, directed by Crawford Young, and Maurizio Mingardi in Milan). Improvisatory techniques are discussed in T. McGee, *Medieval and Renaissance Music: A Performer's Guide* (Toronto, 1985), esp. 191–200, and in L. R. Baratz, 'Improvising on the Spagna Tune', *The American Recorder*, 29 (1988), 141–6, and its sequel, 'Fifteenth Century Improvisation, Take Two: Building a Vocabulary of Embellishments', ibid., 31 (1990), 7–11. Other references from a bibliography supplied to me by Irene Alm, to whom I am much indebted, include Bonnie J. Blackburn, 'On Compositional Process in the Fifteenth Century', JAMS 40 (1987), 210–84; James Haar, *Essays on Italian Poetry and Music in the Renaissance 1350–1600* (Berkeley and Los Angeles, 1986); and Winternitz, *Leonardo da Vinci*

PART II

⁊&

DE PRATICA SEU ARTE TRIPUDII

ON THE PRACTICE OR ART OF DANCING

Notes on the Transcription and Translation

In fifteenth-century Italy, as elsewhere, orthography lacked uniformity. Punctuation was not codified, there was considerable latitude in spelling, and genders were not necessarily respected. Scribal differences between Guglielmo's *De pratica* and the Giovanni Ambrosio version may perhaps be due to copyists of different provenance and training working from the dictation of readers, themselves of diverse origin. A diplomatic transcription of the first pages of both Prefaces shows typical differences (variations in spelling, gender, and punctuation are italicized), although neither of the two scribes remains consistent within his own work.

Guglielmo (Pg)	*Giovanni Ambrosio (Pa)*
PROHOEMIUM INCIPIT:	*PROEMIUM*:

Molte & varie *soño* infra gli humani
& diverse *opinione* nellinvestigare
quale *antica*mente fosse al *mundo*
della musica *inventore.*Impero che
alchuni fermamente tegnano Apollo
potentissimo idio *terreno havere*
prima luso della dolce *ci*thara al
secol ritrovato.Altri vogliano
che uno *anti*quissimo fabro con la
dolce *cõsonantia* di suoi martelli
nellancudine percotendo/prima le
concordantie di tal *scienza ritrovasse.*
Altri di Siringa poeticamente
descriveno:La qual al dolce *mormorio*
delle *transcorrente* acque una certa
melodia & canto formasse.Altri dicono
di Pan *Archadio* pastore:*il* qual per
natural ingegno *congionte insieme* certe
canne artificiosamente composte &
incerate.*et quelle postosi* alla *boccha*
facea col fiato dolce *consonanza/*tal
che le *sue pascente* pecorelle udendo
la dolcezza

Molte & varie *sonno* infra gli humani
& diverse *oppinioni* nellinvestigare
quale *antica*mente fosse al *mondo*
della musica *in ventore.*Impero che
alconi. fermamente tegnano Apollo
potentissimo.idio *Tereno haver*
prima luso.della dolce *Ci*thara al
secol ritrovato..Altri vogliano
c̃h uno *Anti*quissimo fabro con la
dolce *consonancia* di suoi martelli
nella ancodine percotendo prima le
*concordancie.*di tal *sciença ritrovassi:*
Altri di Siringa poeticamente
discriveno [la qual] al dolce *mormoreo*
delle *trasconrente* acque una certa
melodia & canto formasse Altri dicono
di Pan *Arcadio* pastore *el* qual per.
natural ingegno *congionto in sieme* certe
canne artificiosamente composte &
incerate &.*quelli postose* alla *bocha*
facea col fiato.dolce *consonancia* tal
che le *soe pasciente* pecorelle udendo
La dolceça

Orthography

Many words in *De pratica* always appear in an archaic or dialect form: *tegnano*, *bigiogno*, rather than *tengono*, *bisogno*. Erratic, multiform spelling is common (Guglielmo, Guiglielmo, Guilielmo; *Ligiadra*, *Legiadra*, *Lizadra*), and the presence or absence of double letters is inconsistent and often differs from present usage (*sonno* instead of *sono*—'am', 'are'; *fabro* for *fabbro*). In the dance descriptions the number 'two' very often follows the gender of the step: *doi sempii* (masculine), *due continenze* (feminine). No attempt has been made to modernize the spelling in the Italian transcription; footnotes, or the translation itself, should clarify the meaning of words that are obscure because of their spelling.[1] Key words frequently spelt differently from modern usage are: *el* for *il*, *se* (often used instead of the reflexive *si*), *colla* for *con la*, and *del* rather than *dal*. *El* can also be a contraction for *et il*, and *ell*, *ella*, *elli*, *ellei* should read *e l'*[huomo] (or *et il* [huomo]), *et la*, *et li*, *et lei*. 'Is' is distinguished from 'and' (*è* and *e* in modern Italian) by maintaining Pagano's spelling, which is almost always *e* for 'is' and *et*–or the sign &—for 'and' except when *e* is combined with articles as just indicated, and in the introductory poems, where it is elided with *i*. (In the Giovanni Ambrosio copy, a capital *E* seems to indicate 'and'.)

Omissions and contractions

There are surprisingly few occurrences in the *De pratica* manuscript that can be considered 'slips of the pen' and these have either been noted or, in the case of missing letters, added to the transcription in square brackets. Abbreviations have been silently expanded. Other copies of *De pratica*, Giovanni Ambrosio's first of all, have been consulted for scribal ambiguities or omissions.

Punctuation

Guglielmo's scribe, Pagano of Rho, used a variety of signs (still decipherable for the most part): strokes /, one dot ., two dots :, and an abbreviation sign resembling a tilde. His capital letters do not always indicate the beginning of a sentence and full stops are often missing.[2] In the transcription the punctuation has been minimally regularized for legibility. More regularization than I have attempted would have imposed an interpretation on the text that I reserve for the translation. A comma replaces the stroke, and a gap has been left after

---

[1] In the translation of *De pratica* and of documents cited in the introductory chapters, I have standardized the spellings of Guglielmo's and Giovanni Ambrosio's names, modernizing that of the latter (see Ch. 2 n. 13). Where Guglielmo (Pg) has multiple spellings for the names of the *balli*, I have used only one in the translation (that closest to a modern spelling). For those terms, choreographic and other, given in Italian in the translation, a standardized spelling is used (e.g. *ripresa* for *represa*, *rimpresa*).

[2] Pagano's letter 'L' is problematic; it is not easy to distinguish when a capital or small 'L' is intended at the beginning of a word which does not follow a dot.

every sign to space the text. No accents have been introduced anywhere. Since apostrophes were never used, it is not always clear when a letter has been deleted before a vowel, so that *che* ('that', 'which', 'then', 'what', etc.) is often used to mean *ch'è* or *che è* ('who is', 'that is'). In these cases I have added an apostrophe. Apostrophes are also introduced to separate an article from the following noun: e.g. *l'aire*. Today, *nelhumano* would be written *nell'umano*. While maintaining the original spelling, I have decided, as an aid to intelligibility, to separate these and similar words (*nel humano*), just as I have joined *ne i* (*nei*) when Pagano himself has not done so. In Pagano's original and in my transcription, terms like *in contro*, *cio e*, and *in drieto* appear both as one and as two words, and occasionally it has proven difficult to ascertain which was intended. Full stops have been added to the end of a few choreographic descriptions, and, on four occasions, particularly long sections have been split into paragraphs.

Problems of translation

Many of the words in *De pratica* have meanings that differ from their modern or even late sixteenth-century usage. (Florio gives only 'pilgrim' for *peregrino, pellegrino*, whereas Guglielmo's meaning is usually 'rare, choice'.[3] Where dictionaries and comparative texts have proved inadequate for unorthodox spellings, colloquial forms, and archaisms, I have sought the expertise of specialists.

Musical and dance terms having no English equivalents, or whose significance is particular to fifteenth-century Italy, or to the dance-treatises themselves, have not been translated. Some of these are explained in detail in Ch. 4 and all are discussed in the Glossary, where they are listed in their various spellings, and in their singular and plural forms. All the dance steps have been kept in Italian. This is because for some steps (like *continenze*) there is no exact term in English, while for others—where terms do exist—confusion with steps of the same name from other periods and/or countries (such as a Playford 'double' or a French or Burgundian '*simple*') is altogether too possible. (Choreographic and musical terms, whether translated or not, are listed in the Glossary in the original Italian.) Other words, like *virtute* and *liberale*, have been translated literally, with cognates (in this case, 'virtue' and 'liberal'), since these humanistic terms had the same meaning (now archaic) in English and Italian. However, because of the breadth or particularity of their meaning in the Renaissance—and our distance from those modes of thought—they too are commented upon in the Glossary. Thus it will be up to the reader to ascribe the relevant modern significance to Guglielmo's prose.

This I have tried to render in clear and fluent English, preferring, where

---

[3] Cf. *pellegrina* in the *Grande dizionario della lingua italiana*, ed. S. Battaglia and G. B. Squarotti (Turin, 1961–).

possible, a more idiomatic, rather than literal, translation: 'festivity' or 'enter-tainment' for *festa* rather than 'feast'. At the same time, once a word has been translated I have usually repeated the same translation throughout, notwith-standing the literary urge to vary. I have endeavoured to respect the original sentence structure while remaining consistent with modern English. For clar-ity's sake, especially long and complex sentences have, where feasible, been broken up into shorter ones. Ambiguities in the text have been reproduced in the translation despite the temptation to unravel them. The desire for intelligi-bility is particularly acute in the case of Guglielmo's descriptions of Dome-nico's dances, but I have, with a few exceptions, refrained from adding the various missing links and refer the reader to Domenico's treatise.[4] In the end, the criterion that I have followed has been that of trying to reflect in English the sophisticated 'humanistic' style that Guglielmo seems to have so painstakingly sought.

The language in which the choreographies are described is quite straightfor-ward and presents no particular difficulties to the translator. I have maintained the obsessive 'and then', deleted none of the bizarre punctuation,[5] and respected the—at times—ungrammatical sentence structure, so that those who wish to reconstruct the dances have at their disposal all the elements of the original Italian. (Some commas have been added to the translation for the intelligibility of the English. A glance at the Italian will reveal which.) As regards the form of the choreographic instructions, I have preferred the 'direct' style used in both early English dance-manuals and in nineteenth-century American social-dance-books, as well as in square- and folk-dancing today: 'Make three *riprese*', rather than a literal translation of Guglielmo's 'They make three *riprese*'.[6]

The most formidable problems for the translator are, without a doubt, to be found in Books I and II, and notably in the Preface. The syntax, vocabulary, and complex philosophical and theoretical speculations—and the culture in which these are embedded—are particularly resistant to twentieth-century English. Guglielmo undoubtedly had difficulty transferring to the written page concepts with which he was familiar enough when embodied in action. And

---

[4] Any additions, some of which have been included for musical reasons, are in square brackets or footnotes.

[5] In the translation of the choreographies, a dot (.) has been rendered as a semicolon if the sentence which follows is incomplete. Two dots (:) appear only occasionally and they too have been 'translated' as a semicolon, or, on one occasion in *Ingrata*, as a comma. The stroke appears as a comma both in the transcription and the translation, except in the case of *Marchesana*, where syntax has required some of the strokes to be rendered as semicolons.

[6] See, for example, the Playford dances in *The English Dancing Master* (1st edn. 1651; fac. repr., ed. Margaret Dean-Smith, London, 1957); the dances from the Inns of Court (*Dancing in the Inns of Court*, ed. James B. Cunningham, London, 1965); E. Ferrero's *The Art of Dancing* (New York, 1859); and Professor Baron's *Complete Instructor in all the Society Dances of America* (New York, 1881).

his apparent desire to model his work on the examples of contemporary treatises, which were steeped in humanistic thought and terminology and concerned with justifying their worth by following certain conventions,[7] seems at times to have confused what must have been the everyday recognitions of a dancing-master.[8] One cannot help wondering whether he was always clear himself about his meaning.[9] This is particularly frustrating when musical questions, so vital to the dance reconstructor or early music specialist, are discussed. Therefore, as before with the archaic humanistic terms, I have preferred to use—for the most part at least, and English permitting—literal translations of certain concepts, such as 'measure', 'time', and 'concordant voices', because of the possibility of multiple interpretations (listed in the Glossary), and different layers of meaning hidden in the thick foliage of the treatise's apology. Most important, Guglielmo in English will thus be as enigmatic, and as demanding of the reader, as he is—today—in Italian.

A translation of Giovanni Ambrosio's Autobiography appears in App. III without the original Italian since the transcription by F. A. Gallo is readily available.[10] Despite its rather pompous exordium, the journal is extremely repetitive, every entry beginning *Ancora me atrovai* ('I was also present') or *E piu me atrovai* ('Moreover I was present'), and one is sorely tempted to provide, in translation at least, a richer variety of adjectives besides *bello* and *degno* ('beautiful' and 'worthy'). The highly interesting additional chapters from the Giovanni Ambrosio copy (App. I, Italian transcription included), are rendered frustratingly problematic and ambiguous by a particularly ungrammatical Italian.

Given the various difficulties, the Italian text has been included in a facing transcription to permit immediate consultation and to allow the reader the possibility of testing my decisions against the original.

---

[7] See Ch. 1.

[8] See, for example, Ch. 4 for a discussion of the discrepancies in the *balli* mensurations.

[9] Professor Nino Pirrotta expressed to me this particular doubt apropos of Guglielmo's Exercise V.

[10] See Gallo, 'L'autobiografia'.

AD ILLUSTRISSIMUM PRINCIPEM ET EXCELLENTISSIMUM DOMINUM DOMINUM GALEACIUM VICECOMITEM COMITEM PAPIAE & CAETERA:

Gloria sopra ogni gloria alto signore
   Cui studio di prudenza. & di *virtute
   Tira in triumphal carro a sommo honore
Poi che sul piu bel fior di gioventute
   Va dato il ciel belleza. ingegno. & gratia.
   Di quante dote son tra noi vedute
Io come quel che non gia mai si satia
   Servir Sforceschi in quanto ho possa & arte:
   Resarcito ho per voi quel ch'altri stratia.
Dico ch'el danzar sparso in varie carte
   Ho colto in questa opretta. e i suoi fragmenti
   Ch'ora a voi mando per farvene parte. |
Assai son stato cogli spirti attenti
   Qual peregrin per le nocturne valle
   Perso il sentier advien che si sgomenti.
Vedendo a caso poi doppo le spalle
   Un lume d'alta torre indi si spiza
   Per coniectura d'infallibil calle.
Ne si dritta esce d'arco ungaro friza
   Chom'io sentito il raggio di tua fama
   Vengho a te: a cui ogni virtu si driza.
& qual serpente di versatil squama
   Sotto l'incantator ch'el volge e rota:
   Tal a te son se tua bonta mi chiama.
Ma se l'opra d'ornato vi par vota
   Pensate che nei don d'un suo servente
   La fede sol del mandator si nota.
Men degna ella e di voi signor potente
   Questo confesso. pur io non suspetto:
   Che mie ragion per poverta sian vente.
Anzi son certo haura per tal respetto
   Che siati degnato ad accettarla:
   Gloria il mio nome, el cuor sommo diletto.

TO HIS MOST ILLUSTRIOUS PRINCE AND MOST EXCELLENT LORD, LORD GALEAZZO, VISCOUNT AND COUNT OF PAVIA, ETCETERA

Glory to thee, high lord, glory above all glory far,
    Whose study of *virtue[1] and the craft of power
    Draw to supreme honour in triumphal car.
Since heaven to your youth's fair flower
    Has added beauty, grace, and wit,
    What bounteous gifts our lives endower!
I, as one who knows no surfeit
    In serving Sforza with all the skill I may,
    What others rend I have for you reknit.
I mean those dances on various papers stray,
    Here gathered in this little work as many themes,
    Which, to make part of it, I now to you convey.
Brave spirits ever held my high esteem,
    Like the wanderer in the hills at night,
    Who, having lost the path, fears what beseems;
And, turning then by chance, he sees a light
    In a high tower burning, whither at once he hies
    By paths unfailing now to inward sight.
No arrow from the Magyar's bow so swiftly flies
    As I, subject to the beams of your great name,
    Come straight to thee in whom all virtue lies.
Or, as under the charmer's spell made tame,
    The snake of supple skin doth coil and wind,
    So I, when your bounty summon, do the same.
Yet if devoid of grace this book you find —
    But think: of servants' gifts all are aware
    It is but the giver's duty that one minds.
With you, noble lord, its worth cannot compare,
    This I admit. And yet all thoughts decline
    That my words, for lack of substance, are but air.
Nay, that you accept this work of mine
    Is reason certain that no doubt remain;
    My heart shall know delight, my fame shall shine.

---

[1] An asterisk in the transcription and translation indicates the first appearance of a term included in the Glossary.

Vedrete adonque ormai quanto ella parla
    Varij passi. *misura. & come giace
    In due, tre, quattro botte. a iusta farla.
Ben priego almen s'alchuna cosa face
    Del mio, vostra excellenza, el vi sia grato |

    Non vi sdegnati a dir questo mi piace.
Ogni volta non puo pensarsi in stato.
    In regimenti. in dar lege, & iustitia
    Ne contra gli nemici andare armato
Conviene. et questo e quasi altra militia
    Ad un giovenil cuor. tal hor far danze
    Spesso udir *suon, s'el debito non vitia.
Amor vuol la sua parte. et posto ha inanze
    A noi mortali ogni gentil partito
    Per salda scala delle sue speranze.
Di questo il studio mio ve n'ha fornito
    Secundo il suo poter. supplischa fede
    S'el don non e chome esser puo compito.
Pur ch'el vi piaccia, el m'e summa mercede.

I Liber augustas Galeaci faustus ad edes
    Teque mei perfer principis ante pedes.
Hic est: anguigero natus qui caesare: nomen
    Terminet extremi finibus oceani.
Cuius sydereo natura in pectore fixit
    Quidquid in humanis mentibus esse potest.
Hic est: qui Latiam laturus ad aethera gentem
    Illustres magno nomine tollet avos.
Hunc pete parve liber nostri breve pignus amoris.
    & niveam flexo poplite tange manum. |

Dona ferant alij precioso fulva metallo.
    Tinctaque puniceo texta colore vehant.
Non ea nos fortuna iuvat. felixque facultas.
    Quae potes ingenij munera ferto liber.
Et tamen haec claris animum virtutibus augent.
    Solaque ab humano turbine tuta iurent.
Terra prius fruges & stellas exuet aether
    & ruet ad fontes unda reflexa suos:
Quam cultae pereant artes facundaque linguae
    Gratia: quam virtus interitura cadat.
Quod si nobilitas excultis tanta libellis
    Non poteras alio dignior esse viro.
Non est conspicuis praestantior artibus alter:

Here you shall see, then, how is made plain
    *Measure, the various steps, and how lies the key
    In beats two, three, and four, this art to gain.
One thing I humbly beg, if aught there be
    Persuades Your Excellency that thanks he owe,
    He'll not disdain to say 'This pleases me'.
Not every thought upon the state can go;
    On justice, giving laws, or soldiers' pay,
    Nor yet will marching armed against the foe
Serve every turn. Almost another kind of fray
    The young find this. To dance upon occasion,
    To hear *music in due sort won't lead astray.
Love will have her rights, and she positions
    Before us mortals a noble counterpart
    As certain pathway to her own ambitions.
To you these things my study does impart
    As best it may. If the gift proves flawed,
    Make recompense a loyal heart.
That it but please you is my high reward.

Go in good omen, Book, to Galeazzo's stately seat
    And thither lay yourself before my prince's feet.
This is he, born of Caesar's dragon line,
    Whose fame will spread to the farthest ocean's bound,
In whose celestial breast Nature has set
    The sum of what in human minds she can.
This is he will hoist to the heavens the Latin race
    And his famed forebears with his great name exalt.
Thither get thee, little book, poor pledge of my love,
    And touch on bended knee that snowy hand.
Gifts others bear tawny with precious ore
    And stuffs dipped in the Tyrean dye do bring;
Us, no such fortune favours nor such fair means
    So what you may of wit take you in gift,
For its rare virtues do yet the mind endow
    And please when in lone refuge from the crowd.
The earth shall lack its fruits and the sky be sere of stars
    And the bent-back flood break on the spring,
Before the learned arts and fertile grace
    Of speech wither and virtue pining die.
But if there be such worth in books ornate
    No man more worthy of it than are you,
None more outstanding in the foremost arts

Quemáque magis tantus tollat in astra decor.
    Ille manus ad te vultu praetendet amico
      Exceptumáque hilari molliter ore legat.
    Forsitan & blando mitis sermone probabit
      Si nostris aliquis est modo rebus honos.
    Fortunate nimis tantum cui cernere lumen
      Magnanimiáque datur principis ore legi.
    I felix. dominumáque illi committe fidelem.
      Devotum imperijs me sciat esse suis.

[iiiʳ]

GUILIELMI HEBRAEI PISAURIENSIS DE PRATICA SEU ARTE TRIPUDII VULGARE OPUSCULUM INCIPIT:

Dal *harmonia suave il *dolce *canto
    Che per l'audito passa dentro al cuore
    Di gran dolceza nasce un vivo ardore:
    Da cui il danzar poi vien che piace tanto.
Pero chi di tal scienza vuol il vanto
    Convien che sei partite senza errore
    Nel suo concetto apprenda e mostri fuora
    Si come io qui discrivo. insegno. et canto.
Misura e prima. & seco vuol memoria.
    Partir poi di terren con *aire bella.
    Dolce *mainiera, & *movimento & poi
Queste ne dano del danzar la gloria.
    Con dolce gratia, a chi l'ardente stella
    Piu favoreggia con gli ragi suoi.
      E i passi et gesti tuoi
    Sian ben composti et destra tua persona
    Con lo intelletto attento a quel che suona.

Whom abounding grace raises to the stars.
He will to thee reach out with welcome in his face
   And, taking, read soft with smiling lips,
And perchance with mild words flatter that it pleases—
   Should anything of merit lie in our things.
Great good fortune his who meets that gaze
   And is by the prince magnanimous read aloud.
Blithely go, commend me a faithful gentleman
   That he may know me all obedient to his bidding.[2]

HERE BEGINS THE LITTLE WORK IN THE VERNACULAR ON THE PRACTICE OR ART OF DANCING BY GUGLIELMO THE JEW OF PESARO

From smooth *harmony is begot *sweet *song
   Which through the hearing reaches the heart's core.
   From much sweetness is born a lively ardour
   Whence comes then the dance, its pleasure strong.
But who would boast this skill to him belongs
   Should these six chapters without error
   Fix in his mind and show outwardly
   Just as I say here, and teach and make my song:
Measure is foremost and wants with it Memory;
   Partition then of ground, with pleasant *Air;
   Sweet *Manner and *Movement—these the things
   Which give the dance its glory;
With sweet grace in those the fair
   Star most favours with its shining.
     And be thy steps and gesturing
   Well-shaped, thy body's motions featly made,
   And thy wits intent on what is played.

---

[2] This poem seems to me inferior to the preceding one but I have it on better authority that it is on the whole a perfectly competent piece of work, reminiscent in its spirit of Tibullan elegance in modesty and Horatian care in deference. M.S.

[1ᵛ]

PROHOEMIUM INCIPIT:

Molte & varie sonno[a] infra gli humani & diverse opinione nell'investigare quale antichamente fosse al mundo della musica inventore. Impero che alchuni fermamente tegnano Apollo potentissimo idio terreno havere prima l'uso della dolce *cithara al secol ritrovato. Altri vogliano che uno antiquissimo fabro con la dolce *consonantia di suoi martelli nell'ancudine percotendo, prima le *concordantie di tal scienza ritrovasse. Altri di Siringa poeticamente descriveno: La qual al dolce mormorio delle transcorrente acque una certa *melodia & canto formasse. Altri dicono di Pan Archadio pastore: il qual per *natural ingegno congionte insieme certe canne *artificiosamente composte & incerate. et quelle postosi alla boccha facea col fiato dolce consonanza, tal che le sue
[2ʳ] pascente pecorelle udendo la dolcezza | del suo suave suono spesse volte lasciavano il nutritivo cibo: & quasi dalla forza di quella melodia commosse hor in qua, hor in la intorno al suo pastore danzavano, saltavano. Cosi etiandio de infiniti altri anchora potriamo dire & recordare. Ma qual di questi, o altri chi se fusse prima origine, o principio di tal scienza, fu di singular laude & memoria digno.

La qual arte intra le sette non e la minore annumerata. anzi come scienza *liberale se mostra sublime et alta. & da dover seguire come l'altre dignissima. et quasi al humana natura piu che alchuna dell'altre aptissima & conforme: Impero che da quattro *concordanti & principal *voci formata & composta alle nostre quattro principal compositioni correspondente porge ascoltando a tutti nostri sensi singular conforto, quasi si chome ella fusse di nostri spiriti naturalissimo cibo. ne par che si ritruovi al mondo alchuna si cruda & inhumana gente: che al dolce canto & al suave suono d'alchuno *ben *concor-
[2ᵛ] dato instrumento, con | summo piacere non si commuova: si come del famoso Orpheo degnamente si scrive. Il quale con tanta gratia la sua dolce cithara sonando non solamente gli humani spiriti a dolcezza commoveva: m[a] il fiero Plutone & gl'infernali idij & gli animali bruti et ferocissimi leoni coll'altre alpestre fiere, & i sassi & i monti facea per la sua gran dolcezza dalla propria sua natura ad altra piu benigna transmutare. Similmente si scrive dell'antichissimo Amphione: il quale chome vogliano i poeti, alla citta di Thebe col vago suono della sua cithara facea le pietre da gli alti monti scendere: et quelle per se medesme nella fabricatione dell'alte mura miraculosamente comporsi. et di

---

[a] The modern spelling of *sono* ('am, are') is rarely used in *De pratica*.

PREFACE

Many, varied, and diverse are the views of men in their quest to determine who in the world of antiquity was the inventor of music. Thus, some people firmly believe that Apollo, that most powerful Olympian deity,[3] was the first in time to have discovered the use of the sweet-sounding *cithara. Others hold that a smith of long ago, through the sweet-sounding *consonance of his hammers beating on the anvil, first discovered the *harmonies of this science. Others speak poetically of Syrinx, who shaped a particular *melody and song to the sweet murmur of flowing waters. Others name Pan, the Arcadian shepherd, who, with *native wit, joined and *skilfully fashioned and sealed certain reeds together. Lifting them to his lips, he blew such sweet harmonies that his grazing lambs, hearing the sweetness of his pleasant tune, often abandoned their pasture and danced and bounded here and there round their shepherd, as if moved by the power of his melody. Thus could we also describe and call to mind an infinity of others. But whichever of these, or whoever else, was the prime mover or founder of this science, he deserves singular praise and remembrance.

This art is not reckoned the least important of the seven; indeed, as a *liberal science it is clearly sublime and lofty, and as worthy of pursuit as the others. And in some ways it suits and befits human nature more than any other [art] inasmuch as, through the four principal and *concordant *voices[4] of which it is formed and composed (corresponding to our four principal humours),[5] it offers, as we listen, singular comfort to all our senses, as if it were our souls' most natural food. Nor does it seem that there is anyone in the world so uncouth and barbarous as not to be moved to utmost pleasure by the sweet song and the pleasant sound of a *well-tuned instrument. Thus is it truly written of renowned Orpheus that he played his sweet-sounding *cithara* with such grace as to soothe not only the spirits of men, but wild Pluto and the infernal deities, as well as brutish animals, ferocious lions, and other savage beasts. The great sweetness [of music] also transmuted the very nature of rocks and hills into a more kindly one; as in the tale of Amphion of yore who, according to the poets, with the fair sound of his *cithara*, made the stones descend from the high hills and arrange themselves miraculously into the building of the high walls of the city of Thebes. And I could similarly describe

---

[3] Guglielmo has presumably used the term *terreno* (of the earth or world) to distinguish Apollo from the pagan gods of the *under*world, and from the Judaeo-Christian God in Heaven.

[4] Guglielmo may well have intended the four voices known at the time as Cantus, Altus (Contratenor Altus), Tenor, Bassus (Contratenor Bassus).

[5] According to old physiology, the four humours or bodily fluids (yellow bile, blood, black bile, phlegm) determined the four temperaments (choleric or bilious, sanguine, melancholy, phlegmatic), which were also related to the four elements and to the four voices.

molti altri similmente potria narrare: li quali per la dolcezza & virtu di questa vaga & suavissima scienza hanno al mondo fatto singularissimi effetti et mara- vigliosi movimenti: per li quali se comprende di quella essere alla nostra natura & alla compositione delli quatro elementi grandemente colligata. & in gran [3ʳ] parte conforme per la virtu et | potenza della qual gia si commosse il celestiale omnipotente idio dagli humani divotamente pregato: i quali nei sancti sacrificij con alta melodia cantando & con dolci instrumenti & sancti tripudij danzando obtegnevano la domandata gratia: chome gia piu volte si chome si lege il sapientissimo Salamone fece quando contra lui & il suo populo vedeva l'alto idio turbato. & chome anchora fece il glorioso re David: il quale piu volte collo suo amoroso & sancto psalterio & [sic]ᵇ agionto insieme il tribulato populo con festevole & honesto danzare, & col harmonia del dolce canto commovea l'irato & potente idio a piatosa & suavissima pace. Moses anchora principalissimo patriarcha con simil modo placava l'eterno idio con suavi canti: con li quali spesse volte il suo errante populo dalla furiosa & divina vendetta defendeva.

Per li quali exempli & molti altri assai chiaramente si manifesta questa tal virtude & scienza essere di singularissima efficacia, & alla humana generatione [3ᵛ] amicissima & conservativa: senza la quale alchuna lieta | & perfetta vita essere tra gli humani giamai non puote: si chome noi stessi spesse volte proviamo quando con tanto & si fervente studio nutricamo nelle nostre case i vaghi & lieti ucelletti per havere da loro il dolce & suave frutto di suoi amorosi & delettevoli canti: dalla gran maestra di natura in lor creati. Li quali sovente porgono agl'infermi spiriti & alle contristate menti leticia singulare. Le qual cose ci mostrano la grande excellenza & suprema dignitate d'essa scienza. dalla qual l'arte giocunda e[t e]l dolce effetto del danzare e naturalmente proceduto. la qual virtute del danzare non e altro che una actione demostrativa di fuori di movimenti spiritali: li quali si hanno a concordare colle misurate et perfette consonanze d'essa harmonia: che per lo nostro audito alle parti intellective & ai sensi cordiali con diletto descende: dove poi si genera certi dolci commovi- menti: i quali chome contra sua natura ri[n]chiusi, si sforzano quanto possano [4ʳ] di uscire fuori: & farsi in atto manifesti. | Il qual atto da essa dolcezza & melodia tirato alle parti exteriori colla propria persona danzando si dimostra quello quasi con la voce & col harmonia congionto & concordante che [escie]ᶜ dal accordato et dolce canto, overo dall'ascoltante et misurato suono.

Ma perche tal arte e virtuosa contemplatione facilmente non si puo sotto breve parole nel'humano intelletto bene imprimere senza qualche chiara & demostrativa ragione riducendo in praticha et in aperta experienza tutto quello che all'arte del danzare & a tale virtuoso exercitio si conviene. Et per tanto io divotissimo discipulo & fervente imitatore del dignissimo cavaliero messer

---

ᵇ See n. 6 in the translation.
ᶜ Supplied from FN, NY, and S.

many others who, through the sweetness and virtue of this delightful and most pleasurable science, wrought extraordinary changes and marvellous motions in the world. Thus one can understand that [music] is profoundly linked and in great part akin to our nature and to the composition of the four elements. Because of its virtue and power almighty God in heaven was moved by the devout prayers of men who, by singing lofty music, [playing] sweet-sounding instruments, and tripping sacred dances during the holy sacrifices, obtained the grace they had beseeched. We read that wise Solomon did this many times when he saw God on high vexed with him and his people. And so also did glorious King David who, many times, with his lovely and sacred psaltery, drew[6] the troubled people together with festive and decorous dance, and through the harmony of his sweet song moved an irate and powerful God to a merciful and most gentle peace. In the same way Moses, foremost among the patriarchs, placated the Eternal God with pleasant song, often shielding his errant people from wrathful and divine vengeance.

Through these exemplars and many others, this particular virtue and science clearly proves itself to be of the most extraordinary efficacy, and most auspicious and sustaining to the human race; for without it there could never be a joyful and full life for mankind. We ourselves often experience this when, with such very fervent care, we keep pretty and joyous little birds in our homes so as to gather the sweet and pleasant fruit of their lovely and delightful song, begotten in them by Nature's great mastery, which often offers singular gladness to feeble spirits and sorrowing minds. All these things reveal to us the great value and supreme worth of this science, which so naturally ushers in the merry art and sweet effects of the dance. This virtue of the dance is simply an outward manifestation of the movements of the soul, which must accord with the measured and perfect consonances of that harmony which, through our hearing, moves down with delight to our intellect and our affections, where there is then generated certain sweet commotions which, as if pent up unnaturally, struggle mightily to escape and display themselves in action. This action, brought forth by that sweetness and melody through the dancing movement of one's own body, shows itself to be, as it were, joined and concordant with the voice and harmony which emerge from tuneful and sweet singing or from rhythmically played music.

But why this art is worthy of study cannot be easily impressed upon the human intellect in a few words without some clear and conclusive argument, putting into practice and bringing down to plain experience everything that the art of the dance and such a worthy occupation require. Wherefore I, most devoted disciple and fervent follower of that most praiseworthy knight,

[6] The original translates as, '& drawn together the troubled people'. It may be that '&' is a scribal error and should instead read 'ha' (third person singular of the verb 'to have'), which would give us the reading as above.

Domenico da Ferrara nell'arte preditta del danzare doctissimo & singulare quanto dalla sua famosa & prestante doctrina possetti racogliere: Avenga che insofficiente et di basso ingegno a si alta impresa mi ritruovi, non da iactanza overo da gloriosa pompa, ne ancho da prosumptuosa intentione commosso.

[4ᵛ] Ma solamente da amicabili & domestici prieghi d'alchuni | virtuosi & honesti giovani dell'arte preditta cupidi & volontorosi: & quella sapere, et perfettamente intendere. Li quali a me per honestissima amicicia convinctissimi, non possendo io per alchun modo a i suoi persuasivi & honesti prieghi contradire: dispuosi la mente mia quanto alle forze del mio ingegno si concede dovere al lor alto et honesto desiderio in parte satisfare: Mostrando io nella compilatione di questa mia operetta della virtute & arte del danzare alchune opportune & necessarie particelle. Le qual intese & quelle con fermo intelletto ben notate, & alla sua praticha congionte: potra ciaschuno facilmente & con securita in ogni festivo luogho con summa laude danzare, & tal virtute optimamente exercitare. La quale agl'inamorati & generosi cuori et agli animi gentili per celeste inclinatione piu tosto che per *accidentale dispositione e amicissima & conforme. Ma aliena in tutto & mortal inimicha di vitiosi & mechanici plebei: i quali le piu volte con animo corrotto & colla scelerata mente la fano di arte

[5ʳ] liberale & virtuosa sci|enza: adultera & servile: et molte volte anchora alle lor inhoneste concupiscenze sotto specie di honestate la inducono mezana per poter cautamente al effetto d'alchuna sua voluptate danzando pervenire. A i quali quanto piu posso totalmente la niego loro. Ne ponto mi curo che alle sue mani la presente opera pervenga. accio ch'io non sia per alchun tempo alle sue inique & maligne corruptioni efficiente [*sic*: efficiente] & maxima occasione. Ma solamente agli honesti & casti petti, & a chi essa come virtute & licita scienza la desidera, & vuole adoperare con humilissimo & cordiale affetto la racomando. & priegho che quella col mio buon volere lietamente accettando legia. se in quella alchuna particella tralasciata havessi: per la quale meno che perfetta si mostrasse. sottoponendome sempre alla degna correctione del mio honorato et dotto preceptore: & di ciaschun altro in la ditta arte peritissimo et experto. Attenda adoncha et coll'animo giocundo ben racoglia le sue parti, felicemente poi & cun virtu danzando.

Messer Domenico of Ferrara, most learned and outstanding in the aforesaid art of the dance—as can be gathered from his widely known and excellent doctrines—although I find myself unequal to and of small wit for so lofty an undertaking, and prompted neither by insolence nor vainglory nor yet by presumptuous intention, but simply by the amiable and gentle entreaties of some virtuous and upright youths (eager and willing to learn and master to perfection the aforesaid art and closely bound to me by honest friendship), I, being in no way able to deny their persuasive and honest entreaties, resolved, as far as my wits consented, that I had to in part satisfy their lofty and honest desire by presenting—in the compilation of this small work of mine on the virtue and art of dancing—some pertinent and essential elements, which, once grasped and kept firmly in mind, with the addition of practice, will enable everyone to dance with ease and assurance and most commendably on all festive occasions and to exercise this skill in surpassing fashion. This [art of dancing] most favours and befits those whose hearts are loving and generous and those whose spirits are ennobled by a heavenly bent rather than by a *fortuitous inclination. But it is completely alien to, and the mortal enemy of, vile and rude mechanicals[7] who often, with corrupt souls and treacherous minds, turn it from a liberal art and virtuous science into something adulterous and ignoble. And often, in the guise of honour, they even make it pimp for their shameful lewdness so that they may slyly use dancing to satisfy their lust. To such as these, insofar as I am able, I wholly deny my present work, and I wish in no way for it to fall into their hands lest I become at any time the main cause and determinant of their iniquitous and wicked depravity. Therefore I recommend [this work] to the honest and chaste of heart only, and to those who aspire to it [the dance] as a virtue and as a proper science and wish to devote themselves to it with humble and sincere affection. And I beg them to read it, graciously recognizing my good intentions even if I have overlooked any little portion which may render it less than perfect; and ever submitting myself to the valuable criticism of my honoured and learned master and to whomever else is highly skilled and expert in the said art. Therefore, pay heed and with blithe spirit consider well its various parts, thereby dancing happily and virtuously.

[7] 'Mechanical' is used here as a synonym for 'base' and probably as an antonym for the 'liberal' which follows.

[LIBER PRIMUS]

CAPITOLO PRIMO & GENERALE

Qualuncha virtuosamente la scienza & arte dcl danzare con lieto animo & colla mente sincera & ben disposta seguir vuole: bisogna che prima con fermo cuore & con speculante mente & consideratione intenda in generale che cosa sia danzare. ella vera definitione. che altro non e, che un atto demostrativo concordante alla misurata melodia d'alchuna voce overo suono. Il qual atto e composto et colligato con sei regule overo particelle principali. Le qual son queste seguenti, cio e misura. memoria. partir di terreno. aire. mainiera. & movimento corporeo. Le qual sei parti bisogna particularmente et perfettamente intendere & nella mente ben racogliere. Impero che una di queste per alchun modo mancando, non seria l'arte in se perfetta. Unde per haver di quella piu piena intelligenza: mostraremo prima chome se intenda ciaschuna delle preditte parti, et sua natura: & quello che habia ciaschuna adoperare. Le [6ʳ] qual sonno il funda|mento ella via, ella vera introductione a tutta l'arte perfetta del danzare. Diremo adonque prima che cosa sia misura. et pero nota.

CAPITOLO DI MISURA

Misura in questa parte et all'arte del danzare apertinente se intende una dolce & misurata concordanza di voce & di tempo partito con ragione & arte: il qual principalmente consiste nello strumento citharizante o altro suono, il qual in tal modo sia concordante & temperato che tanto sia il suo *v[u]oto, quanto il *pieno, cio e che tanto sia il tenore quanto il contratenore, tal che sia l'un *tempo misuratamente equale all'altro: per lo qual bisogna che la persona che vuole danzare, si regoli et misuri, & a quello perfettamente si concordi nei suoi movimenti si et in tal modo, che i suoi passi siano al ditto tempo et misura perfettamente concordante, & colla ditta misura regulati. et che intenda et [6ᵛ] cognosca qual pie deb|bia andare al pieno, & quale al v[u]oto portando la sua persona libera colli gesti suoi alla ditta misura, et secondo il suono concordante: la qual ci mostra il tempo di *passi *sempij et di passi *doppij & di tutti gli

[BOOK ONE]

INTRODUCTORY CHAPTER

Whoever wishes diligently to pursue the science and art of dancing with a joyful spirit and a sincere and well-disposed mind must first understand, with resolute heart, reflecting mind, and with consideration, what dance is in general and its true definition; which is none other than an outward act which accords with the measured melody of any voice or instrument.[1] This act is composed of and bound to six rules or principal elements which are the following: Measure, Memory, Partitioning the Ground, Air, Manner, and Body Movement. These six elements must be minutely and perfectly grasped and kept well in mind, for if one of these is lacking in any way, the art [of the dance] would not be truly perfect. Therefore, to gain a fuller knowledge of it, we shall show first what is meant by each one of the aforesaid elements, its nature, and how each is to be used. For they are the foundation, the means, and the true introduction to the complete and perfect art of the dance. We shall, then, first speak of what measure is; therefore, take note.

CHAPTER ON MEASURE

Measure,[2] in this part, and as it pertains to the art of dancing, means a sweet and measured accord between sound and rhythm, apportioned with judgement and skill, the nature of which can best be understood through the [playing] of a stringed or other instrument,[3] tuned and tempered in such a way that its *weak [beat] equals the *strong; that is, the tenor is equal to the contratenor so that one *tempo[4] measures the same as the next. Therefore, the person who wishes to dance must regulate and gauge himself, and must so perfectly accord his movements with it and in such a way that his steps will be in perfect accord with the aforesaid tempo and measure and will be regulated by that measure. He must also understand and know which foot should move on the strong [beat] and which on the weak, bearing himself easily, his gestures in accord with the measure and music. [Measure] shows us the timing of *passi *sempii

---

[1] See Glossary for some contemporary definitions of *voce* and *suono*.

[2] See Glossary for various interpretations of measure and *misura*.

[3] According to Tinctoris, *Diffinitorium*, 'rhythmical music' (*musica rithmica*) was made by instruments 'which render the sound by touch'.

[4] See Glossary for a more detailed definition of *tempo*. In this context, a musical unit (similar to a modern bar) is probably intended.

altri tuoi movimenti & atti alla ditta arte condecenti et necessarij, senza la qual
misura serebbeno imperfetti. et questo basti quanto alla misura.

CAPITOLO DI MEMORIA

Intesa la misura et nell'intelletto ben racolta, chome di sopra e detto: e di
bisogno in questo secundo luogho havere una perfetta memoria: cio e una
constante attentione raducendosi alla mente le parti necessarie ad essa memoria,
havendo i sentimenti a se tutti racolti & ben attenti al misurato et concordato
suono. Impero che se quello in alchun modo si mutasse overo allargasse o
astringesse, che colui che fusse nel danzare introdutto, non remanesse per pocha
[7ʳ] avertenza o per manchamento di memoria schernito. Cosi etiandio nel muta|re
di tempi & nelle sue misure in qualuncha *ballo si sia bisogno che a quello
far ricordi di supplire colla buona attentione seguendo colla persona i gesti et
i passi suoi tutte le misure del ditto tempo overo suono ad esso concordante.
Impero che volendo seguire l'arte predicta chome molti fanno transportati piu
tosto & guidati dalla fortuna, che d'alchuna ragione o misura: non si ricordando
qual sia il principio: il mezo: o il fine: remaria chome smemorato: e[t e]l suo
danzare seria imperfetto. et questo basti quanto alla memoria.

CAPITOLO DEL PARTIRE DI TERRENO

Seguita in questo terzo luogho il partire del terreno: il qual summamente e
necessario all'arte perfetta del danzare: nel qual fa di bigiogno optima discre-
tione & fermo intelletto in dovere considerare il luogho ella stanza dove siᵃ
balla: & quella nel suo intelletto ben partire & misurare: Impero che facendo
un ballo o una *bassadanza, e di bigiogno che quando l'huomo si parte dalla
[7ᵛ] donna col | suo tempo danzando, che con quello medesmo tempo la sappia
ritrovare non rompendo il tempo per cagione del terreno o vero per manca-
mento della stanza: La qual fusse al ditto exercitio breve o stretta, dove convien
col propioᵇ ingegno misurare & compartire si & in tal modo il terreno & il

---

ᵃ Orig.: *si* written twice.
ᵇ *Propio* is an archaic spelling of *proprio*.

and *passi *doppii*, and of all your other movements and actions which are fitting and necessary in the aforesaid art [of dancing] which, without measure, would be imperfect. And let this suffice as regards measure.

CHAPTER ON MEMORY

Once measure is understood and firmly imprinted on the mind, as stated above, it is necessary, in second place, to have a perfect memory; that is, constantly trying to recall those elements that need to be remembered, while collecting one's thoughts and paying careful attention to the measured and concordant music so that if it should in any way change, either slowing or quickening, whoever has begun to dance need not be scorned for his lack of forethought or want of memory. Just as, moreover, where there is a change of *tempi* and *misure*[5] in any *ballo*, he must remember to adjust to it most carefully, following all the measures of the aforesaid *tempo*—or its concordant music—with his body, gestures, and steps. For whoever wishes to pursue the aforesaid art as many do—borne along as it were and led by chance rather than by any judgement or measure, not remembering what is the beginning, the middle, or the end—will appear absent-minded, and his dancing will be imperfect. And let this suffice as regards memory.

CHAPTER ON PARTITIONING THE GROUND

The partitioning of the ground follows in third place. This is supremely necessary to the perfect art of dancing, where there is need of keen discernment and unfaltering judgement in taking account of the place and room for dancing, and carefully apportioning and measuring it in one's mind; inasmuch as, while performing a *ballo* or *bassadanza*, when the man leaves [his] lady, dancing to his own time,[6] so must he be able to come back to her in the same time and not get out of time[7] for reasons of space or lack of room. Where it [the room] is short or narrow for the aforesaid activity, it is advisable to use one's wits to measure and partition the ground and dancing area in such a way that with

---

[5] *Misure* in this context seems to refer to the four dance types of which a *ballo* could be composed, each of which had a different tempo as well as a particular metre. The meaning of *tempi*, however, is more ambiguous, although it may be related to *tempus*. See Glossary.

[6] See n. 7 and Glossary for other possible interpretations of *tempo*.

[7] *rompendo il tempo* (literally, 'breaking the time') is probably the opposite of *raccogliere i tempi*: 'picking up' the [different] timings or *tempi*. (See below and n. 12.) Both are concerned with the timing or regulating of one's steps to the music.

luogho dove si balla: che a tutti i tempi colla donna danzando si trovi, & che non gli avanzi ne manchi terreno. Impero che altra misura et altro tempo bigiogna alla stanza stretta et breve: che alla grande et spatiosa, perche il partimento e[t e]l misurato tempo nel luogho stretto e molto piu artificioso & difficile, che non e nel luogho aperto et *largho, dove si puo racogliere i tempi, & facilmente compartire. Bigiogna qui adonche singular & buona advertenza. et questo basti quanto al partire del terreno.

CAPITOLO DELL'AIERE

Bigiogna anchora in questo quarto luogho per adimpire et fare piu perfetta [8ʳ] l'arte preditta un altro | argomentoᶜ et favore chiamato aiere: il qual e un atto de aiereoso presenza et rilevato movimento colla propia persona mostrando con destreza nel danzare un dolce & humanissimo rilevamento. Impero che facendo alchuno nel danzare un sempio, o un doppio, o *ripresa, o *continenza, o *scossi, o *saltarello, e di bigiogno fare alchuno aieroso relevamento & sorgere destramente nel battere di tempi, perche tenendoli bassi senza rilievo & senza aiere, mostraria imperfetto & fuori di sua natura il danzare, ne pareria a i circonstanti degno di gratia & di vera laude. Questo atto adoncha di rilievo e chiamato aiere: bigiogna che con ferma discretione a luogho et tempo necessariamente s'adopri & ponga in praticha: et moderatamente quello dimostri nel danzare i passi & gesti con destra legierezza assai piu grati & di piu piacere. Senza la qual parte seria l'arte preditta simplice & defectiva. Et pertanto a questo ben attenda chi perfettamente vuol danzare. et questo basti quanto all'aiere.

ᶜ Orig.: *augomento*. Correction follows Pa.

every kind of rhythm[8] one is able to dance and keep together with the lady without gaining or losing ground. Thus a different measure and a different timing are required in a narrow and short room than in a large and spacious one, because partitioning the [ground] and [keeping] the measure in a narrow place requires more skill and is much more difficult than in a *wide and open area where one can keep in time and partition [the ground] with ease. Unusual and sound foresight is therefore needed here. And let this suffice as regards partitioning the ground.

CHAPTER ON AIR

In the fourth place a further principle and grace called air is necessary to complete and make the aforesaid art more nearly perfect. This is an act of airy presence and a rising movement with one's body which appears, through nimbleness in the dance, as a sweet and most gentle rising up. Thus, anyone dancing a *sempio* or a *doppio*, a *ripresa* or *continenza*, or *scossi* or *saltarello*, has to lift the body lightly and rise up nimbly on the down-beat,[9] for by keeping [the steps] flat, without rising and without air, dancing would appear imperfect and unnatural. Nor would it seem to the onlookers worthy of favour and sincere praise. This action of rising up, then, is called air and should be employed and put into practice at the right place and time with unfailing discretion; and when [done] with moderation, one's steps and gestures will display nimble lightness, so very pleasing and delightful in the dance. Without this element, the aforesaid art would be plain and faulty. Therefore, whosoever wishes to dance perfectly should mark this well. And let this suffice as regards air.

[8] This can read 'at all timings' (different time units, divisions of time, metres) or 'at every *tempo*' (bar and/or step unit).

[9] Cornazano, under the heading of Manner (V, fos. 3ᵛ–4ʳ), terms this rise *ondeggiare* ('to wave . . . as the waves in the sea', Florio). He instructs the dancer to '*ondeggiare* in the second short step rising gracefully up on that, and with the same grace lower yourself at the third [step] which completes the *doppio*'. He also states, on the other hand (fo. 10ʳ), that *ondeggiare* 'is a measuring the air in the rise' and 'nothing other than a slow rise of the entire body and a quick lowering'. This seems to be a confirmation of Domenico's interpretation of *mainera* (Pd, fo. 1ᵛ) as a movement resembling a gondola riding the little waves in a calm sea, '. . . the little waves rising slowly and lowering themselves quickly'. It is also possible that Cornazano's description of a *bassadanza* step (fos. 10ʳ⁻ᵛ), where the up-beat is 'the first surging [*surgente*] motion', is related to Guglielmo's 'rise up [*sorgere*] nimbly on the down-beat'. It is difficult to know if these diverse explanations are examples of different styles, or an indication of how the embellishment (the rise) was—or could be—applied to different steps. (See, for example, the late 16th-c. *seguito ordinario*, which begins on the toes, and the *continenza* and *passo puntato*, which instead begin flat and end with a brief rising and lowering of the heels.)

CAPITOLO DI MAYNIERA

[8ᵛ]

Anchora nell'arte preditta del danzare bigiogna all'adornamento et perfectione di quella un altro atto overamente regula chiamata mainiera. la quale bigiogna se adopri insieme con l'altre sue parti chome di sopra e ditto. Et questo s'intende che quando alchuno nell'arte del danzare facesse un sempio overo un doppio, che quello secondo accade l'adorni & umbregi con bella mainiera: cioe che dal pie che lui porta il passo sempio o doppio infino ch'el tempo misurato dura, tutto se volti in quel lato colla persona & col pie sinistro o col diritto, col quale lui habia a fare il ditto atto adornato & umbregiato dalla ditta regula chiamata mainiera: la quale nella praticha piu largamente si potra comprendere: senza la quale non haveria la ditta arte la sua naturale & necessaria perfectione. Et per tanto noti bene chiunque a quella pervenire intende. et questo sia a sufficienza quanto a mostrare che cosa sia mainiera.

CAPITOLO DI MOVIMENTO CORPOREO

[9ʳ]

In questa sexta & ultima parte si denota un atto necessario & conclusivo chiamato movimento corporeo: nel quale apertamente si dimostra in atto & in apparenza tutta la perfectione dell'arte & virtute del danzare, el qual bigiogna che sia in se con ogni perfectione misurato. memorioso. airoso. et ben partito. & con dolce mainiera si come di sopra habiam mostrato. Le qual cose sonno molto piu facili & suave a chi dal summo cielo ha la sua natura & complexione gentile a cio disposta & ben proportionata colla sua persona libera. sana. & expedita senza alchuno manchamento di suoi membri: ma giovene. formoso. destro. legiero. & di gratia bene dottato: in cui tutte le preditte parti si possano con piu longa delectatione liberamente exercitando dimostrare. Impero che in persone de suoi membri defectose non possano haver luogho, come sonno [9ᵛ] zoppi. gobbi. stropiati. et simili genti: perche queste tal parti | vogliano & consisteno nello exercitio et movimento corporale. et cosi havemo che cosa sia danzare.

CHAPTER ON MANNER

Furthermore, for the adornment and perfection of the aforesaid art of the dance, another action or rule is needed which is called manner, and it should be employed along with the other elements as mentioned above. This means that when in the art of the dance someone does a *sempio* or a *doppio* he should accordingly adorn it and shade it in comely manner; that is, he should, for the entire duration of the apportioned time,[10] turn his body completely to the same side as the foot with which he takes the *sempio* or *doppio* step (with the left or right foot, whichever he uses for this action), which is [thus] adorned and shaded by the said rule called manner.[11] This will be understood more fully in practice; without it, the said art [of the dance] would lack its natural and requisite perfection. Therefore anyone who wishes to acquire it must mark this well. Now let this suffice to show what manner is.

CHAPTER ON BODY MOVEMENT

In this sixth and last part an essential and final principle called body movement is considered, in which all the perfection of the art and virtue of the dance is clearly demonstrated both in action and appearance. This must itself be perfectly measured, mindful, airy, well-partitioned, and gracious in manner, just as we have shown above. These things are far easier and more amenable for those whose nature and noble make-up have been disposed to it by the heavens above, and whose well-proportioned bodies are pliant, healthy, and agile, with no feebleness of limb; that is, the young, the shapely, the nimble, the lightsome, and those well-endowed with grace, in whom all the aforesaid elements can, through liberal study, be demonstrated with more lasting delight. Thus there is no place for them in persons whose limbs are faulty (like the lame, the hunchbacked, the crippled, and such people), because these particular elements require and have their very essence in exercise and body movement. And there you have what dancing is.

[10] It may be that *tempo* is intended here. In the context this would mean the duration of either a *sempio* or a *doppio*.

[11] Closely related to Guglielmo's shading, and possibly a different name for the same ornament, is Cornazano's *campeggiare*, a term not without ambiguity. (Cennino Cennini uses it to signify 'colorire il campo della pittura', and among Florio's various meanings the most appropriate is probably 'to show, to become well'.) Cornazano says: '. . . se movite el [pede] dritto per fare uno doppio dovete campeggiare sopra el sinistro che rimane in terra, volgendo alquanto la persona a quella parte . . .' (fo. 3ᵛ). '. . . if you move the right [foot] to do a *doppio*, you must *campeggiare* upon the left which stays on the ground, turning the body a little to that part'. To 'that part' should refer to the last direction mentioned in the sentence, that is, the left. On the other hand, Cornazano may have used *quella* to mean 'the former part' as opposed to *questa* ('the latter'), so that the first or right foot (the one that moves) may have been intended. This second interpretation accords with Guglielmo's description of *ombreggiare*.

EXPERIMENTUM [I]

Veduto di sopra & pienamente inteso quanto sia il principale fundamento, elle parti necessarie & appertinenti all'arte preditta del danzare, senza le quale chom'e ditto: non puo alchuno di quella havere perfetta scienza. ne seria tra gli humani intelligenti di laude degna riputata. Hora bigiogna notare alchun altre particelle summamente necessarie: per le qual piu facilmente alla praticha si divegna. perche volendo alchuni fare di se medesmo aperta experienza in cognoscere s'egli intende le sopradette parti: faccia sonare la prima o la secuna misura: o qual si vuole dell'altre ballando in bassadanza overo in saltarello: & pruovi ben prima il partire delle botte over delle voci: che questo bene [10ʳ] intendendo, cognoscera da se stesso se sa danzare | o no. pero che servando bene le ditte misure, & quelle sapendo ben partire et mettere in atto: e segno di buona intelligenza et principio della vera praticha, alla quale fa di bigiogno con queste prove overo experienze se stesso misurando pervenire, le qual danno la via all'uso della perfectione dell'arte preditta, se ben faranno, chome segue execute.

ALIUD EXPERIMENTUM [II]

Un altra regula overo experienza si puo pigliare nel voler per se medesmo alchuno cognoscere quanto lui sia nella ditta scienza overo arte del danzare scientifico & intelligente, in questo modo, cio e che pruovi alchuno voler danzare contra tempo in su la prima overo secuna misura, o in su alchuna dell'altre contra tempo et a tempo. & questa pruova grandemente giova a chi vuole ben imparare: & fa l'intelletto acuto & attento al suono, dove poi piu [10ᵛ] facilmente viene alla perfectione dell'arte preditta: pero che se alchu|no sapra con questa experienza ben ballare contra tempo e segno di buona intelligenza. Impero che ben sapra da puoi alle de [*sic*] debite misure cogliere il tempo. perche ogni cosa per lo suo contrario si cognosce et piu perfettamente s'intende. et questo basti quanto alla secuna regula.

ALIUD EXPERIMENTUM [III]

Puossi anchora in un altro modo far di se medesmo chiara experienza & optima pruova pigliando questa regula, che volendo alchuno ballare un saltarello, pruovi di ballarlo contra tempo colle debite sue misure. et dall'altra parte il

EXERCISE [I]

Having considered the above and fully understood its basic principle and the elements necessary and pertinent to the aforesaid art of the dance (without which, as has been said, no one can have a perfect knowledge of it, nor be considered praiseworthy among men of understanding), we must now take note of some other exceedingly vital particulars which should facilitate putting it into practice. Therefore, anyone wishing to test himself fairly to see if he understands the aforesaid elements should get the first or the second *misura* played (or any of the others he likes) while dancing *bassadanza* or *saltarello*; and well beforehand he should try to scan the beat and the music, because if he masters this well, he will himself understand whether or not he knows how to dance. For closely observing the said *misure* and knowing how to scan and perform them well is the mark of keen intelligence and the beginning of serious practice; to acquire which, one must assess oneself with these tests or exercises; which, if they are well performed—as follows—are the starting-point for the practice of perfection in the aforesaid art.

EXERCISE [II]

Anyone wishing to discover for himself how skilful and knowledgeable he is in the aforesaid science or art of dancing can make use of another rule or exercise in this fashion: that is, he should try dancing counter to the time of [out of phase with] the first or second *misura*, or counter to the time or in time to any other [*misura*]. And this test is extremely profitable to whoever wishes to learn well, and sharpens the wit and makes it attentive to the music; whence one will, with greater ease, acquire perfection in the aforesaid art. For if one can ably dance counter to the time in this exercise, it is a mark of keen intelligence. One will easily know henceforth how to pick up the time[12] of the *misura* in question, since all things are known and more perfectly understood through their opposite. And let this suffice regarding the second rule.

EXERCISE [III]

Yet another way in which one can truly exercise and test oneself reliably is by following this rule: that is, someone wishing to dance a *saltarello* should try to dance it with its proper measures counter to the time while the player, for his

---

[12] See above, n. 7.

sonatore si sforze et pruovi di volerlo mettere nel tempo. Ma lui sia tanto cauto & destro che per alchun modo non si lassi cogliere ad intrare nel tempo. La qual cosa facendo sara manifesto segno di buona pratica & di destreza, & d'essere liberamente signore della sua persona & del suo piede. La quale pruova [11ʳ] e molto necessaria, et perfetta a volere pervenire alla perfectione del | l'arte preditta del danzare.

ALIUD EXPERIMENTUM [IV]

Anchora si puo per lo suo contrario fare un altra experienza in quest'altro modo, che ballando alchuno uno saltarello a tempo & colle sue misure: faccia ch'el sonatore pruovi con ogni ingegno di volerlo cavare del tempo. et colui che balla sia tanto proveduto & destro che mai per alchun modo non si lasci cavare ne uscire del tempo. et questo facendo potra dire havere piena notitia & buona speranza di saper perfettamente ballare. senza le qual experienze, raro si puo saper danzare. et cio basti.

ALIUD EXPERIMENTUM [V]

E[t] nota che tutte queste pruove overo experienze consisteno ad intendere perfettamente la misura, sopra la quale e fundata tutta l'arte preditta del danzare. [11ᵛ] La qual misura se impara et mettesi in praticha mediante le | preditte experienze. Et per tanto se vuole sopra ogn'altra cosa questa perfettamente intendere: perche e cosa molto fructuosa & necessaria. et giova anchora ad ogn'altra scienza alla qual s'apertegna di havere misura. Unde nota che tanta e la sua virtute & perfectione, che qualuncha ha bene la misura secundo le sue regule che son quattro, cio e perfetto magiore. perfetto minore. et imperfetto minore. & *quaternario. et quello tale tochasse il pulso ad uno amalato o alterato di febre cognoscera perfettamente si chome il medico in qual grado batta il polso, avegna che non sappia la qualita della infirmitate, perche scienza separata da questa. Ma basta che intendera se le botte sonno regulate secundo sua ragione o piu, o meno. & questo fa la misura. et assotiglia l'intelletto a molt'altre cose & maximamente all'arte preditta. et questo basti.

part, should strive and try his utmost to get him in time. But he [the dancer] must be so wary and adroit that he in no way lets himself be caught getting in time, the performing of which will be a clear sign of good practice and of adroitness and of unconstrained mastery of his body and his foot. This test is most necessary and perfect if one wishes to attain perfection in the aforesaid art of the dance.

EXERCISE [IV]

One can also do the opposite in another exercise in this other way. The person who is dancing a *saltarello* in time and with its [proper] measures gets the player to try, with all his might, to draw him out of time. The dancer needs to be so alert and adroit that he never allows himself to go or to be drawn out of time in any way. In this fashion he will be able to claim an ample acquaintance with the dance and a good probability of mastering it; [for] without these exercises it is rare to be able to know how to dance. And let that suffice.

EXERCISE [V]

Note that the purpose of all these tests or exercises lies in a perfect understanding of *la misura* [mensuration], which is the foundation of the entire aforesaid art of the dance. Mensuration is learned and put into practice through the aforesaid exercises, wherefore it, above all else, needs to be perfectly understood, since it is something so profitable and necessary, and fosters, besides, every other science where mensuration has a place. Note, therefore, that so great is its virtue and perfection that whoever understands mensuration well (according to its rules, which are four: that is, *perfetto magiore, perfetto minore,* and *imperfetto minore,* and **quaternario*[13]), were he to take the pulse of someone who is sick or feverish, would know as well as a doctor at what rate the pulse was beating, even without knowing the sort of illness (since that is a science [medicine] distinct from this one [dance]); for it would be sufficient for him to discern whether the beat was regular, as it should be, or fast, or slow. This then is mensuration and it sharpens the wits for many other things, but chiefly for the aforesaid art [of the dance]. And let this suffice.

[13] Guglielmo is probably referring to the four prolations. (For a discussion of mensuration and the prolations, see Ch. 4 and Table 1.) Since *quadernaria* is *imperfetto minore,* it would seem that Guglielmo wrote it incorrectly as his fourth prolation instead of '*imperfetto maggiore*'. (The prolations may have been a confusing concept for Guglielmo and his followers, inasmuch as Pa and S confirm the Pg error, while NY has *perfetto maggiore, imperfetto minore* twice, and *quadernaria,* and FN has *perfetto maggiore, perfetto minore,* and *quadernaria.*)

CAPITULUM REGULARE [I]

[12ʳ] Anchora e da notare chome nel sonare sonno due *chiave chiamate | *B. molle. & *B. quadro. et bigiogna quando il sonatore suona che chi vuol ben danzare o bassadanza o saltarello, o che altro si sia, che quello intenda & cognosca se suona per .B. molle, o per .B. quadro. impero che e summamente necessario che i passi & gesti suoi s[i]ano conformi & concordanti a quelle voci. *dolceze. et semituoni o sincopare, che in quella tal misura si suona, cio e o per .B. molle, o per .B. quadro. et quelle ben intendere et seguir colla persona & colli gesti. Et nota che .B. quadro e molto piu airosa la sua misura, che quella di .B. molle. ma e alquanto piu cruda & men dolce. Le qualcose ben intese & poste in praticha danno all'arte preditta del danzare La vera perfectione. et porgeno a chi intende singular dolceza & contentamento.

CAPITULUM REGULARE [II]

Appresso bigiogna intendere et ben notare che chi volesse comporre un ballo [12ᵛ] di nuovo, li conviene havere buona advertenza in pensar prima | s'egli el vuol comporre per .B. molle, o per B. quadro, ritrovando prima colla sua fantasia il tenore overo il suono il qual sia airosa & di perfetta misura, & habia buon *tuono. et guardi anchora il partir del terreno chome di sopra e ditto. et che sopra tutto non li sia alchuno mezo tempo ne altra falsitate. Impero che non seria giusto ne bello. Et bigiogna anchora che sia in tal modo composto et ben misurato con buon aire che lui porgia diletto & piacere ai circonstanti & a chi di tal arte si diletta. & sopra tutto che piaccia alle donne. Impero che tanto si dimostra il danzare esser piu bello quanto piu piace alla moltitudine di resguardanti: i qual danno il suo giudicio piu tosto secundo il piacimento et secundo il suo appetito, che secundo la ragione o l'arte la qual non intendono ne sanno. & questo basti quanto alla compositione del ballo.

RULE [I]

It should be noted furthermore that in playing [music] there are two *chiavi [signatures] called *B molle [B flat] and *B quadro [B natural], and when the player plays, whoever wishes to dance a bassadanza or saltarello (or whatever else) well, must know and recognize if B molle or B quadro is being played, inasmuch as it is of the greatest importance that his steps and gestures conform and accord with those strains, *sweetnesses, semitones, or syncopation[s][14] that are played for a particular misura, that is either in B molle or in B quadro, and to understand and follow them well with body and gesture. Note that the misura[15] of B quadro is far more airy than that of B molle, but it is somewhat coarser and less sweet. If these things are well understood and put into practice, they bestow true perfection on the aforesaid art of the dance and afford those knowledgeable [in it] particular pleasure and contentment.

RULE [II]

Next, it is necessary to understand and mark well that whoever wishes to compose a new ballo should take care to decide first whether he wishes to compose it in B molle or B quadro, using his imagination first to invent the tenor or melody, which should be airy, perfectly measured, and *tuneful. He should then consider the partitioning of the ground—as mentioned above—and [see], above all, that there are no half tempi or other falsities,[16] since this would be neither correct nor comely. Further, it should be so composed and well-measured with fine airiness that it bestow delight and pleasure on the onlookers and on those who take delight in this art. And above all it should please the ladies. For dancing is considered more beautiful the more it pleases the multitude of spectators, who pass judgement according to their pleasure and instinct rather than according to reason or the art which they neither know nor understand. And let this suffice regarding the composition of balli.

[14] The term is not clear in the context. (It is given as a verb in all versions, with the possible exception of NY.) According to Tinctoris, Terminorum, 'a syncopation is a division of some note into (two) parts by an interposed larger note'. S and FN have dolcie (adjective?) instead of dolceze.

[15] Misura seems to refer here to the systems of B molle and B quadro. See chiave in Glossary.

[16] This is puzzling since there are balli, like Domenico's Presoniera (included in De pratica), where the choreography and music explicitly call for a half-tempo.

CAPITULUM REGULARE [III]

La bassadanza bigiogna similmente che sia perfettamente misurata, per alchun [13ʳ] modo non ci sia alchuno mezo te[m]‖po. che altramente seria falsa & di pocho diletto et piacere. si che volendo alchuno comporre bassadanza chome e ditto bigiogna che prima habia buona fantasia a trovare il tenore colle sue parti ben musurate [sic]. et che sopra tutto piaza alla brigata.

CAPITULUM REGULARE [IV]

Appresso per havere piu piena cognitione & intelligenza delle preditte cose, e da notare si chome di sopra nel proemio habiamo fatto mentione, ch'el suono overo canto e principalmente fundato & firmato in quattro voci principali, le qual sonno concordante & conforme alle quattro nostre elementale compositioni, per la qual concordanza havemo l'essere e[t e]l sustentamento del nostro vivere per tal modo & in tal misura che quando per alchuno accidente mancha in noi una di queste quattro sustanze principale chiamate elementi, de li quali siamo composti et formati: subito mancharia la propia vita. Et quando l'una [13ᵛ] parte fusse dall'altra discordante o superante, faria l'essere nostro dive‖nire debile. dispiacevole. & infermo. & riducere la nostra compositione imperfetta. et cosi similmente le quattro voci principali & formative della dolce melodia intrando per lo nostro audito quando hanno le sue debite & misurate concordanze porgeno a i nostri spiriti di singular dolceza una nuova et delectevole vita, per la quale tutti a giocunda *festa par che si commovano. et non solamente ai sani & lieti, ma etiandio ai corpi egri et infermi porge diletto & dolce piacere. Cosi per lo contrario, se alchuna delle preditte voci fusse discordante dall'altre, & non havesse le debite misure, faria & renderia al nostro audito & ai spiriti sensitivi un movimento & alteratione di dispiacere, in modo che quella dolceza che doveria porgere al cuore conforto et notrimento per sua propia natura, si converte in recrescimento & tedio per la discordanza sua. Ma quando hanno perfettamente la sua com[p]ositione consonante & bene accordata colle debite & natural sue misure fanno agli ascoltanti commovere tutti i sensi in [14ʳ] suavis‖sima dolceza, per modo che spesse volte stanno essi fermi & attenti ad odire, sonno da essa dolceza & melodia constretti a fare colla persona alchuni movimenti demostrativi di fuori significando quello che dentro sentono. et non e da farne maraviglia per la ragione sopraditta: si chome si scrive della serena monstro marino, la qual colla dolceza & suavitate del suo canto fa per forza i naviganti adormentare, che non e altro che le quattro virtu principali

RULE [III]

The *bassadanza* must likewise be perfectly measured, [and] on no account should there be any half *tempi*, for otherwise it would be false and offer little delight or pleasure. So anyone wishing to compose a *bassadanza* must first have, as has been said, [a] good imagination to invent the tenor with its well-measured parts. And above all, it should please the assembled company.

RULE [IV]

Next, to gain a more thorough knowledge and understanding of the aforesaid, one should note (as we mentioned above in the Preface) that instrumental or vocal music is chiefly founded and based on four principal voices,[17] which are concordant with and akin to the four elements of which we are composed. In this concord we have our being and the sustenance of our life, in such a way and in such measure that if—by some mishap—one of these four principal substances called elements (of which we are composed and formed) should be lacking, then our life would cease at once. And should one part be in discord with or prevail over another, our being would become weak, displeasing, and feeble, and our make-up would be rendered imperfect. And so likewise, when the four principal voices which form sweet melody have their proper and measured concordances they bring, entering our ears, a new and delectable life of singular sweetness to our spirits; whereby it seems all are roused to merry *festivity. And not only to the healthy and happy does it offer delight and sweet pleasure, but also to the sick and feeble. The opposite is also true: should any of the aforesaid voices be discordant with the others or lack the proper measures, our hearing and our sensitive spirits would be moved and stirred by displeasure so that this sweetness, which should have by its very nature brought comfort and nurture to the heart, would become, because of its discord, irksome and tedious. But when they [the four voices] are so composed as to be in perfect harmony, and accord well with their proper and natural measures, they move all the senses of the listeners with the sweetest pleasure. So that often they [those listening] stand still and prick up their ears, finding themselves compelled by this sweetness and melody to perform some outward movement with their bodies, expressing what they feel within. This is not to be marvelled at for the aforesaid reason. In like manner we read of that sea-monster, the Siren, who through the power of her sweet and soothing song lulled sailors to sleep; and here we simply have the four cardinal virtues,[18]

---

[17] See Preface, nn. 4 and 5.
[18] Could Guglielmo possibly have meant 'principal voices' rather than 'principal virtues'? (See n. 19.)

in quello tanto*d* concordante & conforme ai nostri naturali sentimenti, che commovono et tirano a se i spiriti chome amici naturali, et a se conformi. et non prenda di cio alchuno admiratione, con cio sia cosa ch'el danzare sia tratto & originato da essa melodia chome atto demostrativo della sua propia natura. Senza la qual harmonia overo consonanza, l'arte del danzare niente seria, ne fare si poria. Impero che volendo alchuno danzare senza suono o senza alcuna concordante voce, pensa che piacer seria, o che diletto porgeria a chi danzasse, [14ᵛ] overo a chi ascoltasse. | certo nisuno. Anzi piu tosto demostraria spiacevoleza et matteria, & cosa contra sua natura. Et per tanto diremo essa arte et scienza del danzare esser virtute et scienza naturale composta & naturalmente tratta & cavata della melodia over suono d'alchune concordante voci chome di sopra habiamo ditto. Et pero che essa coll'animo pronto & ben disposto vuole a quella pervenire: bigiogna che tutte le predite parti & capitoli ben noti nella sua mente ben ricoglia, & quella sopra tutto virtuosamente exercitando. Unde ci resta solamente alchuna regula generale apartenente alla conditione & honestate della donna: le qual saranno nel seguente capitolo. et poi mostreremo la sua praticha & arte preditta. et questo basti quanto alla regula.

CAPITULUM REGULARE MULIERUM

Alla giovene donna & virtuosa la quale in tale exercitio et arte se deletta de [15ʳ] apprendere et imparare, se gli conviene havere regula et modo | con piu mode- ranza assai & piu honestade che al huomo. et debia pero tutte le sopradite parti & regule & experienze ben intendere & perfettamente notare, si che sapia la misura & intenda bene il suono, & poi sia a quello attenta et memoriosa, & cognosca il partire del terreno. e[t e]l suo andare sia con debita misura & con honestate airosa. ella sua mainiera sia dolce. moderata. & suave. e[t e]l movimento suo corporeo vuole esser humile & mansueto con un portamento della sua persona degno et signorile. et legiera in sul pie. et i suoi gesti ben formati. et non sia cogli ochi suoi altiera o vagabunda mirando or qua or la chome molte fanno. ma honestamente e[t e]l piu del tempo reguardi la terra. non portando pero chome alchune fanno il capo in seno abasso, ma dritto suso & alla persona respondente, chome quasi per se medesme la natura insegna, & nel suo muovere destra. ligiadra. & continente. perche facendo un sempio overo un doppio bigiogna essere accorta & bene adatta. cosi anchore [*sic*] nelle riprese. contenenze. *riverenza o scossi bigiogna che habia humano. suave. [15ᵛ] & | dolce modo coll'intelletto sempre attento alle concordanze & alle misure,

---

d *Canto* in FN, S, and NY.

so concordant[19] and akin to our natural feelings that they stir our spirits and draw them, with natural affinity, to themselves as friends. And there is nothing here to be astonished at, inasmuch as dancing is drawn and born from this melody as outward show of its true nature; [and] without this harmony or consonance, the art of dancing would be nothing, nor would it be possible to do. Imagine trying to dance without instrumental music or any accompanying voices. What pleasure would there be, or what delight would it offer either the dancer or the listener? None whatever! Rather it would prove to be something unpleasant, foolish, and unnatural. Wherefore we can affirm this art and science of dancing to be a virtue and a natural science, composed and in a natural fashion derived and drawn from the melody or sound of some concordant voices, as we have said above. Therefore, whoever wishes to master it, with a ready and willing spirit, needs to mark well all the previous sections and chapters and keep them firmly in mind. And above all he must practise it virtuously. Whereupon only some general rules remain, which follow in the next chapter, pertaining to the condition and decorum of women. And then we will describe its practice and aforesaid art. And let this suffice regarding this rule.

RULES FOR WOMEN

It behoves the young and virtuous woman, who delights in understanding and learning this discipline and art, to behave and conduct herself with far more discretion and modesty than the man. She therefore should fully understand and observe perfectly the aforesaid elements, rules, and exercises, so that she understands measure and is well skilled in music, and is also attentive and able to remember it, and knows how to partition the ground. Her bearing should have the proper measure and an airy modesty, and her manner should be sweet, discreet, and pleasant. The movement of her body should be humble and meek, and her carriage dignified and stately; her step should be light and her gestures shapely. Nor should her gaze be haughty or roaming (peering here and there as many do), but she should for the most part keep her eyes modestly on the ground; not, however, as some do who sink their head on their breast. Rather, she should carry it upright, aligned with the body, as nature itself—as it were—teaches us. And when she moves she should be nimble, light, and restrained, because when doing a *sempio* or a *doppio* she must be alert and most adaptable. In the same fashion she should also have a gentle, pleasant, and sweet way with her in [performing] *riprese, continenze, *riverenze*, or *scossi*, with her mind constantly intent on the music and the

[19] NY has 'concordant *in that song*'.

si che gli atti suoi e[t] i dolci gesti siano a quelle correspondenti & ben composti. et poi nel fine del ballo lasciata dal huomo con dolce riguardo allui tutta
rivolta faccia una honesta & piatosa riverenza a quella del huomo correspondente. et cosi poi com modesta attitudine si vada a riposare, degli altri notando
gli occorrenti defetti. e[t] gli atti giusti e[t] i movimenti perfetti. Le qual cose
dalla giovene donna ben notate, & quelle con prudente aviso da liei [*sic, passim*]
ben observate, serra dell'arte preditta del danzare laudabilmente dottata &
degna di virtuosa & commendabile fama. & tanto piu, quanto son piu rare le
donne che tal virtute et arte intendino perfettamente. ma piu tosto tale exercitio
usano per certa praticha alla ventura, che per scienza alchuna che in lor sia,
dove spesse volte commettino errore et manchamento, perche ne sonno da chi
intende biasmate. Et per tanto tutti con divoto animo persuado & conforto
[16ʳ] che questa | mia operetta attentamente legiano. Impero che quella non spre-
zando gli porgera suavissimo et virtuoso frutto.

measures [*misure?*], so that her actions and gentle gestures will be well formed and in keeping with them. Then, at the end of the dance, when released by the man, she should, turning her sweet gaze on him alone, make a courteous and tender bow[20] in answer to his. And then, with modest demeanour, she should go to take her ease [whence] to note the flaws of others as they occur as well as their correct actions and perfect movements. If these things are well marked by the young woman, and with careful heed kept well in view, she will become deservedly gifted in the aforesaid art of the dance, and merit a virtuous and commendable reputation. And so much the more considering how rare are the women who are perfectly adept in this virtue and art, since most engage in this activity as a haphazard affair rather than based on any knowledge of theirs, wherefore they often err and make mistakes for which they are reproached by the well-accomplished. Therefore, I would earnestly beseech and prevail upon all to read this little work of mine carefully, for if they do not find it contemptible, it will bear them most sweet and virtuous fruit.

---

[20] While bow is used here, the term *riverenza* is used in the choreographies to indicate a specific step unit.

LIBER SECUNDUS INCIPIT

ARGUMENTUM DISCIPULORUM [I]

Quantuncha desiderosi siamo noi imprendere l'arte del danzare. niente dimeno inanti che nello exercitio di quella ce mettessimo, haveriamo a piacere gli animi nostri fussero schiariti d'alchune cose che contra essa scienza gli pare intendere. Habiamo Guiglielmo apieno inteso quanto diffusamente in commendatione della predicta arte del danzare hai ditto, tenendo quella essere sollenne & vera scienza & arte virtuosissima & naturale. Alla quale sotto brevita responderemo quanto in cio la verita ci dimostra, di che apertamente intendemo esser l'opposito di quello dice di sopra, cognoscendo tal exercitio & arte essere da se indegna et non delettevole a circunstanti chome hai ditto. Conciosia cosa che [16ᵛ] ballando senza | suono dimostra essere una cosa dispiacevole & confusa. et quelli ballano senza di quello pareno chome i pecorelle dentro la mandra. et pareno tutte essere avolupate chome ucelli dentro la rete. & oltra di questo pensa da te stesso quanto essa sia malvagia & ria perche da lei ne descendeno infinite mali & sollicitudine, di che ogni di ne vediamo aperta experienza. & non puoi anchora negare che liei non sia mezana & inducitrice alla voluptate, la cui mediante ne pervengono grandissimi homicidij. discordie & nimicicie, le qual summamente dispiaceno non solo a idio, ma agli mortali. Si che adoncha meritamente diremo non essere degna perfetta ne delectevole chome tu tieni.

RESPONSIO GUILIELMI [I]

Brevemente quanto al mio parvolino ingegno sera possibile respondero a quello voi contra lo exercitio & arte del ballare dicite. Et prima io dico et [17ʳ] confermo essa scienza essere sollenne & virtuosa chome di sopra | havete piu diffusamente veduto, provandovi per vera ragione quella essere cosa naturale & accidentale si chome di sotto intenderite. Et quanto alla prima parte di danzare senza suono: Respondo che siando in un ballo otto o diece persone et ballando quelle coi passi concordatamente & misuratamente insieme senza suono e cosa naturale, et sonando doppo il sonatore & misurando et con-

BOOK TWO

THE PUPILS' CONTENTION [I]

Even though we are eager to learn the art of dancing, nevertheless, before engaging in that [pursuit], we should be pleased to have certain things, which seem to be held against this science, clarified in our minds. We have, Guglielmo, fully understood all that you have said throughout in praise of the aforesaid art of dancing, where you maintain that it is a serious and true science and a most virtuous and natural art; to which we will briefly counter with what seems to us the truth of the matter, which we frankly understand to be the opposite of what you say above, since we know this discipline and art is unworthy in itself and gives no pleasure to the onlookers, as you have claimed; inasmuch as dancing without music proves to be an unpleasant and disorderly thing, and those who dance without it look like a flock of sheep or like birds entangled in a net. You should consider besides how wicked and sinful it[1] is, because it gives rise to infinite evils and distress, of which we see unmistakable examples every day. No more can you deny that it panders and incites to lust. Through it, terrible murders, quarrels, and enmities come about, which are not only exceedingly displeasing to God, but to men as well. Thus we justifiably affirm that it is not, as you maintain, praiseworthy, perfect, or delightful.

GUGLIELMO'S REJOINDER [I]

I shall reply to what you have said against the practice and art of the dance as briefly as my scant wits will allow. And first I say and confirm that this science is serious and virtuous, as you have more fully seen above, going on to prove to you with sound reasoning that it is [both] something natural and artificial,[2] as you will see below. As regards the first point, dancing without music, I reply that when eight or ten people are performing a *ballo*[3] and are dancing without music but with steps which are measured and in accord with each other, this is something natural; whereas, when the player plays and the danc-

---

[1] The pupils, and Guglielmo himself in his Rejoinder [I], refer to the dance—here in its guise as temptress—as 'she'.

[2] See Glossary for meanings of *naturale* and its opposite, *accidentale*.

[3] *Ballo* is used here (and in the following Contentions and Rejoinders) in such a way that it may mean either the particular dance type or the generic term for any sort of dance.

cordando quelli ballano i lor passi col ditto suono e accidentale. Essendo tal
scienza di danzare cosa naturale et accidentale adoncha e perfetta & meritamente
commendativa. Quanto alla secunda parte che da liei ne descendano molti
homicidij. peccati. et altri mali, questo non niegho, & cio quando tal arte e
fatta et exercitata da huomini dissoluti. mechanici. plebei. et voluptuosi. Alli
quali sé bene havete inteso & attentamente letto di sopra gliela prohibischo et
niegho. Ma quando e exercitata da huomini gentili. virtuosi. & honesti, dico
,essa scienza & arte essere buona et virtuosa et di commendatione & laude
[17ᵛ] digna. Et piu | che non solamente gli huomini virtuosi & honesti fa tornare
gentili & pellegrini: ma anchora quegli sonno male acostumati & di vil conditione nati, fa divenir gentili & d'assai: la qual da apertamente a cognoscere la
qualita di tutti. Et questo basti.

ARGUMENTUM DISCIPULORUM [II]

Hora cognosciamo essere vero che essa scienza sia degna & virtuosa chome
hai ditto. Ma se bene ne ricorda habiamo inteso, che in volere haver quella
perfettamente se gli richiede sei cose principali: cio e misura. memoria. partir
di terreno. aiere. mainiera. et movimento corporeo. et maximamente la memoria et misura: Le qual non pocho tra laitre [l'altre] sonno necessarie in questo
exercitio. Et quanto ne facci i petti nostri rimanere di maraviglia, & di admira-
tione pieni, dire nol [non lo] potriamo: perche dan[zan]do noi a tempo et
faciando i passi ordinati & necessarij a quel ballo: et concordanti al suono, che
[18ʳ] ci bigiogna memoria et misura? Ci pareno adoncha | tutte cose superflue. et
senza esse potersi perfettamente ballare. a che fine ce vuoi agiongere queste
superfluitate, le qual summamente dispiaceno ad ogni huomo.

RESPONSIO GUILIELMI [II]

Non habiando voi la vera intelligenza & cognitione della particularitate &
*sottilita dell'arte preditta: le qual manchando non e possibile cognoscere
quella,ᵃ in la perfectione d'essa si richiede: Per tanto niente del vostro dire mi
maraviglio: al quale brevemente rispondo, ch'egli e di necessita a voler essere
l'arte perfetta, ci siano tutte le sei prescritte cose: senza le qual la scienza non
varebbe nulla: et maxime la memoria & misura, le qual servino non solamente
in quest'arte: ma in tutte l'altre liberali. Dimme non e cosa evidente che ballan-
dosi un ballo, et non sapiando cio che deve seguire, quelli ballano non rima-
gnano tutti confusi? Et chome potresti ballare a tempo se non havessi la

---

ᵃ Orig.: *quello*; emendation follows NY.

ers accord and measure their steps to the said music, this is artifice. Since this science of dancing is something [both] natural and artificial, it is perfect and deservedly commendable. As regards the second point, I do not deny that many murders, sins, and other evils come of it; that is, when this art is performed and practised by dissolute, vile, base, and lecherous men to whom —if you have fully understood and carefully read above—I forbid and refuse it. But when it is practised by noble, virtuous, and honest men, I affirm this science and art to be good, virtuous, and worthy of commendation and praise. Moreover, not only does it ennoble and refine virtuous and esteemed men, but even the ill-mannered and the base-born become most noble-minded. Thus it reveals everyone's worth. And let this suffice.

THE PUPILS' CONTENTION [II]

We now know that it is true that this science is worthy and virtuous, as you say. However, if our memory serves us well, we learned that six principal things are required for its perfect acquisition, that is, Measure, Memory, Partitioning the Ground, Air, Manner, and Body Movement—but chiefly Memory and Measure which are, compared to the others, of no small import-ance in this activity. And we cannot say just how this fills our breasts with wonder and amazement, because [if we] dance in time and perform the requi-site steps appointed to that *ballo*, while following the music, what need have we for Memory and Measure? Thus it seems to us that they are both superflu-ous and that one can dance perfectly well without them. To what end do you wish to add these superfluities, which everyone dislikes extremely?

GUGLIELMO'S REJOINDER [II]

Since you do not possess [any] real knowledge and understanding of the particularities and *subtleties of the aforesaid art, lacking which it is impossible for you to understand it in [all] the perfection it requires, nothing of your speech—to which I will briefly reply—surprises me. In order for [the dance] to be a perfect art, it is essential that all the six above-mentioned elements be present (without which it would be worthless as a science), and above all Memory and Measure, which are employed not only in this but in all the other liberal arts. Tell me, is it not obvious that when dancing a *ballo* and not knowing what comes next, the dancers will end up all confused? And how

[18ᵛ] memoria unita al suono? Eccho a|doncha c'e bigiogna et la misura gli e necessaria per fare un passo chome l'altro. et per cognoscere il v[u]oto dal pieno: se[n]za la qual cognitione, impossibile e ballare a tempo.

ARGUMENTUM DISCIPULORUM [III]

In questo non possiamo contradire. & vediamo essergli nell'arte preditta necessarie la memoria ella misura. Faciando adoncha ogni cosa misuratamente et colla memoria: le altre chome mainiera. aiere. & partimento di terreno che ci bigiognano? Del movimento corporeo non diciamo nulla, il quale non si puo contradire perche e dato dalla natura.

RESPO[N]SIO GUILIELMI [III]

Quantunque siete d'animo gentili et tutti pellegrini & virtuosissimi, apertamente comprendo voi non havere mai gustato la sottilita & dolceza di quest'arte: alla quale per manifesta ragione demostraro quanto se gli richieda l'aire ella mainiera, et necessariamente il partimento del terreno. perche facen-
[19ʳ] dose in | un ballo una cosa prolixa in luogho stretto anchor che s'abbia la memoria & misura et non si sappia usare buona & optima descretione al partire del terreno per la stretteza & brevita d'esso luogho, quelli ballano senza tal descritione, sempre rimagneno quasi confusi, perche alchuna volta si trovano longe dalla donna, et alchun altra apresso assai presto piu del dovere. ecco chome il partir del terreno e summamente necessario, vogliamo se gli [se chieda]ᵇ che ce bigiogna l'aire ella mainiera danzando com memoria. misura et partimento di terreno. Dico che danzandosi con queste tre cose, & manchandoci l'aire ella mainiera, parrebbe il danzare essere una cosa cruda et senza alchuno bel gesto et gratia, le qual manchando non mostrarebbe essa arte ne piacevole ne anche delectevole. si che ce sonno necessarie. Altramente de degna sarebbe infecta, et senza alchuna perfectione.

ᵇ Blank space in original. Pa has *se gli se chiada* and S *sel chade*.

could you dance in time if your Memory were not linked to the music? This then is why it is necessary. And Measure is essential to [the dance] in order to make one step like the next and to distinguish the weak [beat] from the strong, [because] without this knowledge it is impossible to dance in time.

THE PUPILS' CONTENTION [III]

We cannot contradict this and we see that Memory and Measure are essential to the aforesaid art. But why, when doing everything according to Measure and Memory, do we need the others—like Manner, Air, and the Partitioning of Ground? As regards Body Movement we have nothing to say because it is a gift of nature and cannot be disputed.

GUGLIELMO'S REJOINDER [III]

Even though you are noble-minded and all valuable and most virtuous [men], it is plain to me that you have never savoured the subtlety and sweetness of this art; and I will prove to you, through clear reasoning, how essential Air, Manner, and, of course, the Partitioning of Ground are to it [the art of the dance]. If those dancing in a confined area do something grand in a *ballo*, even if they apply Memory and Measure but do not know how to use good and perfect judgement in partitioning the ground, due to the narrowness and shortness of the area, they will always end up in confusion, as it were, by dancing without this kind of judgement; because sometimes they will find themselves far from their lady and at other [times] much closer than is seemly. This is why the Partitioning of Ground is exceedingly necessary. Let us imagine that someone should ask what need there is of Air and Manner when dancing with Memory, Measure, and Partitioning of Ground. I affirm that if one dances with these three things but lacks Air and Manner, one's dancing would appear to be a crude affair and quite without fair gesture and grace, lacking which, this art would prove neither pleasurable nor delightful. Hence they are necessary. Otherwise its worth would be sullied and it would be altogether without perfection.

ARGUMENTUM DISCIPULORUM [IV]

Guiglie[l]mo noi concedemo le ditte sei parti requirenti nell'arte del danzare, |
[19ᵛ] chome, memoria et misura, & l'altre delle quale habiamo piu largamente di
sopra [*sic*] parlato, esser necessarie in haver perfettamente la ditta arte. Voriamo
hora intendere da te a che fine et qual necessita ci constringe a far di noi
experienza ballando sempre colle sei prescritte parti chome ci dimostri. Ne
pare questa experienza essere una cosa inaudita et fuori di natura. et piu tosto
di ammovere la volunta & alienare l'intelletto di color volessero imprendere
essa scienza, che indurli a quella. si che ci pare vogli uscire del camino della
verita per provarci. et da scienza degna farla imperfetta.

RESPONSIO GUILIELMI [IV]

Sotto brevita vi rispondo, intendendo provarvi per exempij & vere ragioni
come in havere essa scienza perfecta se gli richiedono et sonno piu necessarij
gli experimenti, et fare di voi experienza, che le sei parti predidette. conciosia
cosa che alienandovi & extrahendovi il sonatore di saltarello in bassadanza &
[20ʳ] di bassadanza in qual si vuole altro | ballo, sempre sareti concordanti a quello
lui suona. et colle ditte parti non e possibile fare nisuna di queste pruove: senza
le qual dico voi ballati piu tosto per praticha che per veruna intelligenza ó
ragione. Et piu che habiando in voi tal pruova & experienza potreti perfettamente danzare Todescho. grecho. schiavo. et morescho. & di qual si vuole
altra natione. & comporre anche balli. Et cosi potrete dire havere la scienza in
perfectione. Et dato che habiati le sei parti gia ditte, non e possibile sapiati fare
nisuna di queste cose senza li ditti experimenti, perche non vi potrebe il sonatore si pocho travagliare, facilmente remaneresti con pocho honore. et ve
acaderia chome al prete di contado, il quale non sapea legere se non al suo libro
incominciando sempre dal principio. Eccho adoncha chome li experimenti gli
bigiognano piu che le sei parti delle quale habiamo parlato.

THE PUPILS' CONTENTION [IV]

Guglielmo, we concede that the said six elements required by the art of dancing (namely, Memory and Measure and the others, of which we have spoken more amply above) are necessary for perfect mastery of the said art. We should now like to understand from you to what end and for what reason we are obliged to practise dancing, always using the six prescribed elements, as you have shown us. This practising appears to be something unheard-of and unnatural, and more likely to take away the desire and alienate the understanding of anyone wishing to learn this science, rather than persuading them to it. Thus it seems to us that you prefer to abandon the path of truth [in order] to put us to the test, and to render a worthy science imperfect.

GUGLIELMO'S REJOINDER [IV]

I shall reply to you briefly with the intention of proving to you by examples and sound reasons that for perfect mastery of this science, exercises and practice are essential and are [even] more necessary than the six aforesaid elements; insofar as, should the player lead you astray and draw you from a *saltarello* into a *bassadanza* or from a *bassadanza* into any other [type of] dance whatsoever, you would always dance according to what he plays. And with the aforesaid elements [only], it is not possible to perform any of these tests; without which, as I say, you would dance more by rote than from any sort of understanding or judgement. Moreover, having mastered such tests and exercises, you will be able to dance German, Greek, Slavonic, and Moorish [dances] perfectly, as well as those of any other country whatsoever; and you will also be able to compose *balli*. Thus you will be able to affirm that you have mastered the science to perfection. But even if you had mastered the six aforesaid elements, it would [still] be impossible for you to know how to perform any of these things without the said exercises, because the player could give you no small trouble and you would, in all likelihood, end up with little repute. You would find yourself in the situation of the country priest who did not know how to read except from his own book, starting from the beginning each time. That is the reason why these exercises are [even] more necessary than the six elements of which we have spoken.

CONCLUSIO GUILIELMI

Voglio ogniun sapia: & maxime quegli nella ditta scienza si dilettano chome |
[20ᵛ] io ho continuato essa scienza o arte anni trenta, per la cui ho cercato le sollenne
&ᶜ degne corte & feste d'italia. E[t] prima quella dello Illustrissimo signore
conte Francescho Sforza duca di Milano, quando sua illustrissima signoria fu
creata Ducha nella intrata d'essa cittade di Milano. & [quel]la dello illustrissimo
signore Marchese Leonello. cio e nelle sue noze in Ferrara. et quelle dello
excelso signore Alexandro Sforza di due moglie in Pesaro. del signore di
Camerino. In Urbino ad due moglie d'esso magnifico conte. In Bologna a
quelle del magnifico messer Santi di Bentevogli. & tra l'altre a quella dello
illustre signore ducha de Cleve, qual fe fare lo prelibato illustrissimo signore
ducha di Milano pur in essa citade. non lasciando da parte quelle alla citta di
Vinegia. et di molt'altri signori & gentilhuomini d'italia. & anchora non mi
pare sappia danzare. & questo dico perche in esse feste & in assai altri luoghi
ho ritrovato molti li quali si tengono maestri, et apena cognoscono il pie dritto
[21ʳ] dal sinistro et si credono in tre giorni esser peritissi|mi. per tanto chi vuol
meritamente esser nomato maestro di quella, gli bigiogna havere le parti principal preditte in essa scienza requirenti. La quale ho trovato sempre esser com-
mendata da tutti i sopraditti & molt'altri di cuore & animo nobili et pellegrini.
Vogli adoncha tu che intendi mostrarla, sforzarti compiacere agli animi di
coloro la gustano, et negarla a quegli per la incapacita & ineptitudine loro la
biasmano & ripruovano. Et di cio in virtu d'esso ne constringo ognun che in
quella intende exercitarsi.

DOCUMENTUM GUILIELMI

Quanto piu posso persuado & priegho tutti quegli intendono seguire lo exercitio del danzare, & tra gli altri gli experti di quello: che ritrovandosi lor per
danzare in qualche luogo: et maximamente unde fossero donne di qual si vuole
stato o conditione, vogliano essere continenti. honesti. & reverenti. perche
acchade el piu delle volte alchuni vedendosi un pocho introdutti in esso danzare
[21ᵛ] prosumere coll'animo dishone|sto. dissoluto. & corrotto esser prosumptuosi
& temerari oltra il dovere. et questi son quegli che di arte dignissima la fanno

---

ᶜ & written twice.

GUGLIELMO'S CONCLUSION

I should like everyone to know, and especially those who delight in the said science, how I have pursued this science or art for thirty years, wherefore I sought out the stately and noble courts and festivities of Italy. Foremost, that of the most illustrious lord, Count Francesco Sforza, Duke of Milan, when, on his entry into the city of Milan, his illustrious lordship was made duke; and that of the most illustrious lord, the Marquis Leonello, at his nuptials in Ferrara; and both weddings in Pesaro of the excellent lord, Alessandro Sforza; and that of the lord of Camerino; [and] both weddings in Urbino of that magnificent count; [and] in Bologna, at that of the magnificent Messer Sante di Bentivoglio; and among the other [festivities], that for the illustrious lord, the Duke of Cleves, which was ordered by the eminent, most illustrious lord, the Duke of Milan, in that same city; not to mention those in the city of Venice and [those] of many other lords and gentlemen in Italy.[4] And still it does not seem to me that people know how to dance.[5] I say this because at these festivities and in various other places, I have met many who consider themselves masters, and they hardly know their right foot from their left, and they believe themselves to be truly expert in three days. Wherefore, whoever wishes to deserve the title of master of the dance needs to have mastered the aforesaid principal elements essential to this science, which I have always found to be praised by all those named above and by many others, noble and rare in heart and mind. Therefore, you who intend to perform it [the dance] should strive to delight the spirits of those who relish it, and refuse it to those who, because of their incapacity and ineptitude, condemn and disapprove of it. And to this, and in virtue of it, I exhort all those who intend to practise this art.

GUGLIELMO'S PRECEPT

To the best of my ability I urge and entreat all those who intend to pursue the discipline of dancing (and even the experts among them) to be temperate, honourable, and reverent when they meet somewhere to dance, especially in the presence of women, whatever their estate or condition. For it often happens that some men, believing themselves a little expert in the dance, take it upon themselves, in a dishonourable, dissolute, and corrupt spirit, to be presumptuous and rash beyond measure. These are the ones who turn this most worthy

---

[4] See App. III for an annotated translation of Giovanni Ambrosio's more extended Autobiography.

[5] This could also read as Guglielmo saying, 'And still it does not seem to me I know how to dance.'

ritornar vile & dishonesta, magiormente non essendo bene doctrinati & acostumati & honesti nel parlare, & sobrij nel lor mangiar & bere, perche la dissolu-
tione & ebrieta sonno destruttrici d'ogni virtu. Pero dato che havessero tutte
le degne parti preditte, & non observassero questo nuovo precepto, non gli
varrebono nulla. Et cosi facendo. seranno amati. honorati. & reveriti in ogni
parte. Et questo basti. Segue adoncha la praticha.[d]

[22ʳ]   Il bel danzar che con virtu s'acquista
                              Per dar piacer all'anima gentile
                              Conforta il cuor & fal piu signorile.
                              & porge con dolceza allegra vista.
                         E 'l senso natural ch'amor contrista
                              Et fal languendo spesso cangiar stile
                              Rinuova le sue forze & fal virile
                              Lieto danzando in amorosa lista.
                         Per sua natura il pellegrin ingegno
                              Che gusta del sonar la melodia
                              Diletto prende & fassi d'honor degno.
                         Pero chi tal virtu imparar disia
                              Disponga la sua mente e[t i]l cuor con degno
                              Seguendo me che mostro altrui la via.
                                   & con quest'opra mia
                              Insegno con vagheza di tal arte
                              La pratica gentil elle sue parte.

---

[d] The lower part of the folio is adorned with the miniature reproduced here as Pl. 3.

art into something vile and shameful, chiefly because they are not well-instructed, mannerly, or modest in their speech, nor sober in their eating and drinking, for dissoluteness and drunkenness are the ruin of every virtue. Thus, even if they had mastered all the worthy elements mentioned above, but were not to observe this new precept, they [the elements] would be worthless to them. But by so doing they will be loved, honoured, and revered everywhere. And let this suffice. Practice now follows.

Fair dancing, which we by effort pay,
   That its pleasure noble souls may beguile,
   Does lift the heart and makes it less servile,
   And with its sweetness does the sight make gay.
Natural feeling, which love makes lackaday
   And often by languishing, change style,
   Renews its strength and makes itself virile
   By merry dancing in love's tourney.
Of their nature, the rarest wits—
   Who relish the playing of music's strains,
   Delight thus obtain and honour merit.
But he who to this virtue would attain
   Must a ready heart and mind outfit,
   Following the way I for the rest make plain.
     And with this work of my brain
   I, while delighting, teach this art's
   Noble practice and its parts.

TAVOLA DI BASSEDANZE[e]

	[D]	REALE [2]	a carte	23
		ALEXANDRESCHA [2 NY]	a carte	23
		GENEVRA [2]	a carte	23
	[D]	MIGNOTTA [amaw^f Pd]	a carte	24
		PIETOSA [2]	a carte	25
		CUPIDO [4^f NY]	a carte	25
		PELLEGRINA [3]	a carte	26
[22^v]	[D]	PHOEBUS [3]	a carte	27
	[D]	DAPHNES [3]	a carte	27
		GIOLIVA [2]	a carte	28
		PATIENTIA [4]	a carte	29
	[D]	FLANDESCHA [2]	a carte	30
		PRINCIPESSA [2^f NY; 3 or 6 S]	a carte	30
		CATERVA [3]	a carte	31

TAVOLA DI BALLI

[D]	ROSTIBOLI GIOIOSO [2]	a carte	32
	DUCH[E]SCHO [3^f]	a carte	32
	LIGIADRA [4]	a carte	33
	COLONESE [6]	a carte	34
[D]	PETIT ROSE [2]	a carte	34
[D]	IOVE [3^ft]	a carte	35
[D]	PRESONIERA [2]	a carte	36
[D]	MARCHESANA [2]	a carte	37
[D]	BELFIORE [3]	a carte	37
[D]	INGRATA [3]	a carte	38
[D]	ANELLO [4]	a carte	39
[D]	GIELOSIA [6]	a carte	39
[D]	BELRIGUARDO [2]	a carte	40
[D]	LEONCELLO [2]	a carte	40
[D]	MERCANCIA [3m 1w Pd]	a carte	41
	GRATIOSO [2]	a carte	42
	SPERO [3]	a carte	42

[e] The information in square brackets is provided for those interested in analysing the sequence and repertoire of the dances, and in comparing these with the chronology and content of other sources (see Gallo, 'Il "ballare lombardo" '). [D] indicates that Guglielmo has attributed the authorship to Domenico. The number in brackets specifies how many dancers the choreography

TABLE OF *BASSEDANZE*†

Alexandresca	127
Caterva	145
Cupido	133
Daphnes	137
Flandesca	141
Genevra	129
Gioliva	139
Mignotta	131
Patienza	139
Pellegrina	135
Phoebus	135
Pietosa	131
Principessa	143
Reale	127

TABLE OF *BALLI*

Anello	161
Belfiore	159
Belriguardo	165
Colonnese	151
Duchesco	147
Gelosia	163
Gratioso	167
Ingrata	159
Iove	153
Legiadra	149
Leoncello	165
Marchesana	157
Mercantia	167
Petit Rose	151
Presoniera	155
Rostiboli Gioioso	147
Spero	169

calls for. (Where Guglielmo is not explicit, another source is included.) A superior 'f' signifies a dance *a la fila* ('in a file'), 'amaw' stands for 'as many as will', and 'm' and 'w' are 'men' and 'woman'.

† The dances have been rearranged in alphabetical order.

QUI COMINCIANO LE BASSE DANZE
DI MESSER DOMENICO ET DI GUIGLIELMO.
& PRIMA UNA BASSADANZA CHIAMATA REALE
IN DOI DI MESSER DOMINICO

In prima doi sempij & quattro doppii. cominciando col pie sinistro. una represa *in sul pie sinistro, & poi vada con doi sempij & un doppio cominciando col pie dritto, & poi faccia doi riprese, una sul pie sinistro et l'altra sul dritto. et poi faccia doi sempii & un doppio partendo col pie sinistro. et poi facciano una riverenza in sul dritto. & poi si *tornino in drieto con doi sempii cominciando col pie dritto, et poi facciano due riprese, una sul sinistro ell'altra sul dritto. et poi facciano quattro continenze in sul pie sinistro.

BASSADANZA CHIAMATA ALEXANDRESCA
COMPOSTA PER GUILIELMO

In prima doi sempii & un doppio cominciando col pie sinistro. et poi diano una *volta tonda con un sempio et un doppio cominciando col pie dritto. et [23^v] poi diano *meza volta in sul pie dritto, tanto | che la donna resti di *sopra l'huomo. et poi faciano doi riprese, una sul sinistro, ell'altra sul dritto. et poi faciano tutto questo un'altra volta, tanto che l'huomo resti al luogho suo. & poi vadano al tondo l'uno drieto all'altro con doi sempii & un doppio, comin-

HERE BEGIN THE *BASSEDANZE*
BY MESSER DOMENICO AND GUGLIELMO.
AND FIRST, A *BASSADANZA* FOR TWO CALLED
REALE[1] BY MESSER DOMENICO

First [do][2] two *sempii* and four *doppii*; beginning with the left foot; a *ripresa* *upon the left foot, and then proceed with two *sempii* and a *doppio* beginning with the right foot, and then do two *riprese*, one on the left foot and the other on the right; and then two *sempii* and a *doppio* starting with the left foot; and then make a *riverenza* upon the right [foot][3]; and then *go back with two *sempii* beginning with the right foot, and then do two *riprese*, one on the left [foot] and the other on the right; and then do four *continenze* [beginning?][4] upon the left foot.

BASSADANZA CALLED *ALEXANDRESCA*[5]
COMPOSED BY GUGLIELMO

First do two *sempii* and a *doppio* beginning with the left foot; and then make a *volta tonda* with a *sempio* and a *doppio*[6] beginning with the right foot; and then make [a][7] *meza volta* upon the right foot, so that the lady finishes *above [to the left of] the man; and then do two *riprese*, one on the left [foot], and the other on the right; and then repeat all this, so that the man finishes in his place; and then go around one behind the other with two *sempii* and a *doppio*,

---

[1] Regal. Domenico does not include this dance in his own treatise.

[2] Guglielmo begins almost all his dances without a verb. In the openings of subsequent choreographies, 'do' appears without square brackets.

[3] Here, and in all the following cases where 'foot' has been added for clarification, the word *pie* appears in the NY and FN versions.

[4] Neither in this nor in other dances (such as *Mignotta*, *Pietosa*, etc.) is it clear if Guglielmo intends all the *continenze* to be performed on the left foot or merely to *begin* on the left foot. Other, probably later, versions of *De pratica* are not enlightening, inasmuch as they change Guglielmo's choreographies, substituting, for example, two *riprese* (left and right) or a *riverenza* (NY, FN, Fol). Domenico almost always specifies *beginning* on the left foot (see below, n. 13). In some instances it seems apparent that the *continenze* would have to have been performed on alternate feet in order to have the left foot free for the following step.

[5] Probably named in honour of Guglielmo's patron Alessandro Sforza.

[6] This unusual *volta tonda* may well be an error, although 'one *sempio* and a *doppio*' is repeated in Pa, NY, and FN. S and Fol simply indicate a *volta del gioioso* which, like the *volta tonda*, is normally performed in *bassadanze misura* with two *sempii* and a *ripresa*.

[7] Here, and in all the choreographies, Guglielmo does not use an article before *meza volta*. See Glossary for possible implications. Henceforth, the article, required by English syntax, is inserted in the translation without square brackets.

ciando col pie sinistro. et poi vadano dall'altra mano con doi sempii et un doppio pur al tondo partendosi col pie dritto. et poi *vadano al contrario l'un dell'altro con doi doppii partendosi col pie sinistro. & poi diano meza volta sul pie dritto. et poi faciano doi riprese, una sul sinistro, ell'altra sul dritto. et una riverenza sul pie sinistro. et poi vadano in contra l'uno all'altro con doi tempi di saltarello, cominciando col pie sinistro. ella donna dia meza volta in sul pie dritto. et poi si pigliano per mano, & facciano due riprese, una sul pie sinistro ell'altra sul dritto con una riverenza in sul pie sinistro.

BASSADANZA CHIAMATA GENEVRA IN DOI.
DI GUILIELMO

[24ʳ] In prima doi sempij et un doppio, et | una reverenza in sul pie dritto cominciando col pie sinistro, & poi torni in drieto con doi sempii & un doppio cominciando col pie dritto. et poi dia meza volta in sul pie dritto tanto che la donna rimangha sopra del huomo. et poi faciano una ripresa in sul pie sinistro. & poi diano una volta tonda con doi sempij & una ripresa in sul pie dritto, cominciando col pie dritto, & poi facciano due continenze. & tutto questo che e ditto di sopra si facia altro tanto, fin che l'huomo ritorni a suo luogho. et poi l'huomo pigli la man dritta della donna: et vadano tondi con doi sempij & un doppio cominciando col pie sinistro. et poi se scambiano le mani, & vadano pur tondi con doi sempij et un doppio cominciando col pie drritto [*sic*]. et poi faciano una riverenza in sul pie sinistro. et poi tornino in drieto con un sempio cominciando col pie sinistro. et poi diano meza volta in sul pie dritto, tanto che rimagneno al contrario l'uno dell'altro. et poi diano una volta tonda con doi sempii cominciando col pie dritto. et poi faciano una ripresa in sul pie [24ᵛ] dritto, & vadano al contrario l'un | dell'altro con doi doppij cominciando col pie sinistro. & poi diano meza volta in sul pie dritto. & faciano due riprese, una sul sinistro ell'altra sul dritto. et poi faciano una riverenza in sul pie sinistro. et poi vegnano in contra l'uno all'altro con doi sempij & un doppio cominciando col pie sinistro. et poi diano una volta tonda con doi sempij & una ripresa cominciando col pie dritto. et faciano una riverenza in sul sinistro, beginning with the left foot; and then go around again in the other direction with two *sempii* and a *doppio* starting with the right foot;[8] and then *advance in opposite directions with two *doppii* starting with the left foot; and then make a *meza volta* on the right foot; and then do two *riprese*, one on the left [foot], and the other on the right; and a *riverenza* on the left foot; and then advance towards one another with two *tempi* of *saltarello*, beginning with the left foot; and the lady makes a *meza volta* upon the right foot; and then take hands, and do two *riprese*, one on the left foot and the other on the right, with a *riverenza* upon the left foot.

BASSADANZA FOR TWO CALLED *GENEVRA*[9]
BY GUGLIELMO

First do two *sempii* and a *doppio* beginning with the left foot, and a *riverenza* upon the right foot, and then go back with two *sempii* and a *doppio* beginning with the right foot; and then make a *meza volta* upon the right foot so that the lady finishes above [to the left of] the man; and then do a *ripresa* upon the left foot; and then make a *volta tonda* with two *sempii* and a *ripresa* upon the right foot; beginning with the right foot, and then do two *continenze*; and repeat all of the above, until the man returns to his place; and then the man takes the right hand of the lady: and both go round with two *sempii* and a *doppio* beginning with the left foot; and then change hands, and go round again with two *sempii* and a *doppio* beginning with the right foot; and then make a *riverenza* upon the left foot; and then go back with a *sempio*[10] beginning with the left foot; and then make a *meza volta* upon the right foot, ending up facing in opposite directions; and then make a *volta tonda* with two *sempii* beginning with the right foot; and then do a *ripresa* upon the right foot,[11] and advance in opposite directions with two *doppii* beginning with the left foot; and then make a *meza volta* upon the right foot; and do two *riprese*, one on the left [foot] and the other on the right; and then make a *riverenza* upon the left foot; and then advance towards one another with two *sempii* and a *doppio* beginning with the left foot; and then make a *volta tonda* with two *sempii* and a *ripresa* beginning with the right foot; and then make a *riverenza* upon the left [foot],

---

[8] NY indicates that while going around, the dancers take hands.

[9] This dance is probably in honour of Ginevra, Alessandro Sforza's illegitimate daughter, who married Sante Bentivoglio in 1454. (See Marrocco, 'Inventory'.)

[10] Confirmed in Pa and FN, while NY specifies two *pasettini* beginning with the right foot. This sequence of one *sempio* (*beginning*? with the left foot) and a *meza volta* followed by a *volta tonda* is most unusual. Not only is the *meza volta* not followed by a *ripresa* on the left foot, but it is not preceded by a step on the right foot.

[11] Guglielmo's punctuation seems to separate the *ripresa* from the *volta tonda*. See *volta tonda* in Glossary.

& in quel tempo della riverenza si tocchano la mano l'uno all'altro. et poi la donna dia meza volta in sul pie dritto. et poi si pigliano per la mano, & faciano due riprese, una sul sinistro, ell'altra sul dritto, & una riverenza in sul pie sinistro.

BASSADANZA CHIAMATA MIGNOTTA ALLA FILA DI MESSER DOMINICO

In prima due continenze in sul pie sinistro. et poi faciano doi sempii & doi doppii cominciando col pie sinistro, & due continenze insul pie sinistro. et poi faciano doi doppij cominciando col pie sinistro, & due continenze insul pie [25ʳ] sinistro, | & due continenze in sul pie sinistro,ᵃ et una ripresa in sul sinistro. et poi faciano un doppio et un sempio & un doppio tornando in dietro cominciando col dritto. et poi diano meza volta in sul pie dritto con due riprese, una sul sinistro ell'altra sul dritto. et due continenze sul pie sinistro. Et poi faciano doi tempi di saltarello cominciando col pie sinistro. et anchora faciano un doppio cominciando col pie sinistro. et poi faciano una ripresa in sul pie dritto. et poi faciano doi doppij insu un pie cominciando col pie sinistro. et una riverenza in sul pie sinistro.

BASSADANZA CHIAMATA PIETOSA IN DOI COMPOSTA PER GUILIELMO

In prima doi passi sempi & uno doppio cominciando col pie sinistro et una ripresa sul pie dritto. ell'huomo facia due continenze sul pie sinistro. et in quel tempo delle continenze, la donna vada dalla man di *sotto del huomo con duoi

---

ᵃ This repetition does not appear in Domenico's own choreography and is probably a scribal slip.

touching one another's hand at the same time; and then the lady makes a *meza volta* upon the right foot; and then take hands, and do two *riprese*, one on the left, and the other on the right, and a *riverenza* upon the left foot.

BASSADANZA IN SINGLE FILE CALLED *MIGNOTTA*[12] BY DOMENICO

First do two *continenze* [beginning][13] upon the left foot; and then do two *sempii* and two *doppii* beginning with the left foot, and two *continenze* [beginning] upon the left foot; and then do two *doppii* beginning with the left foot, and two *continenze* [beginning] upon the left foot,[14] and a *ripresa* upon the left; and then do a *doppio* and a *sempio*[15] and a *doppio* going back beginning with the right [foot]; and then make a *meza volta* upon the right foot with two *riprese*, one on the left [foot] and the other on the right; and two *continenze* [beginning] on the left foot. And then do two *tempi* of *saltarello* beginning with the left foot; and do a *doppio* as well beginning with the left foot; and then do a *ripresa* upon the right foot; and then do two *doppii* upon one [and the same] foot beginning with the left foot;[16] and a *riverenza* upon the left foot.

BASSADANZA FOR TWO CALLED *PIETOSA*[17] COMPOSED BY GUGLIELMO

First do two *passi sempii* and a *doppio* beginning with the left foot and a *ripresa* on the right foot; and the man does two *continenze* [beginning?] on the left foot; and at the same time[18] as the *continenze*, the lady goes to the *lower

[12] Darling. This is the very first dance in NY and Giorgio specifies that it is for two dancers. In Domenico's treatise it is his second *bassadanza* and is presented in two versions. Guglielmo's choreography seems to be based on the 'old' (rather than the 'new') version—*Mignotta vechia*—which is 'for as many as will'.

[13] In Domenico's version, beginning with the left foot is always specified.

[14] '. . . and two *continenze* upon the left foot' is written twice in the original. See n. *a* in the transcription.

[15] Domenico's version reads two *sempii* instead of a *doppio* and a *sempio*.

[16] For '*doppii* upon the same foot', see *doppij* and *contrapassi* in Glossary. See Pd, fo. 27ʳ, for a detailed description of what Domenico intended.

[17] Merciful.

[18] This could also read: 'and during the *tempo* of the *continenze*' (since two *continenze* are performed in one *tempo*). Though a possible interpretation for some dances, it will not work in the case of dances like *Cupido*, *Gioliva*, *Pellegrina*, etc., where the steps in question (for example, two *sempii* and one, two, four, or six *doppii*) last more than one *tempo*. Furthermore, in *Caterva*, the instructions are to take hands 'at the *tempo* of the *riprese*'. In other words, 'during' the *riprese*.

passi sempi, cominciando col pie sinistro. et poi si pigliano per la mano, et
[25v] faciano due riprese, una sul sinistro, ell'altra | sul dritto. & due continenze sul
pie sinistro, & tutto questo che e ditto si faccia altretanto in fin che l'huomo
ritorni al suo luogho. et poi faciano una riverenza in sul pie sinistro. et poi
faciano doi tempi di saltarello cominciando col pie sinistro. et l'huomo facia
una riverenza in sul pie sinistro. et in quel tempo della rivere[n]za, la donna
dia meza volta: et poi vadano al contrario l'uno dell'altro con doi doppij
cominciando col pie sinistro. et poi diano meza volta sul pie dritto. et faciano
due riprese, una sul sinistro ell'altra sul dritto. et una riverenza sul sinistro. et
poi vegnano incontro l'uno dell'altro con due *riprese in galone, una sul sinistro ell'altra sul dritto. et poi si pigliano per la mano, & faciano una ripresa sul
sinistro. et poi diano una volta tonda con doi sempij cominciando col dritto,
& una ripresa sul dritto. et una riverenza sul pie sinistro.

BASSADANZA CHIAMATA CUPIDO ALLA FILA COMPOSTA PER GUILIELMO

In prima doi sempij & doi doppij cominciando col pie sinistro. et poi gli
[26ʳ] huomini diano meza volta in sul pie drit|to, elle donne non si voltino niente.
et poi faciano due riprese, una sul sinistro ell'altra sul dritto. et poi facciano
una riverenza sul pie sinistro. et poi vadino intorno l'uno all'altro, & pigliansi
per la man dritta, et vadano tondi con doi sempij & un doppio cominciando
col pie sinistro. et poi faciano una ripresa in sul pie dritto. Et poi gli huomini
vadano al contrario delle donne con doi doppij cominciando col pie sinistro.
et in quel tempo le donne[b] faciano quattro continenze sul pie sinistro. et poi
diano tutti meza volta sul dritto. et faciano due riprese, una sul sinistro, ell'altra
sul dritto. et una riverenza sul pie sinistro. et poi vegnano incontro[c] l'uno
all'altro con doi sempii cominciando col pie sinistro. et l'huomo dia meza volta
insul pie dritto. et pigliansi per mano, et faciano una ripresa insul pie sinistro.
Et poi diano una volta tonda con doi sempij cominciando col pie dritto, et una
ripresa sul pie dritto. et una riverenza sul pie sinistro.

---

[b] The passage from 'con doi doppij' to 'le donne' is erroneously given twice.
[c] Orig.: *intorno*. Correction follows Pa, FN, and NY.

[other] side of the man[19] with two *passi sempii*, beginning with the left foot; and then take hands, and do two *riprese*, one on the left [foot], and the other on the right; and two *continenze* [beginning?] on the left foot, and repeat all of the above until the man returns to his place; and then make a *riverenza* upon the left foot; and then do two *tempi* of *saltarello* beginning with the left foot; and the man makes a *riverenza* upon the left foot; and at the same time as the *riverenza*, the lady makes a *meza volta*: and then advance in opposite directions with two *doppii* beginning with the left foot; and then make a *meza volta* on the right foot; and do two *riprese*, one on the left [foot] and the other on the right; and a *riverenza* on the left; and then advance towards one another with two **riprese in galone*, one on the left [foot] and the other on the right;[20] and then take hands, and do a *ripresa* on the left [foot]; and then make a *volta tonda* with two *sempii* beginning with the right, and a *ripresa* on the right; and a *riverenza* on the left foot.

BASSADANZA CALLED *CUPIDO*[21] [FOR FOUR][22] IN SINGLE FILE COMPOSED BY GUGLIELMO

First do two *sempii* and two *doppii* beginning with the left foot; and then the men make a *meza volta* upon the right foot, but the ladies do not turn at all; and then do two *riprese*, one on the left [foot] and the other on the right; and then make a *riverenza* on the left foot; and then go around each other, and take right hands, and go round with two *sempii* and a *doppio* beginning with the left foot; and then do a *ripresa* upon the right foot. And then the men advance in the opposite direction to the ladies with two *doppii* beginning with the left foot; and at the same time the ladies do four *continenze* [beginning?] on the left foot; and then everyone makes a *meza volta* on the right [foot]; and do two *riprese*, one on the left [foot], and the other on the right; and a *riverenza* on the left foot; and then advance towards one another with two *sempii* beginning with the left foot; and the men make[23] a *meza volta* upon the right foot; and take hands, and do a *ripresa* upon the left foot. And then make a *volta tonda* with two *sempii* beginning with the right foot, and a *ripresa* on the right foot; and a *riverenza* on the left foot.

---

[19] This may be an error, since the lady is theoretically already on the 'lower' or right side.

[20] At this point in other *bassedanze* (see, for example, *Genevra*, *Cupido*, and *Pellegrina*) the choreography indicates that the lady makes a *meza volta* so as to finish side by side with her partner. It is not known if this ending is an exception.

[21] Cupid.

[22] NY and FN both indicate 'for four' in the title. S (fo. 35ʳ) specifies for six or eight.

[23] The original and all other versions read, 'the *man* makes'.

[26ᵛ]   BASSADANZA CHIAMATA PELLEGRINA IN TRE
          FATTA PER GUILIELMO

In prima doi sempij et doi doppij cominciando col pie sinistro, et poi diano*d*
una meza volta insul pie dritto. et faciano due riprese, una sul sinistro ell'altra
sul dritto: et una riverenza sul pie sinistro. & poi l'huomo piglia la man dritta
della donna & volgiano al tondo con uno sempio & uno doppio cominciando
col pie sinistro. et in quel tempo la donna si volti tonda in quel luogho suo
medesimo, cioe con quelli passi. et poi [l'huomo]*e* pigli la man sinistra
dell'altra donna, et voltandosi tondi con doi sempij & un doppio cominciando
col pie dritto. et quella donna che resta sola, se volta tonda con doi sempij &
un doppio cominciando col pie dritto. & poi vadano al contrario l'uno dall'altro
con doi sempij & doi doppij cominciando col pie sinistro. et poi diano meza
volta sul pie dritto. et facianosi due riprese, una sul sinistro ell'altra sul dritto.
poi vengano l'uno all'altro con doi sempij & uno doppio. cominciando col pie
[27ʳ] sinistro. et poi diano una volta tonda | con doi sempii cominciando col pie
dritto & una ripresa sul pie dritto. et poi vengano in contro l'uno all'altro con
doi sempi cominciando col pie sinistro. & poi le donne diano meza volta sul
pie dritto, et pigliansi per mano, & faciano una ripresa sul sinistro. et poi diano
una volta tonda con doi sempij cominciando col pie diritto, et una ripresa sul
pie dritto, et una riverenza sul sinistro.

          BASSADANZA CHIAMATA PHOEBUS IN TRE
          FATTA PER MESSER DOMINICO

In prima doi sempij & un doppio comminciando [*sic*] col pie sinistro, et poi
una ripresa sul dritto. et questo facciano un'altra volta. et in quel tempo della
ripresa quello*f* di mezo dia meza volta sul dritto. et poi vadano in contrario
uno de gli altri con doi doppij partendosi col pie sinistro, & diano meza volta
sul dritto con doi riprese, una sul sinistro ell'altra sul destro. et poi vegnano
in contro l'uno dell'altro partendosi con doi sempij & doi doppij col pie sinistro
passando in mezo delle donne. et poi diano meza volta sul pie dritto, & faciano

---

d Orig. and Pa: *dia*. Corrected after Fol, FN, and NY.
e Specified in NY.
f Orig. and Pa: *quella* (she; that lady). All other sources have *quello*, necessary for the context.

BASSADANZA FOR THREE CALLED *PELLEGRINA*[24]
COMPOSED BY GUGLIELMO

First do two *sempii* and two *doppii* beginning with the left foot, and then make a[25] *meza volta* upon the right foot; and do two *riprese*, one on the left [foot] and the other on the right; and a *riverenza* on the left foot; and then the man takes the right hand of the lady[26] and they turn around with one[27] *sempio* and a *doppio* beginning with the left foot; and at the same time the [other] lady[28] turns round in place, with those [same] steps; and then the man takes the left hand of the other lady, and they turn round with two *sempii* and a *doppio* beginning with the right foot; and the lady who is left alone turns round with two *sempii* and a *doppio* beginning with the right foot; and then advance in opposite directions with two *sempii* and two *doppii* beginning with the left foot; and then make a *meza volta* on the right foot; and do two *riprese*, one on the left [foot] and the other on the right; then advance towards one another with two *sempii* and a *doppio*; beginning with the left foot; and then make a *volta tonda* with two *sempii* beginning with the right foot and a *ripresa* on the right foot; and then advance towards one another with two *sempii* beginning with the left foot; and then the ladies make a *meza volta* on the right foot, and [all] take hands, and do a *ripresa* on the left [foot]; and then make a *volta tonda* with two *sempii* beginning with the right foot, and a *ripresa* on the right foot, and a *riverenza* on the left.

BASSADANZA FOR THREE CALLED *PHOEBUS*
COMPOSED BY MESSER DOMENICO[29]

First do two *sempii* and a *doppio* beginning with the left foot, and then a *ripresa* on the right [foot]; and do this once again; and at the same time as the *ripresa* the man in the middle makes a *meza volta* on the right [foot]; and then advance in opposite directions with two *doppii* starting with the left foot, and make a *meza volta* on the right [foot] with two *riprese*, one on the left [foot] and the other on the right; and then advance towards one another with two *sempii* and two *doppii* starting[30] with the left foot, the man passing between the ladies;

---

[24] Precious.

[25] This is the only time Guglielmo includes the indefinite article before *meza volta*. (Repeated in Pa; eliminated in FN and NY.)   [26] Fol specifies the hand 'of the one on the right'.

[27] One *sempio* is confirmed in Pa and S, but FN, Fol, and NY substitute two *sempii*.

[28] Fol: 'the one on the left'; NY: the lady 'who is left alone'.   [29] Not included in Pd.

[30] In the original and in Pa, 'starting' occurs earlier in the sentence: 'and then advance towards one another *starting* with two *sempii* and two *doppii* with the left foot'. This is changed in NY and FN to the usual form given here in translation, except that *cominciando* ('beginning') is used instead of 'starting'.

[27ᵛ] due riprese, l'una sul sini|stro & l'altra sul dritto. & una reverenza sul sinistro. et poi diano doi tempi di saltarello cominciando col pie sinistro passando in mezo delle donne. et poi diano meza volta in sul dritto. et poi facciano tre riprese: una sul sinistro ell'altra sul dritto, ell'altra sul sinistro. et poi diano⁸ una volta tonda con doi sempi cominciando col pie dritto & una ripresa sul dritto. Et poi vengano in contro l'uno all'altro con doi sempij cominciando col pie sinistro. elle donne diano meza volta sul dritto. et poi si pigliano tutti tre per mano, & facciano doe riprese, l'una sul sinistro ell'altra sul dritto. et una riverenza sul sinistro.

BASSADANZA CHIAMATA DAPHNES IN TRE DI MESSER DOMENICO

In prima la donna facia due continenze sul pie sinistro, et gli huomini scambiano il luogho cun doi sempij partendo col pie sinistro, cioe quel huomo ch'e *dinanzi passi dinanzi dalla donna. et quello che e da pie passi di dietro dalla [28ʳ] donna. et poi faciano una ripresa sul sinistro. et poi gli | huomini tornino nel luogho suo per la via che si partirono cominciando col pie dritto. et in quel tempo la donna dia una volta tonda con doi sempij partendo col pie dritto. Et poi faciano una ripresa sul pie dritto: et una riverenza sul sinistro. et la donna sola senza gli omini vada tramezando gli huomini a guisa d'un .S. con doi sempij & quattro doppij. poi si pigliano per la mano & faciano due riprese, l'una sul sinistro et l'altra sul dritto. et poi faciano una riverenza sul pie sinistro. et poi gli huomini vadano indrieto con due *riprese in portogalese larghe. et in quel tempo la donna vada innanti con doi sempij et doi doppij, & gli huomini si voltino tondi partendo col pie dritto. et poi faciano una ripresa sul

---

⁸ Orig. and Pa.: *dia*. Corrected after other versions.

and then [all three] make a *meza volta* on the right foot, and do two *riprese*, one on the left [foot] and the other on the right; and a *riverenza* on the left; and then do two *tempi* of *saltarello* beginning with the left foot, the man passing between the ladies; and then make a *meza volta* upon the right [foot]; and then do three *riprese*: one on the left [foot] and the next on the right, and the next on the left;[31] and then make a *volta tonda* with two *sempii* beginning with the right foot and a *ripresa* on the right. And then advance towards one another with two *sempii* beginning with the left foot; and the ladies make a *meza volta* on the right [foot]; and then all three take hands, and do two *riprese*, one on the left [foot] and the other on the right; and a *riverenza* on the left [foot].

BASSADANZA FOR THREE CALLED *DAPHNES*[32] BY MESSER DOMENICO

First the lady does two *continenze* [beginning][33] on the left foot, and the men change places with two *sempii* starting with the left foot, that is the man who is *in front [on the left side] passes in front of the lady; and the one who is at the foot [on the right side] passes behind the lady; and then do a *ripresa* on the left; and then the men return to their places the way they came, beginning with the right foot; and at the same time the lady makes a *volta tonda* with two *sempii* starting with the right foot; and then [all] do a *ripresa* on the right foot; and a *riverenza* on the left; and the lady by herself without the men weaves between the men in the form of an S with two *sempii* and four *doppii*; then take hands and [all three] do two *riprese*, one on the left [foot] and the other on the right; and then make a *riverenza* on the left foot; and then the men go backwards with two slow *Portuguese *riprese*;[34] and at the same time the lady goes forward with two *sempii* and two *doppii*, and the men turn round [make a *volta tonda*] starting with the right foot; and then do a *ripresa* on the right

---

[31] Three *riprese* are often an indication of *riprese in gallone*. (At this point in the choreography, the dancers need to advance towards each other.) See n. 34 and the Glossary.

[32] Daphne.

[33] Clarifications in square brackets are from Domenico's treatise. For a more complete version see Pd, fos. 26^{r-v}.

[34] Two *riprese* done in the time of the lady's two *sempii* and two *doppii* (confirmed in all versions of *De pratica*) would have to be particularly slow. Domenico's version calls for three *riprese* 'in traverso' (obliquely?), the first on the left *gallone* (side, presumably), the next on the right, the next on the left. In Guglielmo's version, the directions for the feet do not seem to follow correctly. Before doing the Portuguese *riprese* the men have made a *ripresa* on the left foot and one on the right and a *riverenza* on the left. Presumably the two Portuguese *riprese* are done with the left and right feet, but then the right foot begins the *volta tonda*. Either three *riprese* are necessary, or the Portuguese *riprese* are performed in a particular way. While there is another problem in *Principessa* (n. 44), there is no discrepancy in *Spero*, which has a sequence of three Portuguese *riprese* performed on alternate feet.

pie dritto. ella donna dia meza volta. et faccia due riprese l'una sul sinistro
ell'altra sul destro. & poi vadano gli huomini incontro alla dona [*sic*] con doi
sempij & doi doppij partendo col pie sinistro. ella donna dia una volta tonda
con quelli medesmi passi, cio e con doi sempij & doi doppij al luogho suo pur
[28ᵛ] col sinistro. et poi gli huomini diano meza | volta sul dritto. et mettano la
donna in mezo. & poi tutti faciano due riprese, l'una sul sinistro ell'altra sul
dritto. et quattro continenze sul pie sinistro. et poi vadano l'uno dietro all'altro
con quattro tempi di saltarello partendo col pie sinistro. Et poi diano meza
volta sul dritto, & una ripresa sul sinistro. et anchora vadano l'uno drieto
all'altro con doi sempij & un doppio partendo col dritto. et poi diano meza
volta sul dritto & una ripresa sul sinistro. et poi diano una volta tonda con doi
sempii partendo col pie dritto. et faciano una ripresa sul dritto: et una riverenza
sul sinistro.

BASSADANZA CHIAMATA GIOLIVA IN DOI FATTA PER GUILIELMO

In prima doi sempij et doi doppij cominciando col pie sinistro. et poi diano
meza volta in sul pie dritto, tanto che la donna resti da man di sopra del
huomo. et poi faciano due riprese, una sul sinistro, l'altra sul dritto, et due
continenze sul sinistro. et poi la donna vada atorno al huomo con doi sempij
[29ʳ] et doi doppij partendosi col sinistro. et in quel | tempo l'huomo stia fermo al
luogho suo. & poi si pigliano per la mano, & faciano due riprese, l'una sul
sinistro, ell'altra sul dritto. et poi l'huomo vada atorno alla donna con doi
sempij & doi doppii cominciando col sinistro. et in quel tempo la donna stia
ferma al luogho suo. et poi faciano due riprese, l'una sul sinistro, ell'altra
sul dritto. et una riverenza sul sinistro. et poi diano doi tempi di saltarello,
cominciando col sinistro. et poi diano meza volta in sul dritto, tanto che
l'huomo resti di sopra la donna. Et poi faciano una ripresa sul sinistro. et poi
diano una volta tonda con doi sempij partendosi col dritto, et una ripresa in
sul dritto. et una riverenza sul sinistro.

BASSADANZA CHIAMATA PATIENZA IN QUATRO DI GUILIELMO

In prima doi sempi & doi doppij cominciando col sinistro, & una riverenza
sul sinistro. et poi vadano al tondo ognuno colla donna sua con doi sempii & un

foot; and the lady makes a *meza volta*; and does two *riprese*, one on the left and the other on the right; and then the men advance towards the lady with two *sempii* and two *doppii* starting with the left foot; and the lady makes a *volta tonda* in place with those same steps, that is with two *sempii* and two *doppii*, also [starting] with the left; and then the men make a *meza volta* on the right; and place the lady in the middle; and then all [three] do two *riprese*, one on the left and the other on the right; and four *continenze* [beginning?] on the left foot; and then advance one behind the other with four *tempi* of *saltarello* starting with the left foot. And then make a *meza volta* on the right, and a *ripresa* on the left; and advance again one behind the other with two *sempii* and a *doppio* starting with the right; and then make a *meza volta* on the right and a *ripresa* on the left; and then make a *volta tonda* with two *sempii* starting with the right foot; and do a *ripresa* on the right: and a *riverenza* on the left.

BASSADANZA FOR TWO CALLED *GIOLIVA*[35] COMPOSED BY GUGLIELMO

First do two *sempii* and two *doppii* beginning with the left foot; and then make a *meza volta* upon the right foot, so that the lady finishes above [to the left of] the man; and then do two *riprese*, one on the left [foot], the other on the right, and two *continenze* [beginning?] on the left; and then the lady goes around the man with two *sempii* and two *doppii* starting with the left; and at the same time the man stands still in place; and then take hands, and do two *riprese*, one on the left [foot], and the other on the right; and then the man goes around the lady with two *sempii* and two *doppii* beginning with the left; and at the same time the lady stands still in place; and then do two *riprese*, one on the left [foot], and the other on the right; and a *riverenza* on the left; and then do two *tempi* of *saltarello*, beginning with the left; and then make a *meza volta* upon the right [foot], so that the man finishes above [to the left of] the lady. And then do a *ripresa* on the left [foot]; and then make a *volta tonda* with two *sempii* starting with the right, and a *ripresa* upon the right; and a *riverenza* on the left.

BASSADANZA FOR FOUR CALLED *PATIENZA*[36] BY GUGLIELMO

First do two *sempii* and two *doppii* beginning with the left, and a *riverenza* on the left [foot]; and then each man goes around with his lady with two *sempii*

---

[35] Blithesome.
[36] Patience.

doppio cominciando col sinistro. Et poi vadano pur tondi, cio e rivoltandose
[29ᵛ] dall'altra mano con doi sempij et un dop|pio cominciando col dritto, tanto che
le donne rimangano al contrario degli huomini. et poi vadano al contrario
l'uno del'altro con doi doppij partendo col sinistro. Et poi diano meza volta
sul dritto. et poi faciano una ripresa sul sinistro et una in sul dritto, & una
riverenza in sul sinistro. Et poi vengano incontro l'uno dell'altro, cominciando
col sinistro facian[d]o quattro tempi di saltarello, cio e tramezando li huomini
colle donne. et poi diano meza volta in sul dritto, et faciano due riprese, l'una
sul sinistro & l'altra sul dritto. et una riverenza sul sinistro. et poi vegnano
incontro l'un dell'altro con doi doppij cominciando col sinistro. et poi le donne
diano meza volta insul dritto. et poi si pigliano tutti quattro per mano, et
faciano due riprese, l'una sul sinistro ell'altra sul dritto, et due continenze insul
sinistro. et poi le donne vadano una dietro all'altra con doi sempij & quattro
doppii, alla guisa di un .S. in torno agli huomini, et stiano ferme. Et quando
le donne sonno tornate al suo luogho, pigliansi per mano, et faciano due
[30ʳ] riprese, una sul sinistro ell'al|tra sul dritto, & due continenze sul sinistro. et
poi il simile faciano gli huomini chome hanno fatto le donne, tanto che gli
huomini ritornano al suo luogho. & poi si pigliano per mano et faciano una
ripresa sul sinistro. et poi diano una volta tonda con doi sempij, cominciando
col dritto. et faciano una ripresa sul dritto & una riverenza sul sinistro.

BASSADANZA CHIAMATA FLANDESCA IN DOI
DI MESSER DOMIN[I]CO

In prima doi passi sempii & un doppio cominciando col sinistro, poi una
ripresa sul dritto, poi due continenze cominciando col sinistro. et poi quattro
continenze cominciando col sinistro. et poi quattro continenze. et poi quattro
tempi di saltarello cominciando col sinistro, et faciano fine dal dritto. Et poi
una ripresa sul sinistro. et poi doi passi sempij, & un doppio, cominciando dal
dritto, et ritornando in drieto. poi faciano due riprese l'una sul dritto, ell'altra
sul sinistro. et puoi [*sic*] due continenze, et poi tre doppij cominciando dal
[30ᵛ] sinistro, | et facendo fine col sinistro. et poi quattro continenze, cominciando
col dritto: et facendo fine al dritto.

and a *doppio* beginning with the left [foot]. And then go round again, that is turning in the other direction with two *sempii* and a *doppio* beginning with the right,[37] so that the ladies and men finish facing in opposite directions; and then advance in opposite directions with two *doppii* starting with the left. And then make a *meza volta* on the right [foot]; and then make a *ripresa* on the left and one upon the right, and a *riverenza* upon the left. And then advance towards one another, beginning with the left [foot], doing four *tempi* of *saltarello*, that is the men and ladies weaving through each other; and then make a *meza volta* upon the right [foot], and do two *riprese*, one on the left [foot] and the other on the right; and a *riverenza* on the left; and then advance towards one another with two *doppii* beginning with the left; and then the ladies make a *meza volta* upon the right [foot]; and then all four take hands, and do two *riprese*, one on the left [foot] and the other on the right, and two *continenze* [beginning?] upon the left; and then the ladies go one behind the other with two *sempii* and four *doppii*, in the form of an S around the men, and stand still. And when the ladies are back in their places, take hands, and do two *riprese*, one on the left [foot] and the other on the right, and two *continenze* [beginning?] on the left; and then the men repeat what the ladies did, until the men return to their places; and then take hands and do a *ripresa* on the left [foot]; and then make a *volta tonda* with two *sempii*, beginning with the right; and do a *ripresa* on the right and a *riverenza* on the left.

BASSADANZA FOR TWO CALLED *FLANDESCA*[38] BY MESSER DOMENICO

First do two *passi sempii* and a *doppio* beginning with the left, then a *ripresa* on the right [foot], then two *continenze* beginning with the left; and then four *continenze* beginning with the left; and then four *continenze*;[39] and then four *tempi* of *saltarello* beginning with the left, and ending with the right. And then a *ripresa* on the left [foot]; and then two *passi sempii*, and a *doppio*, beginning with the right, and going back; then do two *riprese*, one on the right [foot], and the other on the left;[40] and then two *continenze*, and then three *doppii* beginning with the left, and ending with the left; and then four *continenze*, beginning with the right; and ending on the right.[41]

---

[37] NY and FN add 'taking right hands . . . and then taking left hands'.

[38] Flemish [dance]. Not included in Domenico's treatise.

[39] S deletes these last two phrases while in NY and FN they read: 'And then [do] four *riverenze* upon the left foot and then [do] four *continenze*'.

[40] NY and FN have: 'one on the left and the other on the right'.

[41] There are no indications in other versions as to which feet to use. The NY and FN versions end (after the *continenze*) with 'a *riverenza* upon the left foot'.

BASSADANZA CHIAMATA PRINCIPESSA ALLA
FILA FATTA PER GUIGLIELMO

In prima doi sempij & tre doppij partendosi col pie sinistro & poi una riverenza
sul dritto, et da poi tornino in drieto con doi sempij partendosi col dritto. et
poi diano meza volta sul dritto. et una ripresa sul sinistro. et poi diano una
volta tonda con doi sempij cominciando col dritto. et una ripresa sul dritto.
et poi faciano una riverenza sul sinistro. et poi tornino indrieto con un sempio
col sinistro. et poi vadano l'uno drieto all'altro con tre riprese portogalese
cominciando col dritto. et poi diano una volta tonda con doi sempij cominciando col pie dritto & una ripresa sul dritto. & poi diano meza volta sul dritto,
& poi una ripresa sul sinistro ell'altra sul dritto. et una reverenza sul sinistro,
tanto che l'huomo primo rimanga dinanzi chome lui era. et poi vadano con
[31ʳ] tre tempi di *saltarello to|descho. & poi facino una ripresa sul dritto tornando
in drieto. & una ripresa sul sinistro. et poi diano una volta tonda, con doi
sempij cominciando col dritto, & una ripresa sul dritto. et poi faciano due
continenze sul sinistro. et poi doi tempi di saltarello cominciando col sinistro.
et poi diano meza volta sul dritto & una ripresa sul sinistro. et poi tornino in
drieto con un doppio cominciando col pie dritto. et doi sempij cominciando
col sinistro. e[t] poi diano meza volta sul dritto. et poi faciano doi riprese sul
sinistro ell'altra sul dritto, & una riverenza sul sinistro, tanto che l'huomo
primo rimangha dinanzi chom'egli era.

BASSADANZA IN SINGLE FILE CALLED *PRINCIPESSA*[42] COMPOSED BY GUGLIELMO

First do two *sempii* and three *doppii* starting with the left foot and then a *riverenza* on the right, and after that go back with two *sempii* starting with the right; and then make a *meza volta* on the right [foot]; and a *ripresa* on the left; and then make a *volta tonda* with two *sempii* beginning with the right; and a *ripresa* on the right; and then make a *riverenza* on the left; and then go back with one *sempio*[43] with the left; and then advance one behind the other with three Portuguese *riprese* beginning with the right; and then make a *volta tonda* with two *sempii* beginning with the right foot[44] and a *ripresa* on the right; and then make a *meza volta* on the right [foot], and then a *ripresa* on the left and the other [*ripresa*] on the right; and a *riverenza* on the left, so that the first man[45] finishes in front as before; and then advance with three *tempi* of *German *saltarello*;[46] and then do a *ripresa* on the right [foot] going back; and a *ripresa* on the left; and then make a *volta tonda*, with two *sempii* beginning with the right, and a *ripresa* on the right; and then do two *continenze* [beginning?] on the left [foot]; and then two *tempi* of *saltarello* beginning with the left; and then make a *meza volta* on the right [foot] and a *ripresa* on the left; and then go back with a *doppio* beginning with the right foot;[47] and two *sempii* beginning with the left; and then make a *meza volta* on the right [foot]; and then do two *riprese*, [one] on the left and the other on the right, and a *riverenza* on the left, so that the first man finishes in front as before.

---

[42] Princess. NY specifies 'for two' dancers, while S states 'for three or six'.

[43] This is confirmed in all the versions.

[44] The directions for the feet do not seem to follow correctly. If two *sempii* (see n. 43) were made backwards (left, right), then the three *riprese* could follow left, right, left, and the *volta tonda* could thus start on the right. It is not known if Portuguese *riprese* were performed in a particular way. Guglielmo's version of *Daphnes* also has a discrepancy (n. 34); *Caterva* has three on the right foot followed by three on the left; and in *Spero* the feet alternate regularly with each *ripresa*.

[45] This seems to indicate that two men are dancing (perhaps with a lady in the middle?). The same wording is used in the NY and FN versions, which conclude with their typical refrain, specifying: 'the men accompany the ladies to their places', and this despite NY's designation of *Principessa* as a dance 'for two'.

[46] It is not clear what Guglielmo means here: a specific German *saltarello* step? *quadernaria doppii* steps? See '*saltarello todescho*' in the Glossary.

[47] Despite the 'going back' being performed with only one *doppio* (and two *sempii*?), Guglielmo specifies that it should *start* with the right foot. The same expression ('starting' or 'beginning', rather than the usual 'on' or 'with') is used by Guglielmo for the *volte tonde* in *quadernaria* or *piva misura* with which all his *balli* end: those with two *doppii*, starting backwards on the right foot and finishing forward on the left (*Colonnese* and *Gratioso*), and those with only one *doppio*, performed on the left foot (*Duchesco*, *Legiadra*, and *Spero*). Also see *Rostiboli Gioioso* and Guglielmo's version of *Belfiore* (n. 86). The *doppio* 'beginning with the left' in *Caterva* may simply be an oversight.

BASSADANZA CHIAMATA CATERVA IN TRE
DI GUILIELMO

Inn [sic] prima doi sempij cominciando col pie sinistro & due continenze sul
sinistro & un doppio cominciando col sinistro. et poi diano una volta tonda
con doi sempij cominciando col dritto: et una ripresa sul dritto, una riverenza
[31ᵛ] in sul sinistro. & poi vadano uno drieto l'altro | alla fila con doi sempii & doi
doppij cominciando col sinistro. & poi faciano una ripresa sul dritto & una
riverenza sul sinistro, et anchora vadano alla fila uno drieto l'altro con sei
tempi di saltarello todescho cominciando col sinistro, faciano una ripresa sul
sinistro. et in quel tempo faciando la ripresa, si piglino tutti per la mano, &
poi faciano tre riprese portugalese sul pie dritto. et poi il simile sul sinistro. et
poi diano una volta tonda con doi sempi cominciando col dritto. & una ripresa
sul dritto, due continenze sul sinistro, quattro tempi di saltarello todescho,
cio e battendo i tempi allo *inanci, et meza volta sul dritto. & due riprese, una
sul sinistro ell'altra sul dritto: una riverenza sul sinistro. et poi faciano quattro
tempi di saltarello cominciando col sinistro. et poi diano meza volta in sul
dritto: una ripresa sul sinistro. et poi diano una volta tonda con doi sempij,
cominciando col dritto, una ripresa sul dritto, una riverenza sul sinistro.

FINITE LE BASSEDANZE COMINCIANO I BALLI
DE LI PREDITTI

BASSADANZA FOR THREE CALLED *CATERVA*[48]
BY GUGLIELMO

First do two *sempii* beginning with the left foot and two *continenze* [beginning?] on the left and a *doppio* beginning with the left;[49] and then make a *volta tonda* with two *sempii* beginning with the right; and a *ripresa* on the right, a *riverenza* upon the left; and then advance one behind the other in single file with two *sempii* and two *doppii* beginning with the left; and then do a *ripresa* on the right [foot] and a *riverenza* on the left, and again advance in single file one behind the other with six *tempi* of German *saltarello*[50] beginning with the left, and do a *ripresa* on the left; and at the same time as the *ripresa*, all take hands, and then do three Portuguese *riprese* on the right foot; and then the same on the left; and then make a *volta tonda* with two *sempii* beginning with the right; and a *ripresa* on the right, two *continenze* [beginning?] on the left, four *tempi* of German *saltarello*, that is beating the *tempi* *ahead [starting on the up-beat?],[51] and a *meza volta* on the right [foot]; and two *riprese*, one on the left and the other on the right; a *riverenza* on the left; and then do four *tempi* of *saltarello* beginning with the left; and then make a *meza volta* upon the right [foot]; a *ripresa* on the left; and then make a *volta tonda* with two *sempii*, beginning with the right, a *ripresa* on the right, a *riverenza* on the left.

HAVING FINISHED THE *BASSEDANZE*, THE *BALLI*
BY THE AFORESAID [COMPOSERS] BEGIN

[48] A Company of Fellows.

[49] See n. 47.

[50] See n. 46.

[51] *Battere il tempo* means beating time. *Allo inanci* could also mean 'forward'. The NY version states 'non [not] battendo all'innanzi' and FN confirms this with 'non battendo tempo all'innanzi'. S on the other hand has 'baptino alla mano i tempi' (beating the *tempi* with the hand?), all of which are equally obscure.

[32ʳ] BALLO CHIAMATO ROSTIBOLI GIOIOSO IN DOI COMPOSTO PER MESSER DOMINICO

In prima due riprese, l'una sul sinistro ell'altra sul dritto. et poi l'huomo se parta dalla donna con doi sempij et doi doppij cominciando col pie sinistro. & poi faccia due riprese, una sul sinistro ell'altra sul dritto. et in quel tempo la donna anchora faccia le riprese insieme con l'huomo. et poi l'huomo faccia anchora doi sempij & doi doppij, & poi doi riprese, l'una sul sinistro ell'altra sul dritto, & l'huom[o] si fermi. et poi la donna faccia tutto quello ha fatto l'huomo. et poi si pigliano per mano, & facciano due riprese, l'una sul sinistro ell'altra sul dritto. et poi facciano doi sempii & tre doppij cominciando col sinistro. et poi diano una volta tonda con doi sempij cominciando col pie dritto, & una ripresa sul dritto. et tutto questo facciano un'altra fiata. et poi faciano sedici tempi di saltarello cominciando col pie sinistro. et poi si fermano, et l'huomo faccia uno schosso, ella donna gli responda. et l'huomo vada inanzi [32ᵛ] con un doppio | partendo col sinistro. ella donna facia un scosso, ell'huomo gli responda, et vada la donna apresso l'huomo partendosi col sinistro. & faccia un passo doppio, elli schossi altri tanto con un doppio chome ditto.

BALLO CHIAMATO DUCHESCO IN TRE ALLA FILA DI GUILIELMO

In prima quindici tempi di saltarello cominciando col pie sinistro. et poi se fermino. et poi diano una volta tonda con doi sempij partendo col pie dritto, et una ripresa sul dritto, et una reverenza sul sinistro. ella donna che e in mezo vada tramezando gli huomini a guisa d'un .S. con doi sempij & sei doppij partendo col sinistro, tanto che lei ritorni al suo luogho. et gli huomini in quel tempo stia[no]ʰ fermi. et quando la dona e gionta al luogho suo facciano due riprese, l'una sul sinistro ell'altra sul dritto. et una riverenza sul sinistro. et poi

---

ʰ In the original, *stia*, the last word in the line, is followed by a dash (a hyphen) indicating that it is incomplete.

BALLO FOR TWO CALLED *ROSTIBOLI GIOIOSO*[52] COMPOSED BY MESSER DOMENICO

First do two *riprese*, one on the left [foot] and the other on the right; and then the man leaves the lady with two *sempii* and two *doppii* beginning with the left foot; and then he does two *riprese*, one on the left [foot] and the other on the right; and at the same time the lady also does the *riprese* together with the man; and then the man again does two *sempii* and two *doppii*, and then two *riprese*, one on the left [foot] and the other on the right, and the man stops; and then the lady does everything the man did; and then take hands, and do two *riprese*, one on the left [foot] and the other on the right; and then do two *sempii* and three *doppii* beginning with the left; and then make a *volta tonda* with two *sempii* beginning with the right foot, and a *ripresa* on the right; and do all of this once again; and then do sixteen *tempi* of *saltarello* beginning with the left foot; and then stop, and the man does a *scosso*, and the lady replies; and the man goes forward with a *doppio* starting with the left;[53] and the lady does a *scosso*, and the man replies, and the lady goes up to the man starting with the left, and does a *passo doppio*, and the *scossi* yet again with a *doppio* as described [above].

BALLO CALLED *DUCHESCO*[54] FOR THREE IN SINGLE FILE BY GUGLIELMO

First do fifteen *tempi* of *saltarello* beginning with the left foot; and then stop; and then make a *volta tonda* with two *sempii* starting with the right foot, and a *ripresa* on the right, and a *riverenza* on the left; and the lady who is in the middle weaves around the men in the form of an S with two *sempii* and six *doppii* starting with the left, until she is back in her place; and at the same time the men stand still; and when the lady has reached her place [all?] do two *riprese*, one on the left [foot] and the other on the right; and a *riverenza* on the

---

[52] *Rostiboli Gioioso* is an Italian version of a dance known in France as 'Rotî bouilli' (the roasts and boiled [meats]), and as 'Rusty Bully' or 'Roty buly' in England. In the versions in NY, in M (for three), and in FN (for two), it appears simply as *Gioioso* (*Joyous; Blithe*). There is no version of the *ballo* in Domenico's own treatise and no extant music except in Pa. NY̅ has the most complete and detailed description, and also includes a 'Spanish' *Gioioso* and a version for three dancers. S's version for three (similar to NY's) is called 'el gioioso'; another *Gioioso* for two is included in the list of *balli* composed by Domenico, but is headed *Rotiboli* in the actual description. For a detailed account of the dance see Heartz, 'A 15th-Century Ballo'. Other references in Ch. 1 n. 36, Ch. 2 n. 55, and Ch. 3.

[53] See n. 47.

[54] Ducal. According to Gallo, 'Il "ballare lombardo"', this first *ballo* may have been composed by Guglielmo to commemorate Francesco Sforza's entry into Milan as Duke. No music is preserved.

quel huomo che e di nanci vada in contro alla dona con doi tempi di saltarello todescho, et tocchi la mano alla donna. et quel huomo che e di drieto faccia il [33ʳ] simile che ha fatto il | primo. e[t] gliⁱ huomini si fermano, & poi la donna vada tramezando gli huomini con quatro tempi di *piva a guisa d'un .S. et poi vadano l'uno drieto all'altro, cio e alla fila con doi sempij et doi doppij partendo col sinistro, et una riverenza sul sinistro. et poi si fermino. ella donna faccia uno schosso, & gli huomini respondano. et la donna dia unaʲ volta tonda partendo col sinistro. et gli huomini faciano un schosso, ella donna gli responda. et poi gli huomini diano una volta tonda sul sinistro cominciando col sinistro. et poi ancho la donna dia una volta tonda con un doppio partendo col pie sinistro.

BALLO CHIAMATO LEGIADRA IN QUATRO DI GUILIELMO

In prima sedici tempi di saltarello, et poi si fermino. ella coppia prima dia meza volta insul pie dritto et faciano due riprese, una sul sinistro, ell'altra sul dritto. et in quel tempo delle riprese la coppia di drieto faciano quattro continenze in sul sinistro. et poi vengano in contra l'uno dell'altro con doi sempij [33ᵛ] & doi doppij | cominciando col sinistro, cio e passando l'una coppia nel mezo dell'altra. et poi diano meza volta sul pie dritto. et faciano due riprese, l'una sul sinistro ell'altra sul dritto. et poi facciano quattro con[t]inenze sul sinistro. et poi vadano incontroᵏ l'un all'altro con doi sempij & doi doppij partendo col sinistro, cio e tramezando l'una coppia dentro l'altra. et poi diano meza volta sul dritto. et poi facciano due riprese, l'una sul sinistro l'altra sul dritto. & poi faciano doi schossi l'una coppia insieme ell'altra gli risponda. et poi vadano un huomo incontro la donna del compagno con un tempo di saltarello todesco cominciando col sinistro. et cosi vada l'altra donna del compagno con quel medesmo. et poi facciano tre riprese sul dritto, et poi diano una volta tonda con un doppio cominciando col sinistro, cio e l'huomo vada al luogho della donna. ella donna con quegli passi medesmi al luogho del huomo. et tutto questo che e detto faciano l'altro huomo coll'altra donna, tanto che ognuno si ritruovi col suo compagno. et poi gli huomini vadano atorno le [34ʳ] donne con doi | tempi di piva. et poi la donna vada intorno al huomo con doi altri tempi di piva. et poi si fermi l'una coppia & faccia uno schosso ell'altra coppia gli risponda. et diano una volta tonda cominciando col pie sinistro con un doppio.

ⁱ Orig.: *egli.*
ʲ *Una* is written twice.
ᵏ Orig.: *intorno.* Corrected after all other versions (cf. *Cupido,* n. *c*).

left; and then the man who is in front advances towards the lady with two *tempi* of German *saltarello*, and touches the lady's hand; and the man who is behind does the same as the first; and the men stop, and then the lady weaves around the men with four *tempi* of **piva* in the form of an S; and then advance one behind the other, that is in single file with two *sempii* and two *doppii* starting with the left, and a *riverenza* on the left; and then stop; and the lady does a *scosso*, and the men reply; and the lady makes a *volta tonda* starting with the left; and the men do a *scosso*, and the lady replies; and then the men make a *volta tonda* on the left beginning with the left;[55] and then the lady also makes a *volta tonda* with a *doppio* starting with the left foot.[56]

BALLO FOR FOUR CALLED *LEGIADRA*[57]
BY GUGLIELMO

First do sixteen *tempi* of *saltarello*, and then stop; and the first couple makes a *meza volta* upon the right foot and does[58] two *riprese*, one on the left [foot], and the other on the right; and at the same time as the *riprese* the couple that is behind does four *continenze* [beginning?] upon the left; and then advance towards one another with two *sempii* and two *doppii* beginning with the left, that is one couple passing through the other; and then make a *meza volta* on the right foot; and do two *riprese*, one on the left and the other on the right; and then do four *continenze* [beginning?] on the left; and then advance towards one another with two *sempii* and two *doppii* starting with the left, that is one couple weaving through the other; and then make a *meza volta* on the right [foot]; and then do two *riprese*, one on the left, the other on the right; and then do two *scossi*, [first] one couple and the other replies; and then one man advances towards his companion's lady with one *tempo* of German *saltarello* beginning with the left; and the companion's lady does the same; and then they do three *riprese* [beginning?] on the right [foot],[59] and then they make a *volta tonda* with a *doppio* beginning with the left,[60] that is the man goes to the lady's place; and the lady, with the same steps, goes to the man's place; and the other man and lady do everything that has been described, so that everyone ends up with his own partner; and then the men go around the ladies with two *tempi* of *piva*; and then the lady goes around the man[61] with two more *tempi* of *piva*; and then one couple stops and does a *scosso* and the other couple replies; and make a *volta tonda* with a *doppio* beginning with the left foot.

[55] In FN this passage reads 'upon the left foot, beginning with the left foot'.
[56] See n. 47.
[57] Fair One.
[58] Plural in original and in other versions.
[59] NY and FN specify the feet for these *riprese*: right, left, right.
[60] See n. 47.
[61] NY corrects this to: 'then the *ladies* go around their *men*'.

BALLO CHIAMATO COLONESE IN SEI
COMPOSTO PER GUILIELMO

In prima sedici tempi di saltarello, et poi si fermano. et quella coppia ch'e di dietro vada con doi sempij et quattro doppij partendo col pie sinistro, cioe tramezando le due coppie, tanto che la coppia di drieto si truovi dinanti a tutti. ella donna si truovi dalla man di sopra del huomo. et in quel tempo che la coppia di drieto fa questo, quella di mezo vada al tondo con doi sempij et un doppio partendo col sinistro, cio e pigliandosi colla man dritta ognuno. et poi in quel tempo medesmo vadano pur al tondo con doi sempi, & un doppio partendo col pie dritto, et poi facciano una riverenza in sul sinistro. et cosi [34ᵛ] faccia la coppia di mezo chome ha fatto quell'ultima, | cio e con doi sempij & quattro doppij. et in quel tempo che quegli di drieto vanno, la coppia di mezo vada sempre al tondo¹ con doi sempij & un doppio chome e ditto, tanto che le donne si truovano tutte da la man di sopra, elle coppie si truovano tutte a s[u]oi luoghi chome stavano in prima. et poi se fermano tutti ad un tempo. et poi vadano intorno alle donne loro con tre tempi di piva. et in quel tempo le donne stiano ferme, et poi facciano quello hanno fatto gli huomini, cio e quegli tre tempi di piva. et poi tutti tre gli huomini facciano un schosso ad un tempo insieme, elle donne gli respondano. et poi gli huomini elle donne si *tirano in drieto con un doppio partendo col pie dritto. et poi vengano in contro l'uno all'altro con un doppio partendo col sinistro, cio e voltandosi tondo tutti quanti.

BALLO CHIAMATO PETIT ROSE IN DOI
DI MESSER DOMINICO

In prima sedici tempi di piva, & poi si fermano. et l'huomo faccia un schosso, [35ʳ] ella donna gli risponda. et poi | l'huomo dia una volta tonda cominciando col

---

¹ Orig.: *sopra al sicondo* (above [to the left of] the second [couple]), which is confusing since the middle and second couples are the same. Correction follows Pa and FN.

BALLO FOR SIX CALLED *COLONNESE*[62]
COMPOSED BY GUGLIELMO

First do sixteen *tempi* of *saltarello*, and then stop; and the rear couple advances with two *sempii* and four *doppii* starting with the left foot, that is weaving through the two [other] couples, until the rear couple ends up in front of everyone; and the lady finishes on the upper [left] side of the man; and at the same time that the rear couple is doing this, the middle couple goes around with two *sempii* and a *doppio* starting with the left, that is everyone taking right hands; and then at the same time [that the rear couple is still moving] they go around again[63] with two *sempii*, and a *doppio* starting with the right foot, and then they make a *riverenza* upon the left; and the middle couple now does what the last [couple] did, that is with two *sempii* and four *doppii*; and at the same time as those at the rear advance, the [new] middle couple continues to go round with two *sempii* and a *doppio* as was described [above], so that the ladies all finish on the upper [left] side, and the couples are all in their places as they were in the beginning; and then everyone stops at the same time;[64] and then [the men] go around their ladies with three *tempi* of *piva*; and at the same time the ladies stand still; and then they do the same as the men, that is those three *tempi* of *piva*; and then all three men do a *scosso* together at the same time, and the ladies reply; and then the men and the ladies *draw back with a *doppio* starting with the right foot;[65] and then they advance towards one another with a *doppio* starting with the left, that is everybody turning round [doing a *volta tonda*].

BALLO FOR TWO CALLED *PETIT ROSE*[66]
BY MESSER DOMENICO

First do sixteen *tempi* of *piva*, and then stop; and the man does a *scosso*, and the lady replies; and then the man makes a *volta tonda* beginning with the left

[62] Marrocco, 'Inventory', points out that the Siena version of *Colonnese* includes the dedication, 'Composed for My Lady Sveva of the Colonna family'. Sveva Colonna was Alessandro Sforza's second wife. (See Ch. 2 n. 11 and Biographical Notes.)

[63] NY specifies 'taking left hands'.

[64] For a clearer and more complete description see the NY version. The choreography must be repeated a third time (as the repeat numeral in the music suggests) in order for the three couples to end up in their starting positions.

[65] See n. 47.

[66] Not included in Domenico's treatise. No music is preserved. The version in NY, called *Pettirosso* ([Robin] Redbreast), is more detailed. Crane, *Materials*, points out (92) that the NY title is similar to that of the French-Burgundian *basse danse*, *Le petit roysin*. (See also *Petit Riense*, App. II, n. 17.)

sinistro. et similmente faccia la donna. et pos [*sic:* poi] si pigliano per mano et vadano faciando tre doppij cominciando sul sinistro. et per ogni doppio se ritiri in drieto col dritto, et poi col sinistro. et poi si fermino. Et poi l'huomo dia meza volta l'uno al contrario dell'altro con doi tempi di saltarello, cio e ch'el primo tempo vada di longho, ell'altro si vadano a tocchare la mano.

BALLO CHIAMATO IOVE IN TRE A LA FILA
DI MESSER DOMINICO

In prima facciano t[r]e tempi di saltarello todescho cominciando col pie senestro [*sic*]. et poi facciano la *volta del gioioso. et poi altro tanto quel medesmo. Et poi quel dinanti si volti verso la donna tochandogli la mano dritta con un passo doppio. ella donna vada nel luogho del huomo. et l'huomo vada nel luogho della donna senza firmarsi. et quel huomo vada con un altro passo doppio tocchando la man sinistra all'altr'huomo scambiandosi li luoghi. et poi la donna se rivolta con un altro passo doppio tocchando la man dritta al [35ᵛ] huomo, & schambiando li luoghi. et chosi | quel huomo di dietro vada inanti voltandosi inverso la donna: & vadala a trovare con un passo doppio. ella donna il simil faccia verso l'huomo tocchandosi la man dritta, & schambiandosi li luoghi. et poi tocchi la man mancha all'altr'huomo. andandolo a trovare con un passo doppio per uno schambiando li luoghi. et poi la donna se volti, & vadansi a trovare con un passo doppio tocchandosi la man dritta. et quello ch'era di drieto vada innanti. et poi vadano doi altri passi sempij & un doppio. et poi faciano tre tempi di piva a spinapesce tramezandose l'uno all'altro tanto che torni ognuno al luogho suo, et poi faciano un schosso, & poi quattro tempi

[foot]; and the lady does the same;[67] and then take hands and advance doing three *doppii* beginning on the left; and for every *doppio* draw back with the right, and then with the left; and then stop. And then the man makes a *meza volta* [and then advance] in opposite directions with two *tempi* of *saltarello*, that is during the first *tempo* go[68] lengthwise [straight ahead?],[69] and at the other [*tempo*] advance to touch hands.

BALLO CALLED *IOVE*[70] FOR THREE IN SINGLE FILE BY MESSER DOMENICO

First do three *tempi* of German *saltarello* beginning with the left foot; and then do the **volta del gioioso*; and then the same again. And then the man in front turns towards the lady with a *passo doppio* touching her right hand; and the lady goes to the man's place; and the man goes to the lady's place without stopping; and that [same] man advances with another *passo doppio* touching the left hand of the other man, changing places; and then the lady turns around with another *passo doppio* touching the man's right hand, and changing places;[71] and in like manner the man in the rear goes forward, turning towards the lady; and he goes up to her with a *passo doppio*; and the lady does the same towards the man, touching right hands, and changing places; and then [he][72] touches left hands with the other man; going up to him with a *passo doppio* each, changing places; and then the lady turns, and they go up to each other with a *passo doppio* touching right hands; and the one who was in the rear goes in front;[73] and then [all three] advance two more *passi sempii* and a *doppio*; and then do three *tempi* of *piva* in herringbone fashion, weaving around one another until everyone gets back to his place, and then do a *scosso*,[74] and then four

---

[67] At this point, according to the NY version, the lady does a *scosso*, the man replies, and then she makes a *volta tonda*.

[68] The verb is third person singular in the original and in Pa but plural in NY and FN.

[69] The same expression is used again in *Gratioso*. However, when the figure is repeated, Guglielmo instructs the lady to go 'towards' the man. In the NY version of *Gratioso*, the phrase is substituted with 'adirittura de la stanzio', i.e. 'straight in the room'.

[70] Jove. See Domenico's more detailed version, called *Jupiter*, in Pd.

[71] At this point S inserts 'and ends up in the middle in her place. And then in single file all do two *sciempij* and one *doppio*'. Giorgio's version is similar: 'so that the man who was in front ends up in the rear and the one in the rear ends up in front and the lady is once again in the middle. Then advance all together one behind the other with two *passi sempii* and one *doppio*'. This addition of two *sempii* and a *doppio* seems to be confirmed by Guglielmo a few lines later when he writes 'and then advance two *more passi sempii* and a *doppio*'.

[72] No personal pronoun is specified in the original. If the same choreography is followed as before, so that all three end up in their original places (see NY and S), then this should read 'he'. However, FN has 'and then the lady'.

[73] At this point, according to Domenico and Giorgio, the men have returned to their original places.

[74] Missing in Domenico's version. Is this a preparatory *movimento*? (See Glossary.)

di saltarello, cioe gli huomini, ma la donna ne facia doi, et stia ferma. et l'huomo dinanti di quegli quattro ne facia doi inanti et doi voltandosi in drieto passando presso a la donna, & andando al luogho del huomo di drieto. & quel di drieto vada a quel dinanti, andando dall'altro lato della donna. et poi la donna faccia una volta tonda nel suo luogho. et poi faccia[no]*'''* altri quattro
[36^r] tempi di saltarello simili a quelli che hanno fatto | ognuno tornando al suo luogho. et poi l'homo dinanti faccia meza volta con una reverenza tocchando la mano alla donna. et poi la donna si volti verso l'altr'huomo tocchandogli la mano e[t] l'huomo*''* faciando una riverenza.

BALLO CHIAMATO PRESONIERA IN DOI
DI MESSER DOMINICO

In prima due continenze incominciando dal pie sinistro. et poi facciano tre passi sempij & un doppio cominciando dal sinistro, et poi faciando fine dal dritto. poi una riverenza sul sinistro. et questo si faccia due volte. poi l'huomo lassi la donna faciando doi passi sempij cominciando dal sinistro. et poi faccia doi doppij col sinistro verso la donna. et poi la donna si parta faciendo doi passi sempij cominciando col pie dritto & doi doppij col pie dritto. Poi la donna e[t] l'huomo si muovino insieme faciendo doi passi sempij & due continenze cominciando col sinistro, et remanendo la donna dal canto di sopra dal huomo. Et poi la donna si parta dal huomo con doi passi sempij cominciando dal
[36^v] sinistro. et poi faccia doi doppij sul sinistro voltandosi col | viso verso l'huomo, & fermisi la donna, et poi l'huomo si parta facendo doi passi sempij cominciando dal dritto, & poi doi doppij dal dritto. et poi l'huomo ella donna si movano insieme facendo doi passi sempij cominciando col sinistro. et poi facia due continenze remanendo dal canto di sopra. et poi si pigliano per la mano facendo quattro tempi di saltarello todescho, cio e andando un passo doppio

---

''' See n. 75 in the translation.
'' Confirmed in Pa, although the meaning is not altogether clear. S inserts the word *gli* ('to her', in this case): 'et luomo *gli* fa una riverentia'.

tempi of *saltarello*, that is the men, but the lady does [only] two of them, and [then] stands still; and the man in front does two of the four [*tempi* of *saltarello*] forward and two turning back passing next to the lady, and going to the rear man's place; and the one [man] in the rear goes to the one [man] in front, going on the other side of the lady; and then the lady makes a *volta tonda* in place; and then do[75] four more *tempi* of *saltarello* like those done before[76] every one returning to his place; and then the man in front makes a *meza volta* with a *riverenza* touching the lady's hand; and then the lady turns towards the other man touching his hand and the man making [makes her?] a *riverenza*.[77]

BALLO FOR TWO CALLED *PRESONIERA*[78]
BY MESSER DOMENICO

First do two *continenze* beginning with the left foot; and then do three *passi sempii* and a *doppio* beginning with the left, and then ending with the right; then a *riverenza* on the left; and do this twice; then the man leaves the lady doing two *passi sempii* beginning with the left; and then [he] does two *doppii* with the left[79] towards the lady; and then the lady sets off doing two *passi sempii* beginning with the right foot and two *doppii* with the right foot. Then the lady and the man move together doing two *passi sempii* and two *continenze* beginning with the left, and the lady finishes on the upper [left] side of the man. And then the lady leaves the man with two *passi sempii* beginning with the left; and then [she] does two *doppii* on the left turning to face the man, and [then] the lady stops, and then the man sets off doing two *passi sempii* beginning with the right, and then two *doppii* with the right;[80] and then the man and the lady move together doing two *passi sempii* beginning with the left; and then do[81] two *continenze*, [the man] finishing on the upper [left] side; and then take hands doing four *tempi* of German *saltarello*, that is doing one *passo doppio* and

---

[75] Original and FN have *faccia* (third person singular), as if only the lady does the four *tempi* of *saltarello*. Pa and NY have *facciano*.

[76] Pd and NY specify that the lady's *volta tonda* is also repeated.

[77] See n. *n* in the transcription.

[78] Prisoner. See Domenico's version (Pd) for a more complete and detailed description.

[79] Three *doppii* taken with the same foot can indicate, in Domenico's *balli*, that they should be performed in two *tempi*. Lo Monaco and Vinciguerra, 'Il passo doppio', have pointed out that these *doppii*-on-the-same-foot are, in later treatises, often called *contrapassi*. Indeed, the FN version substitutes two *contrapassi* for Guglielmo's two *doppii*, while the NY description calls for three *contrapassi*.

[80] This time Guglielmo does not use *con* ('with') or *su* ('on') as before, but *dal*, which always follows 'beginning' or 'ending'. However, a comparison with Domenico's choreography makes clear that this is either a scribal error or a use of *dal* as 'on'.

[81] Singular in original. Compare with the first description of this section. Both times Pd, NY, and FN substitute a *riverenza*—performed by both the man and the lady—for the *continenze*.

& una ripresa per tempo di saltarello. & fermansi. et tirandosi poi in dietro
l'huomo faccia un movimento, ella donna gli risponda, lasciandosi et tirandosi
in dietro guardandosi per lo viso, & facendo tre passetti sul dritto per uno, &
fermansi. et poi la donna faccia un movimento e[t] l'huomo gli risponda
tirandosi anchora indrieto con tre passetti cominciando dal dritto. et al terzo
passetto piglise il tempo del saltarello andando incontro l'uno all'altro un
tempo di saltarello cominciando dal sinistro. et piglians[i] per la mano con doi
altri tempi di saltarello cominciando dal dritto, & poi un doppio sul dritto.

BALLO CHIAMATO MARCHESANA IN DOI
DI MESSER DOMINICO

[37ʳ] In prima dodici passi doppij tri per pie cominciando dal sinistro, et facendo
fine sul dritto. da poi l'huomo lassi la donna, & partisi con doi doppi cominciando dal sinistro. et poi la donna facia il simile, apresso l'huomo piglia la
donna per mano et faciano insieme due riprese, l'una sul sinistro ell'altra sul
dritto, apresso l'huomo lassi la man sinistra da la donna, et pigli la destra volto
con volto, et vadano intorno doi passi sempij & un doppio cominciando dal
sinistro. et apresso si lassino la mano dritta. faciando una ripresa sul dritto, &
poi si pigliano per la mano sinistra faciando al tondo do[i] passi sempij et un
doppio cominciando dal sinistro. et poi faciano una ripresa sul dritto, & vadano
da poi al contrario l'uno dell'altro con doi doppi. et poi tutti doi si voltino in
meza volta sul pie dritto, & faciano due riprese l'una sul sinistro l'altra sul
dritto. et poi faciano quattro continenze cominciando dal sinistro et finiendo
dal dritto. et poi l'huomo facia un movimento, ella donna gli responda. et poi
[37ᵛ] faciano un doppio per uno al incontro sul sinistro, apresso la donna facia | un
movimento et l'huomo gli risponda. et poi faciano doi doppij sul sinistro l'uno
incontro l'altro. et al terzo se voltino tutti doi con un *salto sul pie dretto
[dritto].

a *ripresa* for each *tempo* of *saltarello*; and stop; and then drawing back the man does a *movimento* and the lady replies, dropping hands and drawing back facing each other, and doing three *passetti*, each [beginning] with the right, and stop; and then the lady does a *movimento* and the man replies, [both] drawing back again with three *passetti* beginning with the right; and at the third *passetto* get into *saltarello* rhythm advancing towards one another [with] one *tempo* of *saltarello* beginning with the left; and taking hands [advance] with two more *tempi* of *saltarello* beginning with the right, and then a *doppio* on the right.

BALLO FOR TWO CALLED *MARCHESANA*[82] BY MESSER DOMENICO

First do twelve *passi doppii*, three with each foot beginning with the left, and finishing on the right;[83] after this the man leaves the lady, and sets off with two *doppii* beginning with the left; and then the lady does the same; next the man takes the lady by the hand and together they do two *riprese*, one on the left [foot] and the other on the right; next the man drops the lady's left hand, and takes the right, facing one another; and [then] go around two *passi sempii* and a *doppio* beginning with the left; and next drop right hands; doing a *ripresa* on the right [foot], and then take left hands going around two *passi sempii* and a *doppio* beginning with the left; and then do a *ripresa* on the right, and after this advance in opposite directions with two *doppii*; and then both turn a *meza volta* on the right foot, and do two *riprese*, one on the left [foot], the other on the right; and then do four *continenze* beginning with the left and ending with the right; and then the man does a *movimento* and the lady replies; and then do a *doppio* each, towards one another, on the left [foot]; next the lady does a *movimento* and the man replies; and then do two *doppii* on the left [foot] towards one another; and on the third both turn with a *salto* on the right foot.[84]

---

[82] Marchioness.

[83] The NY version reads 'sixteen *contrapassi*, that is four with each foot'.

[84] In Domenico's version, the first of these final *doppii* is taken forward (on the left foot), while the second (also on the left), is done turning, after which the dancers leap on to ('saltando su') the right foot and take a *posada* (pause). Therefore, Guglielmo's 'on the third' may refer to the third *tempo* of music rather than to a third *doppio*.

BALLO CHIAMATO BELFIORE IN TRE
COMPOSTO PER MESSER DOMENICO

In prima dodici tempi di piva tutti tre insieme. et fermisi il primo, et poi si mova con un passo doppio cominciando dal sinistro. et nel fine del passo doppio riduca, [*sic*] il pie dritto al stanco, et fermasi. et poi cosi facia il secondo et il terzo. et il primo poi facia un movimento, et poi il secundo gli responda, et il simile il terzo. et poi il primo faccia una volta tonda cio e un passo doppio cominciando dal sinistro. et il simil facia il secundo & anche il terzo, l'uno apresso l'altro. et il primo poi si muova, et faccia doi passi doppii sul sinistro, et uno sempio sul dretto andando dal canto drieto dei compagni, & truovasi cosi al paro di sotto di compagni, et fermansi. et il secundo facia il simile, et fermasi come l'altro. et il terzo si muova con quattro passi doppi sul [38ʳ] sinistro, pur dal canto di drie|to. et quello che rimane apresso colui che fa li quattro doppij preditti, facia un doppio dal canto di sotto pur di drieto rimanendo pur al pari. et quello che fa i quattro doppii, nel fine del quarto vada nel lu[o]gho di colui & fermansi tutti doi. & appresso quel di mezo faccia tre tempi di piva, et un passo sempio circundando quello dalla man dritta andando drieto & passando per mezo a doi compagni, & rimanga di sopra.

BALLO CHIAMATO INGRATA IN TRE
DI MESSER DOMENICO

In prima nove tempi di saltarello tutti tre insieme, et fermansi. et poi la donna si mova al inanci con quattro sempii cominciando dal pie sinistro, & fermansi. apresso gli huomini faciano il simile. et vadano inanzi al pari della donna. et

BALLO FOR THREE CALLED *BELFIORE*[85]
COMPOSED BY MESSER DOMENICO

First all three do twelve *tempi* of *piva* together; and the first one stops, and then he moves with a *passo doppio* beginning with the left;[86] and at the end of the *passo doppio* he brings the right foot up to the left, and stops; and then the second does the same and [also] the third; and the first then does a *movimento*, and then the second replies, and likewise the third; and then the first makes a *volta tonda*, that is a *passo doppio* beginning with the left;[87] and the second does the same and also the third, one after the other; and the first then moves, and does two *passi doppii* on the left [foot], and one *sempio* on the right[88] going behind his companions, thus ending below [on the right?] in line with his companions, and [then] he stops; and the second does the same, and stops like the other [the first]; and the third moves with four *passi doppii* on the left [foot],[89] also going behind; and the one who is next to the one who did the aforesaid four *doppii*, does a *doppio* to the lower [right?] side, also [going] behind [and] finishing in line as well; and the one who does the four *doppii*, at the end of the fourth goes in the other's place and both stop; and next the one in the middle does three *tempi* of *piva*, and a *passo sempio* encircling the one who is on the right-side, going behind and passing between the two companions, and finishes above.[90]

BALLO FOR THREE CALLED *INGRATA*[91]
BY MESSER DOMENICO

First all three do nine *tempi* of *saltarello* together, and stop; and then the lady moves forward with four *sempii* beginning with the left foot, and she stops; next the men do the same; advancing and coming abreast of the lady; and next

[85] Fair Flower. Gallo, 'Il "ballare lombardo" ', 61, points out that Belfiore was the name of a palace near Ferrara, one of the residences of the Este family. While Domenico choreographs this *ballo* for two men and one lady, neither Guglielmo nor Giorgio specifies 'lady' or 'man', indicating instead only the first, second, or third 'one' (masculine or common gender). The music for *Belfiore* is in Pd only.

[86] See n. 47.

[87] In Domenico's version the *volta tonda* is done with 'four small *sempii* beginning with the left foot'.

[88] NY has the *doppii* 'beginning on the left foot', while the *sempio* is with the right. Domenico specifies three *doppii* on the left.

[89] NY again specifies 'beginning on the left foot'. Domenico confirms the same three *doppii* as before and then adds another *doppio*.

[90] To the left, or in front.

[91] The Ingrate. The NY version offers some clarification, but for the most detailed and complete description, see Pd.

apresso la donna subito se volti in meza volta con doi passi sempij cominciando col pie sinistro, & voltandosi dal lato mancho, facendo poi quattro tempi di saltarello al innanzi. et gli huomini faciano quel medesimo. et poi si voltino [38ᵛ] tutti tre sul pie dritto dagando meza volta volto con vol‖to. et facendo due riprese larghe, una sul sinistro & l'altra sul dritto. et poi si mova la donna del suo luogo andando contro a gli huomini. & il simile faciano gli huomini contra la donna faciendo doi passi sempij & un doppio comincian[d]o col sinistro, sequitando con una volta in bassadanza cominciando a far la volta col dritto, et poi anchora faciano doi sempij & un doppio cominciando dal sinistro facendo una medesma volta secundo che di sopra e ditto. Apresso gli huomini et la donna secundo che si ritrovano faciano quattro passi doppij cominciando dal sinistro, et finiendo dal dritto. Apresso se voltino tutti ad un tempo: et rimangano voltati volto con volto voltandosi sul lato dritto, et facendo una ripresa sul sinistro, et un altra sul dritto, andando poi l'uno contra l'altro, cioe la donna facendo sei tempi di saltarello ciaschuno. cio e facendo un doppio sul sinistro et una ripresa sul dritto in drieto a guisa di piva: et poi gli huomini fermino et rimangano tutti ad essere in tre. et la donna vada circundando gli [39ʳ] huomini con sei tempi di saltarello cominciando col sinistro et finien‖do dal dritto andando prima circundando quel di sopra cominciando dal lato di fuori, & intrando poi per mezo, et circundi l'altro compagno. & poi il primo huomo facia una volta quando la donna il circunda andando drieto allei. e[t i]l simile facia il compagno trovandosi tutti al suo luogho.

BALLO CHIAMATO ANELLO IN QUATTRO DI MESSER DOMENICO

In prima otto tempi di saltarello cominciando dal pie sinistro & finiendo dal dritto. et all'ultimo tempo, cio e fatti li sette, gli huomini lassino le mani alle donne, & rimangano in quadro, cio e gli huomini incontro l'uno all'altro, et il simile faciano le donne, et fermansi. a presso gli huomini faciano un movimento, et le donne gli rispondeno. et poi gli huominj si cambieno con doi

the lady immediately turns a *meza volta* with two *passi sempii* beginning with the left foot, turning to the left side, then doing four *tempi* of *saltarello* forward; and the men do the same; and then all three turn on the right foot making a *meza volta*; [ending] face to face; and doing two slow *riprese*,[92] one on the left [foot] and the other on the right; and then the lady moves from her place advancing towards the men; and the men do the same towards the lady doing two *passi sempii* and a *doppio* beginning with the left, followed by a *volta* in *bassadanza* [*misura*][93] beginning the *volta* with the right [foot], and then do two more *sempii* and a *doppio* beginning with the left doing the same *volta* as described above. Next the men and the lady according to where they have ended up do four *passi doppii* beginning with the left, and ending with the right.[94] Next all turn at the same time, finishing face to face, turning to the right side, and doing a *ripresa* on the left [foot], and another on the right, advancing then towards one another, that is [towards] the lady, doing six *tempi* of *saltarello* each; that is doing a *doppio* on the left and a *ripresa* on the right afterwards in *piva* fashion;[95] and then the men stop and all finish in a threesome; and the lady circles round the men with six *tempi* of *saltarello* beginning with the left [foot] and finishing with the right, first encircling the man who is above [on the left] beginning on the outside, and then going into the middle, and encircling the other companion; and then the first man does a *volta* when the lady circles round him following[96] her; and his companion does the same, everyone ending in place.

BALLO FOR FOUR CALLED *ANELLO*[97]
BY MESSER DOMENICO

First do eight *tempi* of *saltarello* beginning with the left foot and finishing with the right; and at the last *tempo*, that is having done seven, the men drop the ladies' hands, and [all four] finish in a square, that is the men facing one another, and the ladies do the same, and [all] stop; next the men do a *movimento*, and the ladies reply; and then the men change [places] with two *tempi* of

---

[92] Domenico makes clear in his description that the *ballo* has thus far been in *saltarello* and *quadernaria misure*. The *riprese* begin a *bassadanza* section.

[93] Confirmed in all other versions. Only Domenico specifies a *volta tonda*.

[94] NY specifies 'the lady *in su* [up, to the top] and the men *in giu* [down, to the foot]'. Pd has the men and lady doing the four *doppii* '*al contrario*' (advancing in opposite directions).

[95] A more idiomatic translation is 'a *doppio* on the left followed by a *ripresa*'. But the original 'et una ripresa in drieto' is not clear and could also be interpreted as being performed backwards instead of afterwards. Domenico describes the step as two *sempii* and two *riprese*. An example of *doppii* followed by a *ripresa* 'in *piva* fashion' can be found in Domenico's *Tesara*. See also *Presoniera*'s German *saltarello*, which consists of 'one *passo doppio* and a *ripresa* for each *tempo* of *saltarello*'.

[96] It is not clear if *andando drieto* means following or going behind. (See also *Alexandresca*.)

[97] Ring. For a more precise description, see Pd, which is also the only source for the music.

tempi di saltarello cominciando col pie sinistro & dando meza volta dal canto dritto a ricontro l'uno all'altro. et poi se trovino in quadro. a presso le donne facciano un movimento e[t] gli° huomini gli rispondino. et poi si scambino con quel medesmo che hanna [*sic*] fatto gli huomini, et pur si trovino in [39ᵛ] quadro. et poi | tutti insieme faciano un movimento: apresso gli huomini faciano una volta tonda voltandosi dal lato mancho. et poi le donne facino il simile, et fermansi. Apresso gli huomini se partino & vadano drieto a suoi compagni con quattro tempi di piva partendosi col sinistro et finiendo dal dritto, cambiandosi le poste, et ritrovansi pur in quadro. et poi le donne faciano il simile. et truovansi tutte alle lor poste. Apresso gli huomini faciano un movimento, elle donne gli rispondano. et questo si fa due volte.

BALLO CHIAMATO GELOSIA IN SEI DI MESSER DOMENICO

In prima faciano tutti otto tempi di saltarello facendo a doi a doi, cio e un huomo & una donna per coppia & fermansi. Apresso l'huomo ch'e di sopra si parta dalla donna sua compagna et vada a trovare la compagniaᵖ secunda, cio e quella di mezo con tre passi doppij sul pie sinistro, et una riverenza tocchando la mano a quella donna. et poi l'huomo suo compagno ch'e in mezo se parta [40ʳ] con un passo doppio sul pie sinistro, et | vada a trovare quella donna che e rimas[t]a di sopra. & poi l'huomo primo seguendo con doi passi vada a trovare sul pie sinistro l'altra donna che e di sotto alla terza coppia. e[t] l'huomo che e compagno a quella di sotto se parta con un passo doppio sul pie sinistro, & vada a trovare quella di mezo. et poi quel primo huomo vada per di drieto da quella donna con doi tempi di piva cominciando col sinistro et vada di sotto alla donna. et apresso si partino tutti insieme con quattro tempi di *piva todescha, et fermansi. et apresso la coppia di nanci dia una volta tonda. ella coppia secuna poi responda. et poi il simile faccia la terza. et poi fatto questo se piglino per la mano sinistra et facino doi passi sempij sul pie sinistro, cambiandosi posta per posta. et poi si cambino le mani, et faciano anchora il simile. et apresso, quello ch'era il primo, sia drieto, et quello ch'era drieto sia il secundo. et quello ch'era il secundo sia il primo.

° Orig.: *egli*, followed by a dash (hyphen), and *huomini* on the next line. Pa has & *li homini*.
ᵖ The spelling of *compagna* as *compagnia* is used by Giovanni Ambrosio in the preceding phrase, 'dalla donna sua compagnia'. Here, however, he uses the word *coppia*, confirmed in FN and NY.

saltarello beginning with the left foot and making a *meza volta* to the right side to face one another; and then finish in a square; next the ladies do a *movimento* and the men reply; and then they change [places] in the same way as the men did, and also finish in a square; and then all do a *movimento* together: next the men make a *volta tonda* turning to the left side; and then the ladies do the same, and stop. Next the men set off and go behind their partners with four *tempi* of *piva* starting with the left [foot] and ending with the right, changing places, and finishing in a square again; and then the ladies do the same; both finishing in their places. Next the men do a *movimento*, and the ladies reply; and this is done twice.

BALLO FOR SIX CALLED *GELOSIA*[98]
BY MESSER DOMENICO

First everyone does eight *tempi* of *saltarello* two by two, that is a man and lady in each couple, and stop. Next the man who is above [at the head] leaves the lady who is his partner and goes up to the second lady, that is the one in the middle, with three *passi doppii* on the left foot, and a *riverenza* touching her hand; and then her partner who is the man in the middle sets off with a *passo doppio* on the left foot, and goes up to the lady who has remained above [at the head]; and then the first man continuing with two *passi* [*doppii*] on the left foot goes up to the other lady who is below [at the foot] in the third couple;[99] and the man who is the foot lady's partner sets off with a *passo doppio* on the left foot, and goes up to the lady in the middle; and then the first man goes behind that lady with two *tempi* of *piva* beginning with the left [foot] and he goes below[100] the lady; and next all set off together with four *tempi* of *German piva*, and [then] stop; and next the head couple makes a *volta tonda*; and the second couple then replies; and then the third does the same; and then this done take left hands [with your partner] and do two *passi sempii* [starting?] on the left foot, changing places; and then change hands, and do the same again; and next, the man who was the first, is at the foot, and the man who was at the foot is second; and the one who was second is first.

---

[98] Jealousy. For clarification, see Domenico's description. The version in NY provides interesting variations.

[99] In Domenico's version, three *doppii* and a *riverenza* are repeated. NY substitutes three *contrapassi* and a *riverenza* both times.

[100] *Sotto* (on the right) may be an error, since Domenico clearly states that the man ends on the lady's left side.

BALLO CHIAMATO BELRIGUARDO IN DOI
DI MESSER DOMINICO

[40ᵛ] In prima quindici tempi di saltarello | et fermasi. et poi faccia[no]*q* quattro doppij cominciando dal pie sinistro. Apresso faciano tre doppij sul sinistro, & doi sempi dal dritto. et poi doi riprese, l'una sul sinistro et l'altra sul dritto. Apresso faciano doi tempi di saltarello cominciando dal sinistro con due altre riprese l'una sul sinistro ell'altra sul dritto. et anchora faciano doi tempi di saltarello con due riprese, l'una sul sinistro ell'altra sul dritto. et poi facciano doi passi sempij et un doppio cominciando dal sinistro, et una ripresa sul dritto. Et poi quattro continenze.

BALLO CHIAMATO LEONCELLO IN DOI
DI MESSER DOMENICO

In prima facciano tre passi doppij su un pie cominciando dal sinistro. et poi tre altri sul dritto et altri tre sul sinistro. A presso faciano doi movimenti, prima l'huomo et poi la donna. et poi si parta l'huomo & vada per dinanti alla donna col pie dretto facendo un doppio et meza volta dal lato dritto. Et apresso la donna facia un movimento, et l'huomo gli risponda, et poi faccia la volta.
[41ʳ] et poi l'huomo si parta con quattro passi sempij comincian|do dal sinistro & un doppio. et la donna vada a trovarlo con quei passi medesmi. Apresso l'huomo faccia tre doppij su un pie cio e sul sinistro. et poi la donna gli vada drieto con quelli medesmi passi. l'huomo facia doi sempij & doi doppij cominciando dal sinistro: & poi la donna faccia il simile. Et apresso si pigliano per mano & faciano doi riprese l'una sul sinistro ell'altra sul dritto. et poi faciano doi sempij & doi doppij cominciando dal pie sinistro, finiendo dal deritto. et poi due riprese l'una sul sinistro & l'altra sul dritto. et po[i] l'huomo faccia un movimento, ella donna gli risponda.

---

q Singular also in Pa but plural in NY and FN.

BALLO FOR TWO CALLED *BELRIGUARDO*[101]
BY MESSER DOMENICO

First do fifteen *tempi* of *saltarello* and stop; and then do four *doppii* beginning with the left foot. Next do three *doppii* on the left,[102] and two *sempii* [beginning] with the right; and then two *riprese*, one on the left [foot] and the other on the right. Next do two *tempi* of *saltarello* beginning with the left, with two more *riprese*, one on the left [foot] and the other on the right; and again do two *tempi* of *saltarello*, with two *riprese*, one on the left [foot] and the other on the right; and then do two *passi sempii* and a *doppio* beginning with the left, and a ripresa on the right. And then four *continenze*.

BALLO FOR TWO CALLED *LEONCELLO*[103]
BY MESSER DOMENICO

First do three *passi doppii* on one [and the same] foot beginning [*sic*] with the left; and then three others on the right and another three on the left. Next do two *movimenti*, first the man and then the lady; and then the man sets off and goes in front of the lady doing a *doppio* with the right foot and a *meza volta* to the right side. And next the lady does a *movimento*, and the man replies; and then [she] does [a *doppio* and] the [*meza*] *volta*;[104] and then the man sets off with four *passi sempii*, beginning with the left, and a *doppio*; and the lady goes up to him with those same steps. Next the man does three *doppii* on one [and the same] foot, that is on the left; and then the lady follows him with those same steps; the man does two *sempii* and two *doppii* beginning with the left; and then the lady does the same. And next take hands and do two *riprese*, one on the left [foot] and the other on the right; and then do two *sempii* and two *doppii* beginning with the left foot, finishing with the right; and then two *riprese*, one on the left [foot] and the other on the right; and then the man does a *movimento*, and the lady replies.

[101] *Belriguardo*, meaning 'beautiful view', was, like *Belfiore*, the name of an Este villa near Ferrara. See Domenico's version in his treatise, where it is the very first dance. (It is followed by another version for three dancers.) See n. 103.

[102] FN and NY substitute four *contrapassi*, which are repeated after the following two *sempii* (performed right, left). Domenico's version, instead, has three more *doppii*, this time 'upon the right foot', reported also in Pa ('beginning with the right').

[103] Probably dedicated to Leonello d'Este. According to Gallo, 'Il "ballare lombardo" ', Domenico composed both *Belriguardo*, his first *ballo*, and *Leoncello*, his second, during the early part of his career when he was in Ferrara at the Este court. For a more detailed and complete description, see Domenico's version—*Lionzello vechio*—in Pd, where it is followed by 'New Leoncello', a version for three dancers.

[104] See versions in Pd and NY.

BALLO CHIAMATO MERCANTIA
DI MESSER DOMENICO

In prima faciano undici tempi [di saltarello tucti]' quattro insieme, & vada la
donna con un huomo, & gli altri doi insieme: ella donna sia nella coppia di
sopra & fermansi. Apresso gli huomini che sonno di drieto si acolgano' con
sei riprese intraverso, l'uno se alargha a man sinestra ell'altro a mane [*sic*]
dritta. Apresso la donna dia meza volta dal lato mancho. ell'huomo suo com-
[41ᵛ] pagno vada inanti con tre doppij cominciando | dal pie sinistro, et la donna
venga a rimanere cogli altri doi huomini in triangolo. et apresso l'huomo che
e a man dritta se parta con doi passi sempij & un doppio cominciando col pie
sinistro, & vada a tocchare la mano alla donna, et poi se volti a man dritta con
doi sempij, & un doppio, cominciando col dritto, & ritorni al suo luogho, dove
lui era. Apresso il suo compagno che e a man sinistra faccia il simile. et nota
che la donna vuole dare una volta tonda, quando il primo huomo gli [h]a
tocchato la mano. et cosi faccia quel medesmo al huomo secundo. Apresso
quel huomo che e di sopra dia meza volta dal lato dritto. & poi gli huomini
che sonno di sotto si piglino per la mano et facciano doi sempij & un doppio
col pie dritto inanti, & scambiasi le poste. apresso quel huomo che e di sopra
si parta con doi tempi di saltarello cominciando col sinistro et finiendo dal
dritto. et vadase apresso la donna. et poi subito la donna se volti verso l'huomo,
et l'huomo gli tocchi la mano con una riverenza sul sinistro. et apresso quel
[42ʳ] medesimo huomo vada da man sinistra della | donna. & vada a pigliare l'huomo
ch'e da man dritta con doi sempij & un doppio cominciando col dritto. et quel
ch'era a man sinistra vada a pigliare la donna con quelli medesmi passi, &
rimanga lui colla donna.

BALLO CHIAMATO GRATIOSO IN DOI
COMPOSTO PER GUIGLIELMO

In prima vadano insieme con tre tempi di saltarello todescho cominciando col
pie sinistro, et poi si fermino. Et poi l'huomo vada dalla man di sotto, [d]ella'
donna con un doppio partendosi col pie dritto. et in quel mezo la dona stia
ferma. et tutta questa parte. et tutto questo medesmo faciando un'altra volta"

' Supplied from Pa and NY.
' See n. 106 in the translation.
' Pa has 'di la donna'.
" Scribal repetition. Pa has '& Tucta questa parte midesima facciano unaltra volta'.

BALLO CALLED *MERCANTIA*[105]
BY MESSER DOMENICO

First [all] four do eleven *tempi* [of *saltarello*] together, and the lady goes with one of the men, and the two other men together; and the lady should be in the leading couple; and stop. Next the men who are behind draw together[106] with six sideways *riprese*, one [of the men] widening out to the left side and the other to the right side. Next the lady makes a *meza volta* to the left side; and the man who is her partner goes forward with three *doppii* beginning with the left foot, and the lady comes to end up in a triangle with the two other men; and next the man who is on the right side sets off with two *passi sempii* and a *doppio* beginning with the left foot, and goes to touch the lady's hand, and then he turns to the right side with two *sempii*, and a *doppio*, beginning with the right [foot], and returns to his place, where he was. Next his companion who is on the left side does the same; and note that the lady should make a *volta tonda*, when the first man has touched her hand; and she should do the same with the second man. Next the man who is above [in front] makes a *meza volta* to the right side; and then the men who are below [behind] take hands and do two *sempii* and a *doppio* with the right foot forward, and change places; next the man who is above [in front] sets off with two *tempi* of *saltarello* beginning with the left [foot] and finishing with the right; and goes up to the lady; and then the lady immediately turns towards the man, and the man touches her hand making a *riverenza* on the left [foot]; and next that same man passes by the left side of the lady with two *sempii* and a *doppio* beginning with the right [foot]; and joins the man who is on the right side; and the man who was on the left side goes to join the lady with those same steps, and he ends up with the lady.

BALLO FOR TWO CALLED *GRATIOSO*[107]
COMPOSED BY GUGLIELMO

First advance together with three *tempi* of German *saltarello* beginning with the left foot, and then stop. And then the man goes to the lower [right] side of the lady with a *doppio* starting with the right foot; and in the meantime the lady stands still; and do all this part again so that the man finishes in his place,

[105] Merchandise; Seller of Wares. Compare with Domenico's more complete and detailed description in Pd.

[106] This is almost certainly an error (repeated in Pa, NY, and FN). The men, according to Domenico's version in Pd, '*si alargano*', they 'separate from one another'.

[107] Gracious.

tanto che l'huomo rimanga al suo luogho, et po[i] si fermano. Et poi l'huomo si parta dalla donna con doi tempi di saltarello todescho, et doi sempij et un doppio partendosi col pie sinistro, et poi si fermi. et poi la donna vada a ritrovare l'huomo con quegli passi medesmi. et poi si partino insieme con doi sempij et doi doppij partendosi col pie sinistro, cioe l'huomo vada di longho ella donna vada intorno tanto che ritorni al suo luogho. et poi si voltino con [42ᵛ] doi riprese, l'una sul | sinistro ell'altra sul dritto, & poi faciano una continenza. et poi faciano doi sempij et doi doppij partendosi col pie sinistro, cioe l'huomo vada al tondo ella donna vada inverso l'huomo con quelli passi medesmi. et poi si piglino insieme et faciano due riprese l'una sul sinistro ell'altra sul dritto. et poi facciano doi continenze. et poi l'huomo vada intorno la donna con tre tempi di piva & poi stia fermo. et poi l'huomo dia un scosso, ella donna gli risponda. et poi si tirano indrieto con un doppio cominciando col pie dritto. et poi diano una volta tonda con uno doppio cominciando dal pie sinistro.

BALLO CHIAMATO SPERO IN TRE
COMPOSTO PER GUILIELMO

In prima quattro doppij in todescho, battendo il tempo inanti, et poi si fermano. et poi quello di mezo si parte dalle donne con doi sempij et un doppio partendo col pie sinistro. Et in quel tempo le donne stiano ferme. et poi tutte due le donne vadano apresso l'huomo con doi sempij & un doppio partendo col pie sinistro. et in quel tempo di quel doppio l'huo|mo si volti [43ʳ] con un doppio al contrario delle donne cominciando dal pie dritto. et poi vadano al contrario l'uno dell'altro con doi tempi di saltarello todescho bat-

and then stop. And then the man leaves the lady with two *tempi* of German *saltarello*, and two *sempii* and a *doppio* starting with the left foot, and then he stops; and then the lady goes up to the man with those same steps; and then set off together with two *sempii* and two *doppii* starting with the left foot, that is the man goes straight[108] and the lady goes around so that [she] returns to her place; and then [both] turn with two *riprese*, one on the left [foot] and the other on the right, and then do one *continenza*;[109] and then do two *sempii* and two *doppii* starting with the left foot, that is the man goes around and the lady goes towards the man with those same steps; and then join [hands] and do two *riprese*, one on the left [foot] and the other on the right; and then do two *continenze*; and then the man goes around the lady with three *tempi* of *piva* and then he stands still;[110] and then the man makes a *scosso*, and the lady replies; and then [both] draw back with a *doppio* beginning with the right foot; and then make a *volta tonda* with a *doppio* beginning with the left foot.[111]

BALLO FOR THREE CALLED *SPERO*[112]
COMPOSED BY GUGLIELMO

First do four *doppii* in German [*saltarello?*],[113] beating the *tempo* ahead [starting on the up-beat?],[114] and then stop; and then the man in the middle leaves the ladies with two *sempii* and a *doppio* starting with the left foot. And at the same time the ladies stand still; and then both ladies go up to the man with two *sempii* and a *doppio* starting with the left foot; and at the same time as that *doppio* the man turns with a *doppio* in the opposite direction to the ladies beginning with the right foot; and then advance in opposite directions with two *tempi* of German *saltarello* beating the *tempo* in *gallone* [starting the *tempo*

---

[108] See n. 69.

[109] The Pa version has two *continenze*, while S confirms the one. When this part of the choreography is repeated below, Guglielmo also has two *continenze*. NY and FN substitute a *riverenza*.

[110] Pa adds, 'And the lady does the same and they stop'. This is confirmed in all the other versions as well as in the music.

[111] See n. 47.

[112] Hope. In modern Italian the sole meaning of *spero* is 'I hope'. But in Guglielmo's time it also meant 'hope', 'mirror', and 'sphere'. It is possible that *La speranza* ('Hope'), performed in 1459 in Florence (see Ch. 3 n. 6), is the same dance as *Spero*. NY and FN, against all likelihood, attribute the *ballo* to Domenico.

[113] The NY version changes this to 'four *tempi* of German *saltarello*'. Since the music appears to be in *saltarello misura*, and not in *quadernaria* (see musical transcription), German [*saltarello?*] in this case may mean *quadernaria doppii* performed to *saltarello* music.

[114] Confirmed in all versions. See *Caterva* and n. 51.

tendo il tempo in gallone. et poi vegnano in contra l'uno all'altro con quattro tempi di saltarello partendo col pie sinistro, cioe passando l'huomo per mezo delle donne. Et poi diano meza volta sul pie dritto. Et poi faciano due riprese, l'una sul sinistro ell'altra sul dritto. poi faciano una riverenza sul sinistro. poi si tira indrieto con un sempio sul pie sinistro. poi vengano incontra l'uno all'altro con tre riprese in portogalese comin[c]iando sul pie dritto. Et poi le donne diano meza volta sul pie dritto, et mettano l'huomo in mezo, et faciano una ripresa sul pie sinistro. poi dano tutti tre una volta tonda in bassadanza con doi sempij cominciando dal pie dritto. et poi faciano una riverenza sul pie sinistro. Et poi quello di mezo piglia la donna ch'e da la man dritta colla man dritto, et vadano al tondo con tre tempi di piva cominciando col pie sinistro.

[43ᵛ] et poi piglia la donna ch'e alla man sinistra et vadano al tondo | con tre tempi di piva partendo col pie dritto. et poi l'huomo faccia uno schosso et le due donne gli respondano insieme. et l'huomo dia una volta tonda con un doppio cominciando dal pie sinistro. et poi le due donne insieme danno una volta tonda con un doppio cominciando dal pie sinistro.

FINIS

to the side?];[115] and then advance towards one another with four *tempi* of *saltarello* starting with the left foot, that is the man passing between the ladies. And then make a *meza volta* on the right foot. And then do two *riprese*, one on the left [foot] and the other on the right; then make a *riverenza* on the left; then draw back with a *sempio*[116] on the left foot; then come towards one another with three Portuguese *riprese* beginning on the right foot. And then the ladies make a *meza volta* on the right foot, and put the man in the middle, and [all three][117] do a *ripresa* on the left foot; then all three make a *volta tonda* in *bassadanza* [*misura*] with two *sempii* beginning with the right foot;[118] and then make a *riverenza* on the left foot. And then the man in the middle takes the lady who is on his right side by the right hand, and they go around with three *tempi* of *piva* beginning with the left foot; and then he takes the lady who is on his left side and they go around with three *tempi* of *piva* starting with the right foot; and then the man makes a *scosso* and the two ladies reply together; and the man makes a *volta tonda* with a *doppio* beginning with the left foot; and then both ladies make a *volta tonda* together with a *doppio* beginning with the left foot.[119]

FINIS

[115] The different instructions here and in *Caterva* for how to 'beat the *tempo*' in German *saltarello* seem to reflect different *misure*. Beating 'ahead' apparently refers to *quadernaria doppii* performed to *saltarello* music (and in *Caterva* to *bassadanza* music), while here, beating 'to the side' refers to *saltarello doppii* performed to *quadernaria* music. (*Saltarello* and *bassadanza misure* begin on the up-beat, *quadernaria* on the down-beat.) The term is further obscured by our not knowing how Guglielmo did the German *saltarello* step, although it may conceivably have ended with a little *ripresa* to the side. See Glossary. Giorgio at this point in the choreography adds a *meza volta*.

[116] The verb is singular in the original and in Pa but plural in FN and NY. Rather than specifying a *passo sempio*, the NY version says, 'and draw back the left foot'. This may indicate a weight change performed during an up-beat, rather than a step-unit with a duration of half a *tempo* or bar.

[117] Specified in NY.

[118] Guglielmo has omitted 'and a *ripresa*', included in Pa, NY, and FN.

[119] See n. 47.

CANZON MORALE DI MARIO PHILELFO AD HONORE
ET LAUDE DI MAESTRO GUILIELMO HEBREO

Qual fama hormai qual gloria sia di Alceo:
   De chi l'antiquita tanto ha cantato?
   Del dolce cloma? et claro Timotheo?
Che se Terpandro fusse ben rinato:
   Seria da men: se ben quel bon Cradia:
   De quel: de chi questo volume e honorato.
Tanto e suave & angelica harmonia
   Nel dolce suon di Guiglielmo hebreo.
   Tanto e nel bel danzar la lizadria.
L'arme faria riporre al Machabeo.
   A Salamon il senno, & al re Davit.
   Humiliare il crudel Heuristeo.
Faria danzar se ben fusse Judit.
   & Socrate & Aristotel con Platone
   & se alchun piu sever nacque degit.
Faria danzando inamorar Catone.
   & inclinar Diana a sua corea.
   Lassar la degna impresa a Scipione.
Faria inclinar al suo danzar Panthea
   & Tomire. Orithia. con Antiopa.
   Coll'aspra et forte & gran Pantasilea.
Per costui mancha fama al prisco Iopa.
   O qualunque altro mai fu sotto il cielo.
   In Libia o in la grande Asia o nella Europa.
Per costui e vinto quel che fu con Belo.
   Con Agenor. con Cadmo. et quanti a Thebe.
   & s'altri hebbe quest'arte dal gran Delo.
Piante non fur mai tante in tutta glebe:
   Diverse in frutti in fronde in seme in fiori.
   Tante canne palustre intorno a Bebe:

ᵛ The folio numbers for the Ode, and for the following balli tunes, have been added subsequently, by another hand.

A MORAL ODE BY MARIO FILELFO IN HONOUR AND PRAISE OF MASTER GUGLIELMO THE JEW[1]

What fame survives, what glory has Alcaeus,[2]
    He whom the ancients sang amain?
    What has sweet Cloma? What name Timotheus?
For were Terpander to return again
    He'd small appear—even good Cradia comparing—
    To him for whom this book does honour gain.
The angelic harmony is so entrancing
    In the sweet strains of the Jew Guglielmus;
    Such beauty is there in fair dancing
It would sheathe the sword of Maccabeus,
    Get Solomon his lore to cast away,
    And make the cruel inventor David blush.
Though it were Judith, she should the dance obey;
    Socrates, great Aristotle, and Plato,
    Or any born with graver minds than they.
It would to love, while dancing, convert Cato,
    Make Diana to its chorus condescend,
    And Scipio all his gallantry forgo.
Panthea, to the dance, herself would lend,
    And Tomyris, Orithyia, and Antiope
    With the fell Penthesilea would bend.
For his, old Iopas' fame declines away
    Or that of any man that ever was
    In Europe, Libya, or in wide Cathay.
For him yields place who stood with Belos;
    With Agenor, with Cadmus, and those at Thebes,
    And all who learned this art of Delos.
Never such wealth of plants in all the glebes,
    Diverse in fruit, in frond, in seed, in flower,
    Never round Boebe so many marsh reeds

---

[1] Previously published in Italian in O. Kinkeldey, 'A Jewish Dancing Master of the Renaissance', in *Studies in Jewish Bibliography . . . in Memory of Abraham Freidus* (New York, 1929).

[2] Filelfo's honorific intent is clear, but in comparing Guglielmo to better and lesser known Greek sages and poets, mythological figures, and mythic (or otherwise) kings of the Eastern Mediterranean, he casts his net wider than this translator's capacity to annotate. The 're Davit' of line 11 is certainly King David, but is, for example, the 'Phitia' of line 47 Phidias, the renowned Athenian sculptor? M.S.

Quanti son stati triumphanti honori:
   Ch'[h]a ricevuto pel suo bel danzare
   Da r[e]i. da duchi. marchesi. & signori.
Che non so chome si potessen fare
   Tante harmonie col son: quante con l'arte
   De mano in man costu[i] sa minutare.
Tal non fu Apollo in suon, ne in guerra Marte.
   Mercurio in lyra. o Palla in lanificio:
   In cavalcar quei che nasenno a Sparte:
Quant e celebre lui nel exercitio
   D'ingegno e[t] corpo in musica trovato:
   Del qual nasce il danzar per l'opificio.
Qual Dicearcho o Aristoxen mai nato?
   O Tamiras? Philamon? o Tirteo?
   Qual Phemio mai fu si glorificato?
Qual di Modoco il dolce Corcireo?
   O Polimnesto? o Phitia? o Pericleto?
   Qual hiagni al tempo del popul Judeo?

[45ʳ]   Regula non fu mai d'altro Apotheto.
   Ne helego ne comarcho ne Schemon.
   Dio [duo]. & trimele. & ogni suo epitheto.
Fata da Polinesto, ne cepion:
   Che non habia costui contubernale
   Qual Glaucho olimpo. o Marsia o'l grande harion.
Il qual per gloria e gia fatto immortale.
   & vivera fin ch'el mondo lontana.
   Tanto ha fatto in virtu suo capitale.
Il suo danzar non e d'industria humana
   Ma d'ingegno celeste, & saper divo.
   Senza aparenza simulata et vana.
D'ogni inconveniente non men schivo:
   Che Citharea de vergini vestali.
   D'ogni indecoro passo altiero et privo.
Non son si destre l'aquile in lor ali
   Quanto e l'agilita di Guiglielmo:
   Le virtu cui si pon creder fatali.
Ma non fu Hector si destro soto l'elmo:
   Quanto e costui in l'arte sua excellente.
   Tra gli altri qual fra gli altri paraschelmo.
Molte madonne illustre & eminente
   Di mortale ha fatte parer Diane.
   Mia figlia Theodora novamente.

As have been the triumphant rewards
   That for his fair dancing he has had regale
   From kings, dukes, marquises, and lords.
Nay, I knew not that music could avail
   As many harmonies as his skill
   From hand to hand allows him to retail.
Not Apollo for music, nor Mars at the kill,
   Not Mercury's lyre, nor the loom when Pallas plies,
   Nor the Sparta-born for their horse-drill
Were famed as he is in that exercise
   Of body and of mind in music found
   From which, through industry, the dance has rise.
What Dichearchos or Aristoxenus in all time's bound?
   Or Thamyras? Philemon? or Tyrtaeus?
   What Phemius' name did ever so resound?
Or the sweet Corcyrean Demodocus?
   Or Polymnestus? or Phitias? Or Pericletes?
   In the time of the Hebrews what Hyagnis?
No rule is there of any Apothetes,
   Or Helegos, or Comarchos, or Schemon—
   Duo or triharmonic or such as these—
Given by Polymnestes or Cepion
   With which this man is not at home and cordial
   As Olympian Glaucus, Marsyas, or great Arion.
His fame so great, by now he is made immortal
   And will last longer than the world has durance,
   So much he has done with an art so capital.
His dance is not of human provenance -
   But comes of heavenly wit and fire divine
   And has no false or vain appearance.
Of disagreeables there is no more sign
   Than with the gittern of the virgin vestal,
   Nor any step indecorous to repine.
The eagle on the wing shows not so well
   As Guglielmo when he's nimbly tripping—
   Whose skill can seem the outcome of a spell.
Hector in his helm less deftly stepping
   Than this man in his art so excellent
   Among all others, all others far outstripping.
He makes women, noble and eminent,
   To seem Diana's self, who were but human;
   My daughter Theodora the most recent.

[45ᵛ]

Che non fur mai ne greche ne Romane
  Che equipararse possano a coloro
  Che porte han per sapere a lui le mane.
De per dio donche il nobile lavoro
  Che se contien nell'opera d'un tanto:
  Vogliatilo estimare quasi un thesoro:
E[t] & [*sic*] rimirarlo ben da ogni canto.
  [C]he quando tutto ben transcorso harete
  Mai sciese in terra un huom di simil vanto.
Ne mai ne andera alchun che passi lethe.

EXCRIPSIT PAGANUS RAUDENSIS .V°. NONAS
OCTOBRES ANNO A NATALI CHRISTIANO
M°CCCC°LXIII. MEDIOLANI. REGNANTE FRANCISCO
SPHORTIA MEDIOLANENSIUM INCLYTO DUCE
QUARTO. Vale qui legisti.

QUI SEQUITANO I BALLI NOTATI[w]

---

[w] A hand with its index finger pointing towards the next page has been drawn at the end of the line.

Never a woman was there, Greek or Roman,
    Could ever of those be a neighbour
    Who held out hands for guidance from this man.
Wherefore, by God's grace, the noble labour
    Which does, in part, within this work reside;
    Prize it as treasure I ask as favour
And admire it well from every side.
    And when you have perused from end to end—
    No earthly man had juster claim to pride
Nor ever any such that shall over Lethe wend.

PAGANO OF RHO FINISHED WRITING THIS ON THE
FIFTH NONES [11th] OF OCTOBER,[3] AD 1463 IN MILAN IN
THE REIGN OF FRANCESCO SFORZA DECREED
FOURTH DUKE OF MILAN. Farewell to the reader.

THE NOTATIONS OF THE *BALLI* FOLLOW

[3] In the month of October, the nones fall on the seventh (rather than the fifth) day of the month.

I Balli Notati
Transcription of Music, with Commentary

Notes on the Transcription

IN transcribing *De pratica*'s musical notations I have attempted to correlate music and choreographic descriptions by the appropriate placement of barlines (none in the original), and by reduction of note-values according to the *misura* in question. The *balli* tunes are transcribed by sections (marked with Roman numerals), and a synthesis of the choreography, also by sections, follows. All discrepancies between music and choreography are reported in the commentaries. Only the tunes as notated in the Pg version of *De pratica* are transcribed. This is not a critical edition, but other sources are cited when their variants seem interesting or significant. (Pertinent choreographic information from other treatises is included as well.) A facsimile of the original notation appears below each transcription for purposes of study, comparison, and evaluation, and to encourage the reader to look for different solutions. Four additional tunes from Pa are transcribed and included in App. II.

The tunes, with the exception of *Belriguardo*, have been transcribed in the treble clef rather than in the original alto clef. The commentaries report all original mensural and proportion signs and explain the time signatures used in the transcriptions. All editorial additions and corrections are noted. The scribe was sometimes careless about the point of division; discrepancies have not been noted. See Ch. 4 for further information on mensuration, the four *misure*, and the transcription of mensural and proportion signs, *piva*, German *saltarello* and *piva*, *doppii* 'on' or 'upon' the same foot, and the introductory *saltarello*.

For ease of consultation a list of the *balli* tunes, arranged in alphabetical order with page numbers, follows.

Abbreviations

Step (and other) abbreviations used in the notation of the choreographies. The duration of each step (as specified in Pd and V) is indicated in brackets.

bd	*bassadanza misura*
c	*continenza* (½ *tempo*)
d	*doppio* (1 *tempo*)
ft	foot
mis	*misura*
mov	*movimento, movimenti* (½ *tempo*)
mv	*meza volta* (see Glossary)
(mv)	*meza volta* performed during the up-beat
p	*passo di natura* (natural step)
quad	*quadernaria misura*
r	*ripresa* (1 *tempo*)
R	*riverenza* (1 *tempo*)
s	*sempio* (½ *tempo*)
t	*tempo, tempi*
vt	*volta tonda* (2 *tempi* in *bassadanza misura*; see Glossary)

Steps following a stroke / are performed simultaneously with those preceding the stroke. Additional information is bracketed.

Balli Tunes

*Amoroso	242
Belriguardo	184
Colonnese	204
Gelosia	190
*Gioioso [Rostiboli], El	246
Gratioso	202
Ingrata	194
Iove	188
Legiadra	206
Leoncello	186
Marchesana	198
Mercantia	196
*Petit Vriens [Riense]	244
Pizocara	192
Presoniera	182
*[Rostiboli] Gioioso	246
Spero	200
*Voltati in ça Rosina	240

*Appendix II

PRESONIERA

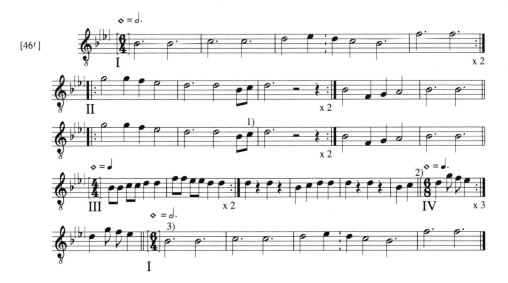

[46ʳ]

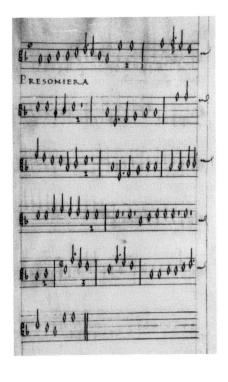

PRESONIERA

CHOREOGRAPHY

Guglielmo (Pg)

I. cc sss d R x2
II. ss dd(on the same ft) x2 ⎫
    sscc   ⎬ x2
III. 4 t German saltarello
    mov mov 3 passetti x2
      (the 2nd time 3rd passetto
      initiates the saltarello)
IV. 3 t saltarello + 1 doppio

Domenico (Pd)

I. 4½ t bd x2
II. 2½ t bd: ss dd(on the same ft) x2 ⎫
    (mv) 2 t bd: ssR   ⎬ x2
III. 8 t piva
    mov mov 4 passetti x2
IV. mov, 4 t saltarello

Presoniera

Concordances: Pd (*Prexonera*), Pa (*Prisonera*). Pa is notated a fourth lower, with a signature of Bb, corresponding to Eb in the transcription.

Remarks: I–II. Pg's ☉ (9/4) seems mistaken; I have followed Pd's ₵ , which corresponds to the instructions for 4½ *tempi* of *bassadanza* for the first section. Pa has ○ (3/4); the section is notated in *breves*, which Pa occasionally uses (rather than *semibreves*) for *bassadanza misura*. Whereas both music and choreography take up 2½ *tempi*, the half-*tempo* rest in II, bar 3 is unaccountable. (The 2 *doppii* 'on the same foot', which last, theoretically, 1½ *tempi*, are replaced in NY by 3 *contrapassi*, which take up 2 *tempi*.)

III. No mensural sign in Pg; the notation suggests *misura quadernaria*, which concords with Pg's instructions for German *saltarello* (saltarello in *misura quadernaria*). ○ in Pd, indicating change of *misura* to *piva* (see n. 2, c). The final bar corresponds to Pg's instructions to begin the *saltarello* with the third step. It does not accord, however, with Pd's choreography, which calls for 4 *passetti* both times. (See the last 2 bars of the version in Pa, which are repeated, in n. 2, a.) A proportional sign '3' in Pa indicates that this section should be played proportionately faster than the preceding *bassadanza* section. The apparent 6/8 metre suggests that German *saltarello* in this context probably means one *quadernaria doppio* performed to 2 *tempi* of *saltarello* music. If transcribed, however, in *quadernaria*, in triplets (see n. 2, b), this section corresponds in *misura* to those in Pd and Pg, and to the choreographic instructions for German *saltarello* (saltarello *doppii* performed in *misura quadernaria*). Perhaps this is what Domenico is trying to suggest with the sign ○:

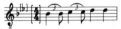

Pd's choreography of 8 *tempi* of *piva* requires a different barring (see n. 2, c).

IV. ₵ in all sources.

Notes on the music:

1) Orig.: 2 *minimae*; emendation follows bar 2 above and Pd.

2) Variant version of III in Pa (transposed):

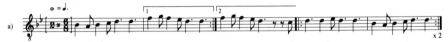

The last note of the first half is eliminated in the repeat because of the rests. The division line occurs just before the rests; theoretically, the final repeat should begin here.

Alternative transcription:

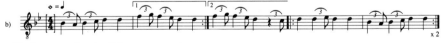

Variant version in Pd:

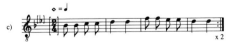

3) Headed 'Intrata' in Pd; section omitted in Pa.

BELRIGUARDO

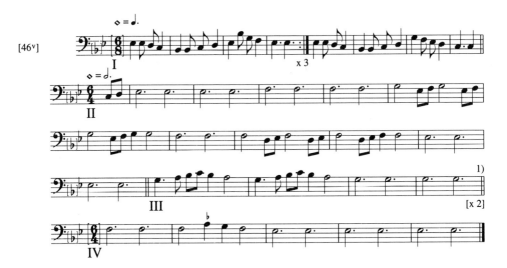

[46ᵛ]

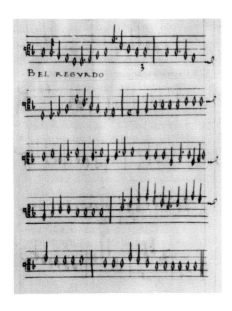

B EL REGVRDO

CHOREOGRAPHY

Guglielmo (Pg)

I. 15 t saltarello
II. dddd ddd(on left ft) ss
    [ddd(on right ft)] rr
III. 2 t saltarello rr x2
IV. ss d r cccc

Domenico (Pd)

I. 11 t saltarello
II. bd: dddd ddd(upon left ft) ss
    ddd(upon right ft) rr
III. mov, 2 t slow saltarello rr
IV. 5 t bd: ss d r cc R

Belriguardo

Concordances: Pd, V (transposed a fifth higher, without flat), Pa. The Eb signature (signed one space lower in Pd) implies a Bb.

Remarks: I. No mensural sign in any version, though all choreographies specify *salta-rello*. In Pa all the pairs of *minimae* are written as *minima, semiminima*. As the first of these notes is dotted, a 3/2, 3/4 metre seems to emerge. Pg indicates 15 *tempi*. The extra bar of music may be for an introduction and a *movimento* with which to initiate the *saltarello*. Pd's choreography specifies 11 *tempi* of *saltarello*, which requires a repeat numeral of '2' rather than '3'.

II. C. There is a discrepancy between musical *tempi* and step-units. Pg has 10 step-units and Pd 13; there are 11 bars of music. Pg's description leaves out (probably a scribal omission) 3 *doppii* 'on the right foot' (see Pd's choreography). These are indicated as *contrapassi* in the NY version. If the 3 *doppii* 'on the same foot' are performed in 2 bars of music, as 3 *contrapassi*, then the steps and music match.

III. No mensural sign in any version, and so *bassadanza misura* may well continue. This would seem to be confirmed by Pd's instructions for 'slow *saltarello*' and by the presence of *riprese* (steps which are found most often in *bassadanza* and *quadernaria misure*). However, the notation of the first 2 bars is problematic, for if transcribed literally, the result is a *saltarello* in 9/8.

It is not clear if this was intended, and if so, how and why the *saltarello* would have been performed in this way. The transcription given here is one possible interpretation.

IV. Pd specifies *bassadanza misura*.

V has a fifth section, marked 'Intrata', consisting of the first 6 notes of the introductory *saltarello*.

Note on the music:
1) The repeat numeral is missing in Pg, but specified in other sources and necessary for the choreography.

LEONCELLO

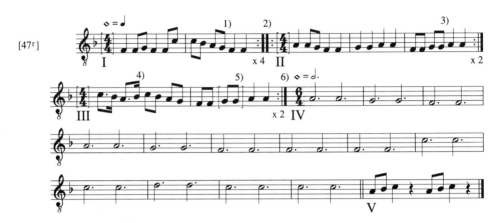

[47^r]

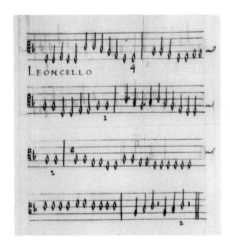

LEONCELLO

CHOREOGRAPHY

Guglielmo (Pg)

I. ddd(on one ft*) ddd* ddd*
    (*V: 3 contrapassi)
    mov mov d mv
    mov mov [d?] mv
II. ssss d x2
III. ddd(on one ft*) x2
IV. ssdd x2; rr ss dd rr
V. mov mov

Domenico (Pd) (Lionzello vechio)

I. 6 t saltarello in mis quad
    mov mov 1 t slow saltarello mv
    [2 mov?] 1 t slow saltarello mv
II. ssss d x2
III. ddd(on left ft) in quad x2
IV. 3 t bd: ssdd x2; 7 t bd: rr [ss] dd rr
V. 2 t quad: 2 mov

Leoncello

Concordances: Pd, V (no flat), Pa.

Remarks: I. No mensural sign in any version. Pd specifies *misura quadernaria*. Pg's choreography of 3 *doppii* 'on the same foot' needs 2 bars of music (V has 3 *contrapassi*). Nine *doppii* would therefore require 3 playings of the section. Two *movimenti* and a *doppio* also need 2 bars and, if repeated, require 2 additional playings of this section, a total of 5 playings as indicated by Pd. (However, Pd's choreography has no repeat of the last *movimenti* section, probably an oversight, and therefore requires only 4 playings.) Pa and V indicate 3 playings (9 *doppii*), and then Pa gives another phrase—to be played twice—to which the *movimenti* and *doppio* may be performed (see n. 2). The *meze volte* are, presumably, performed during up-beats.

II. No mensural sign in any version; appears to continue in *quadernaria*.

III. Pd specifies *quadernaria misura*.

V. In *Lionzello vechio*, Pd specifies 2 *tempi* and *quadernaria misura*, an exception to his own rule that a *movimento* lasts a half-*tempo* (in *bassadanza misura*?). Since there is no *misura* indicated in *Lionzello novo*, it is conceivable that *bassadanza* continues. (It is not clear whether the black *semiminimae* are the up-beat to the *movimento*, or the first beat of the bar.) Pg's repeat number '2' is superfluous. V ends with a few notes of the introduction, marked 'Intrata'.

Notes on the music:

1) Pa:

2) Additional phrase in Pa:

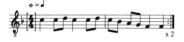

3) *Semibrevis, semibrevis* in Pa; cf. bar 2 of n. 6.
4) The first 4 notes are *minimae* in V.
5) Missing notes supplied from Pd and V.
6) Version of III in Pa:

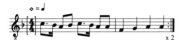

IOVE

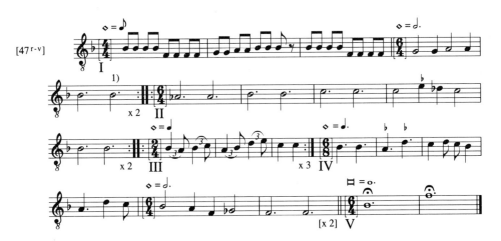

[47 r-v]

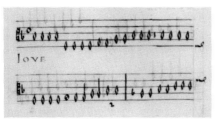

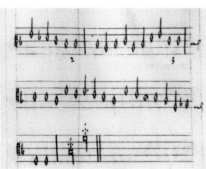

CHOREOGRAPHY

Guglielmo (Pg)

I. 3 t German saltarello ⎫
   volta del gioioso   ⎬ x2
                         ⎭
II. ddd [ssd] ddd ssd
III. 3 t piva [x3?]
IV. 1 scosso, 4 t saltarello, vt,
    4 t saltarello [vt?]
V. mv, R x2

Domenico (Pd)

I. 3 t saltarello in quad ⎫
   vt in bd (2 t)   ⎬ x2
                          ⎭
II. 5 t bd: ddd ssd x2
III. 9 t piva
IV. 4 t saltarello, 2 t bd: vt x2
V. mv, R x2

Iove

Concordances: Pd (*Jupiter*), Pa, V (*Giove*; flat in III only).

Remarks: The curious flats in section II (present in all sources), together with those in IV, bar 2 (found only in Pd and V), should perhaps be applied throughout (II–IV).

I. ○ (3/4) in all versions, indicating German *saltarello*, i.e. *saltarello* in *misura quaderna-ria*. For the last 2 bars: ⊙ in Pg, ℂ in Pa and Pd, no sign in V; Pd specifies *bassadanza misura*.

II. No mensural sign, indicating that the previous *misura* continues; Pd confirms *bassadanza*.

III. Pd and V have ₵3, indicating a change from *bassadanza* to *piva* with a pro-portional increase in speed, suggesting a transcription in 2/4 with triplets. Pg's choreo-graphy does not specify, as does Pd's, that the 3 *tempi* of *piva* should be played 3 times.

IV. ℂ in Pd and V. All choreographies specify *saltarello*. At bar 5, ⊙ (9/4) in Pg, Pa, and Pd probably indicates a change to *bassadanza misura* (specified in Pd); V's ○ may be a scribal error. The repeat numeral is lacking in all sources except Pa, but a repeat is indicated in the choreography.

V. No mensural sign; *misura* not specified in the choreographies, and presumably *bassadanza* continues. The dots above the final *longae*, which correspond to the final *riverenze*, are almost certainly a kind of fermata, indicating that the notes can be held as long as necessary. V ends with 4 notes, marked 'Intrata', from the introductory German *saltarello*.

Note on the music:
1) A dotted *semibrevis* in Pa replaces Pg's 2 *semibreves*.

GELOSIA

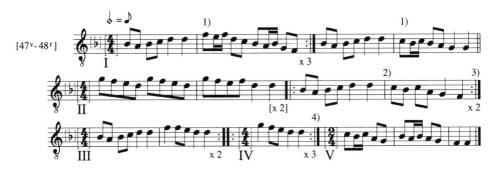

[47ᵛ-48ʳ]

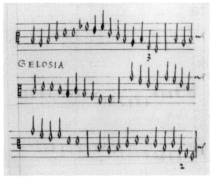

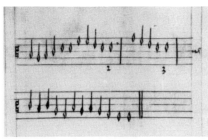

CHOREOGRAPHY

Guglielmo (Pg, Pa)

I. 8 t saltarello
II. ddd(on left ft) R d
    2 passi [doppii] (on left ft)
    d, 2 t piva
III. 4 t German piva
IV. vt x3
V. ss (on left ft) x2

Giorgio (NY)

I. 6 t German saltarello
II. 3 contrapassi R/d x2
    1 doppio
III. 8 t piva
IV. R x3
V. 3 t piva x2

Domenico (Pd)

I. 6 t slow saltarello in mis quad
II. ddd(on left ft) R in mis quad ⎫
    1 saltarello in quad/   ⎬ x2
    1 saltarello   ⎭
III. 8 t piva
IV. mv in 1 t piva x3
V. sss x2 mv

Gelosia

Concordances: Pd (*Giloxia*), Pa. All versions give a flat before the first F, which probably indicates F natural; a B flat signature has been added to avoid diminished fifths and tritones.

Remarks: No mensural sign in any version.

I. Pd specifies *saltarello in misura quadernaria*, NY German *saltarello*. Pg's choreography calls for 8 *tempi* of *saltarello*. Both Pd's and NY's choreographies have only 6 *tempi*, which requires changing the repeat numeral from '3' to '2'.

II. Pd's choreography gives *misura quadernaria*. Pa has a repeat numeral '2' for the first half of this section only. If combined with Pg's repeated second half, there is a total of 8 bars of music, which in part matches the choreography (seemingly incomplete) as described in Pg and Pa. The last bar allows for the 2 *tempi* of *piva* in Pg's choreography, as well as for the one *saltarello* in Pd. Pd's repeat numeral '2' indicates that the entire section is to be repeated. (NY's choreography appears to be slightly different and might require placing the repeat numeral at the end of bar 3.)

III. Pg's choreography indicates 4 *tempi* of German *piva* (i.e. *piva doppii* in *quadernaria misura*). Pd and NY specify 8 *tempi* of *piva*, which would call for barring in 2/4.

IV. *Misura* not specified in Pg. It is not clear how the *volta tonda* is to be done: with a *doppio* in *quadernaria*? with 2 *tempi* of *piva* in *quadernaria*? Pd calls for a *meza volta* in one *tempo* of *piva*, but if the music is barred in 2/4, this would result in 2 *tempi* of *piva*.

V. NY, which has different steps, specifies *piva misura*. Pd appears to give a repeat numeral '5', probably a scribal error. It is not clear how either Pg's or Pd's steps (*quadernaria*?) fit the music (*piva*?). The choreography in NY requires this section to be repeated.

Notes on the music:
1) Orig.: *semibrevis* (also in Pa).
2) A line in Pd, added by a later hand, is not a division line.
3) II, bars 3–4 in Pa:

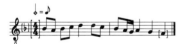

4) Sections III–IV in Pa:

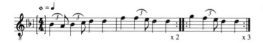

PIZOCARA

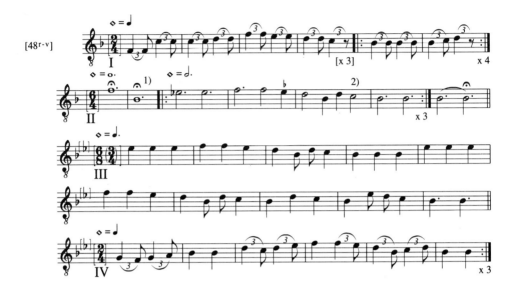

[48r-v]

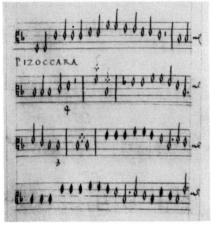

PIZOCCARA

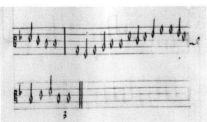

CHOREOGRAPHY

Domenico (Pd)

I. 12 t piva
　　4 t piva x2
II. R(1 t) 14 t bd: r ss 11 doppii r
III. 9 t saltarello
IV. rr 4 t piva x3

Siena

I. 12 t saltarello
　　4 t piva
II. R(?) ss 12 doppii R(?)
III. 8 t saltarello
IV. rr 4 t piva x3(?)

Pizocara

Concordances: Pa, Pd. Since no choreography is given in any of the redactions of *De pratica*, with the exception of a very abridged version in S (synopsis included), the transcription is based on Pd's choreography.

Remarks: I. No mensural sign in any source. Pd's choreography specifies *piva*, transcribed here in 2/4 with triplets to differentiate it from the *saltarello* of III. The first repeat numeral is supplied from Pd and Pa.

II. No mensural sign in Pg; Pa and Pd have C; Pd specifies *bassadanza*. The *signa congruentiae* apparently indicate that the *semibreves*, corresponding to the *riverenza* and *ripresa*, should be held as long as necessary; in the last bar the *signum* seems to join the 2 notes. Pd repeats the first 2 bars 5 times, with no repeat of the following 4 bars.

III. No mensural sign in any version. Pd specifies 9 *tempi* of *saltarello*. In *prolatio maior* each blackened *semibrevis* is imperfect and has the value of 2 *minimae*, while the white is perfect and lasts 3 *minimae* (see Ch. 4).

IV. No mensural sign in Pg and Pa. Pd specifies *piva misura* and has a proportion sign '3', which indicates a proportional increase in tempo from the preceding *saltarello misura* and suggests a transcription in 2/4 with triplets.

Notes on the music:
1) Pd has D, without *signum*.
2) *Minima* in all versions.

INGRATA

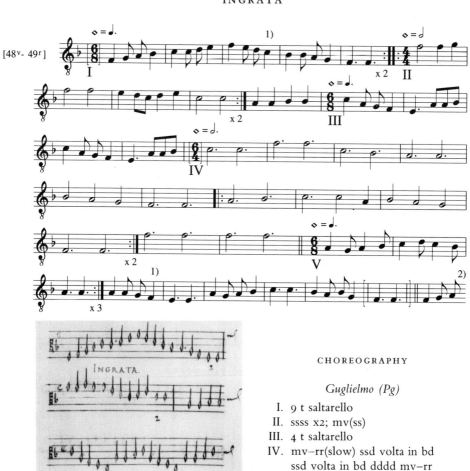

[48ᵛ- 49ʳ]

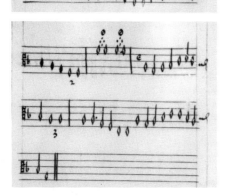

CHOREOGRAPHY

Guglielmo (Pg)

I. 9 t saltarello
II. ssss x2; mv(ss)
III. 4 t saltarello
IV. mv–rr(slow) ssd volta in bd
     ssd volta in bd dddd mv–rr
V. 6 t saltarello (d+r in piva fashion)
    6 t saltarello

Domenico (Pd)

I. 9 t saltarello
II. quad: ssss x2; mv(ss) and mov
III. 4 t saltarello
IV. 16 t bd: mv–rr ssd vt(ssr)
     ssd vt(ssr) dddd mv–rr
V. 15 t mis quad: ssrr x3
    3 t piva, 2 t piva, mov

Ingrata

Concordances: Pa, Pd.

Remarks: I. C in Pa and Pd. The choreography calls for only 9 *tempi* of *saltarello*; the extra bar may well be for an introduction and a *movimento* with which to initiate the *saltarello*.

II. C . Unless the repeat is omitted, there is a discrepancy between the choreographic instructions for 4 *sempii* done twice (a total of 4 *tempi*) and the music, which, if barred in 4/4 according to the mensuration (Pd specifies *quadernaria*) and repeated, results in 8 *tempi*. (If this section were to be transcribed $\circ = \,\bullet\!\!\!\!\!/$, then it could be repeated. In this case, however, the final bar would consist of only 2 beats or a half-*tempo*, insufficient for 2 *sempii*.)

III. C. No division line in any version to indicate either the beginning or the end of the *saltarello* section.

IV. Pd specifies *bassadanza* and Pg's choreography implies it. The last 2 bars have the sign ⊙ (corresponding to 9/4) and what appear to be *signa congruentiae*. There is no choreographic explanation for the change. Pa gives a *signum* for each note, Pd for the first and third notes. Pg's *signa* join the first 2 and the last 2 notes and are probably correct since they result in 2 *tempi*, corresponding to the choreography.

V. C, also in Pa. Pd has C3 to indicate the change of tempo after *bassadanza*, suggesting a transcription in 2/4 with triplets. Pg specifies 6 *tempi* of *saltarello* 'in *piva* fashion', followed by a final *saltarello*. The *saltarello* 'in *piva* fashion' is specified here as a *quadernaria doppio* (done to 2 bars of *saltarello* music) and a *ripresa* (one bar), as in *Tesara* (Pd). There are 9 *tempi* of music for 6 steps. Pd, on the other hand, calls for 15 *tempi* of *misura quadernaria*—which should probably read *piva* instead, the first part *quadernaria* steps performed to *piva* music. The bracketed notes appear only in Pa, necessary for Pg's 6 *tempi* of *saltarello* (Pd's choreography calls for 5 *tempi* of *piva*).

Notes on the music:

1) *Minima* in all 3 versions.

2) These notes appear in Pd only and are the beginning of the introductory *saltarello*. Is this why Pd ends with a *movimento* even though the choreography does not suggest repeating the *saltarello*?

MERCANTIA

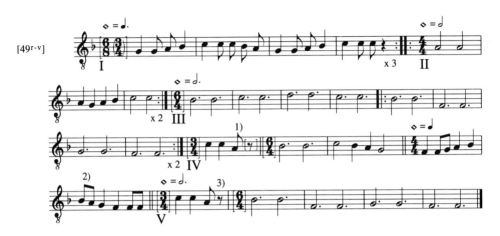

[49r-v]

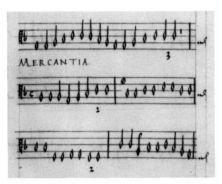

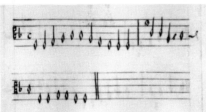

MERCANTIA

CHOREOGRAPHY

Guglielmo (Pg)

I. 11 t [saltarello: NY]
II. 6 riprese
III. mv ddd
     ssd ssd/vt x2
IV. mv ssd 2 t saltarello
V. lady turns, R [ ] ssd

Domenico (Pd)

I. mov + 11 t saltarello
II. 6 riprese in mis quad
III. 4 t bd: mv(1 t) ddd
     8 t bd: ssd ssd/vt x2
IV. mv 2 t saltarello, 2 t saltarello
V. mv/r; 4 t bd: R(1 t) cc ssd/vt(ssr)

Mercantia

Concordances: Pa, Pd, V (without flat).

Remarks: I. No mensural sign in Pg or Pa; O (3/4) in Pd and V. I have preferred a transcription in 6/8 because it reflects the typical *saltarello* rhythm. The extra bar of music is presumably introductory and allows for a *movimento* with which to initiate the *saltarello* (11 *tempi*).

III. ⊙ (9/4) in Pg, an error for the C of the other versions. Pd specifies *bassadanza misura*.

IV. The first bar corresponds to the man's *meza volta* and seems to be in 3/4. However, it can also be considered as a half-*tempo* in *bassadanza misura* since the preceding *bassadanza* appears to continue after the 3 notes (no division line in any version). The choreography that follows in all sources is 2 *sempii* and a *doppio* (with the exception of Pd, which specifies 2 *tempi* of *saltarello*), thus confirming the supposition of *bassadanza misura*. In bar 4 all versions have C for *quadernaria*, while all the choreographies indicate *saltarello*, without specifying German *saltarello* or *saltarello* in *quadernaria*. If barred in 6/8 (*saltarello*), there would be more than 2½ bars of music.

V. Pg has ⊙, again an error for the C in the other sources. No division line following the first bar. Pd specifies *bassadanza* for the last 4 *tempi*. Discrepancy between Pg's choreography of only 3 *tempi* and the music, owing, probably, to the omission of 2 *continenze*.

Pd and V close with a repeat of the first 7 notes of I, marked 'Intrata' in V.

Notes on the music:

1) In Pa the *fusa* is followed by a rest. V has a white flagged minim and a *minima* rest, Pd a *semiminima* and a *semiminima* rest.

2) Orig.: *semibrevis* (also in Pa).

3) Pa lacks the rest. V's last note is a *minima*.

MARCHESANA

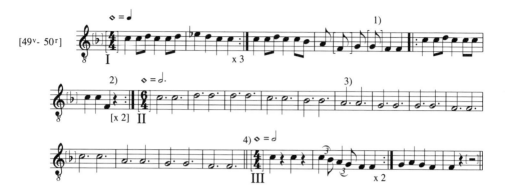

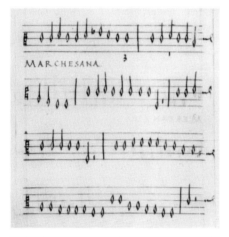

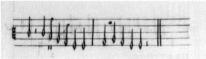

CHOREOGRAPHY

Guglielmo (Pg)

I. 12 doppii (3 per ft)
   dd x2
II. rr ssd r ssd r dd rr cccc
III. mov mov d x2; d(d?) salto

Domenico (Pd)

I. 8 t saltarello in mis quad
   3 frapamenti, 1 t saltarello [in mis
   quad] x2
II. 12½ t bd: rr ssd r ssd s dd rr cc
III. mis quad: mov mov d x2; d salto,
   posada

Marchesana

Concordances: Pa (with flat signature), Pd (without clef or signature). Bonnie Blackburn commented that the absence of signature in Pg and of signature and clef in Pd suggest that the notation was made deliberately unspecific to accommodate playing it in F or C. The Eb in bar 2 would become Bb if read in the soprano clef. See also n. 3.

Remarks: I.   in Pa; Pd specifies *misura quadernaria*. Pg's choreography of 12 *doppii* corresponds to the first 2 sections because every group of 3 *doppii* 'on each foot' lasts 2 *tempi*.

II. O in Pa (notated in *breves*) and Pd, which specifies *bassadanza misura*. Pa has a repeat numeral '1' followed by 2 additional bars (see n. 4), making 15, rather than 13, bars of music, while the choreography indicates 14 step-units. Pd's choreography specifies 12½ step-units in 12½ *tempi*. In no version is the correspondence between steps and music clear.

III. Pd specifies *misura quadernaria*. Pa's alternative reading (see n. 4) has **C**.

Notes on the music:

1) The notes in square brackets, missing also in Pd, are supplied from Pa.

2) *Minima* in all versions, with incorrect *minima* rest in the repeat. In Pa, where the repeat is indicated by a numeral, and not written out as in Pg, there is no rest.

3) In Pg and Pd this note is preceded by a sharp, in this case indicating *mi* after a previous *fa*—here Bb, but if read in the soprano clef, F.

4) 2 additional bars in Pa lead directly into a different version of III (the note marked with an asterisk is a *brevis* in the original):

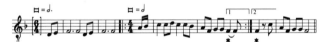

SPERO

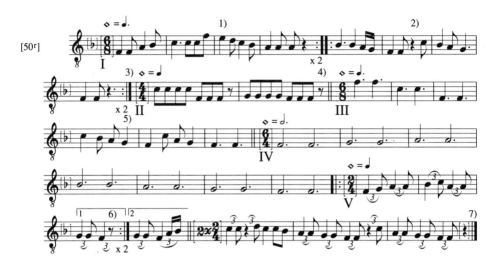

[50r]

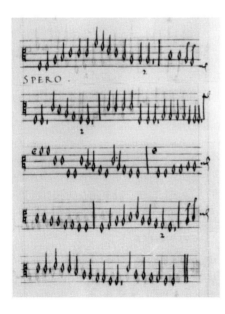

SPERO .

CHOREOGRAPHY

Guglielmo (Pg)

I. 4 doppii 'in German' [saltarello: NY]
    ssd x2
II. 2 t German saltarello
III. 4 t saltarello
IV. rr R s rrr r ss[r] R
V. 3 t piva x2
    2 scossi dd

Spero

Concordances: Pa (with flat signature).

Remarks: I. C in Pa. While the music suggests *saltarello misura*, the choreography (first part) specifies German *saltarello* (usually, *saltarello* in *quadernaria misura*; see n. 3 for a transcription). It is possible that Guglielmo intended *quadernaria doppii* performed to *saltarello* music. In this case (4 *quadernaria doppii* in 8 bars of music), each *doppio* would require 2 bars of music (2 × 6/8).

II. C in Pa.

III. C in both sources. The choreography calls for 4, not 6 *tempi* of *saltarello*.

IV. ⊙ in both sources, indicating a proportional change between the *saltarello misura* (III) and *bassadanza*, suggested by the choreography. (Pa notates this section in *breves* and III in *semibreves*.) There seems to be another discrepancy in this section: 7 bars of music for 9½ step-units. (It is possible that the *sempio* is taken merely as a change of weight and foot during the up-beat prior to the following *ripresa*.) Comparing Pg's choreography and the version in NY, it seems probable that Pg omitted a *ripresa* from the *volta tonda* at the end of the section, which would bring the step-units up to 10(½).

V. No mensural sign in either source; Pg specifies *piva*. Notated in *semibreves* and *minimae* in Pa. Transcribed in 2/4 to differentiate it from the *saltarello* in III and also because of its melodic and choregraphic affinity to the *piva* endings of other *balli* composed by Guglielmo (*Colonnese, Gratioso, Legiadra*), all of which have a definite 2/4 character. The second part probably continues in *piva misura*. As in other *piva* endings, the 2 *scossi* and *doppii* are probably *quadernaria* steps performed to *piva* music. The alternative version in Pa (n. 7) is closer melodically to the endings of *Legiadra* and *Gratioso*; the division line after the third beat of the second bar is probably a scribal slip.

Notes on the music:

1) Orig.: *minima; semibrevis* in Pa.

2) The *semibrevis* rest is perfect in this mensuration, yet Pg seems to treat it as imperfect (also in the second part of section V).

3) The notation of section I in Pa eliminates the problematic rests. It is transcribed here in *quadernaria* as 4/4 with triplets, as is suggested by the choreography.

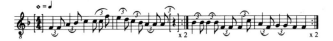

4) Orig.: *semibrevis* rests in both bars; corrected after Pa.

5) This and last note in following bar are *minimae* in Pa.

6) Orig.: *semibrevis* rest, in both sources. Pa omits the division line and the repeat numeral.

7) Alternative version in Pa (ignoring a dot of division after the second note):

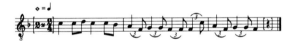

GRATIOSO

[50ᵛ]

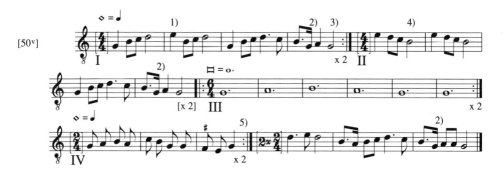

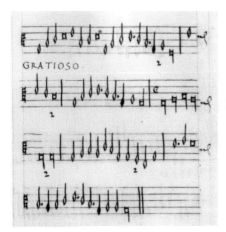

GRATIOSO.

CHOREOGRAPHY

Guglielmo (Pg)

I. 3 t German saltarello d x2
II. 2 t German saltarello ssd x2
III. ss dd rr c[c] ss dd rr cc
IV. 3 t piva [lady repeats?], scosso x2, dd

Gratioso

Concordances: Pa. Compare endings with those of *Colonnese*, *Spero*, and *Legiadra*. In Pa all sections are set off by double division lines, with 'bis dicitur' instead of the repeat numeral '2'. All sections end in *longae* (transcribed here as *breves* except in III). Is it possible that Guglielmo/Giovanni Ambrosio was experimenting with a notation for his own *balli* that differed from that of Domenico? Bonnie Blackburn has suggested that, because of its chanson-like opening and cadential structure, it might be derived from a chanson, thus accounting for its different notation.

Remarks: I. What looks like O corrected to C in Pa. The choreography (German *saltarello*) and notation suggest *quadernaria*.

   II. No mensural sign in either source. Choreography specifies German *saltarello*. Pa writes out the first bar twice and places 'bis dicitur' at the beginning of the line, indicating that the whole section, not just the first bar (as indicated in Pg's choreography), is to be repeated. This concords with the repeat in the choreography.

   III. C. The music has 12 bars, but the choreography (with only one *continenza*) has 11½ step-units. The NY and FN versions resolve this discrepancy by substituting a *riverenza* for the *continenza*.

   IV. No mensural sign in either source; choreography specifies *piva misura*. The repeat numeral suggests that a repeat in the choreography has been overlooked. No change of *misura* is indicated in bar 4, although the choreography suggests *quadernaria* steps to *piva* music. If barred as in the first part of this section, there would be twice as much music as step-units. See the endings of *Spero*, *Colonnese*, *Legiadra*, and [*Rostiboli*] *Gioioso*.

Notes on the music:
1) 2 *minimae* in Pa.
2) 2 *fusae* (A, G) followed by 2 *minimae* in Pa (cf. the end of IV in Pa's notation, n. 5).
3) Orig.: F. Corrected in Pa.
4) *Longa* in Pa (also in repeat).
5) Pa's version:

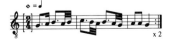

COLONNESE

[50ᵛ- 51ʳ]

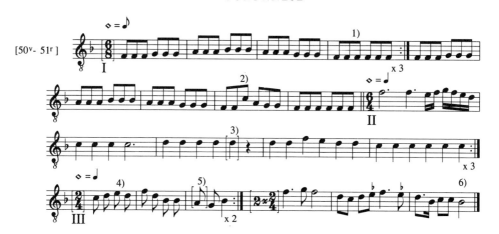

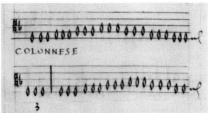

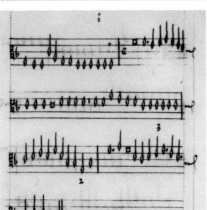

CHOREOGRAPHY

Guglielmo (Pg)

I. 16 t saltarello
II. ss dddd/ssd ssd R x2
III. 3 t piva x2, scosso x2, dd

Colonnese

Concordances: Pa. Compare endings with those of *Spero*, *Legiadra*, and *Gratioso*.

Remarks: I. No mensural sign in either source; choreography specifies 16 *tempi* of *saltarello*. One extra bar of music is presumably introductory and allows for a *movimento* with which to initiate the *saltarello*.

II. **C**; *bassadanza* is suggested by the choreography and notation. The choreography calls for only one repetition; if the third couple also repeats the steps of this section (to the third playing), the couples will end up in their starting positions, as they are instructed to do.

III. No mensural sign in either source; choreography specifies *piva misura*. In the second section there is no indication that the *misura* has changed, but unless barred in this way, twice as much music as step-units results. The choreography suggests *quadernaria* steps to *piva* music. (See the endings of *Spero*, *Gratioso*, *Legiadra*, [*Rostiboli*] *Gioioso*.)

Notes on the music:

1) Pa has a division line here, with the repeat numeral, and then continues with the third note of the penultimate bar (2). For this notation to provide 17 bars, the following transcription is necessary:

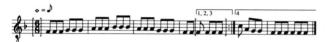

2) Orig.: C and A *minimae*; corrected after Pa.
3) Missing note (also in Pa) supplied following *Legiadra*, II, bar 4.
4) It is unclear if flats were intended in this section.
5) Missing note supplied from Pa.
6) Orig.: *longa* (also in Pa).

LEGIADRA

[51ʳ⁻ᵛ]

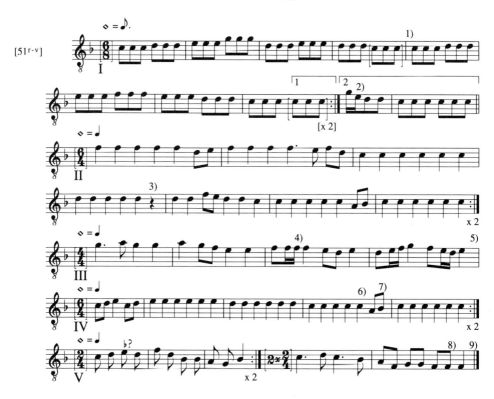

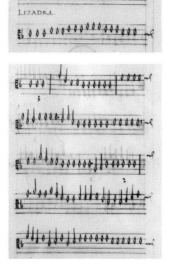

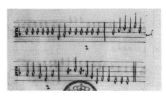

LIZADRA.

CHOREOGRAPHY

Guglielmo (Pg)

I.   16 t saltarello
II. rr/cccc ss dd rr cccc ss dd rr
III. 2 (4?) scossi, 1 (2?) t German
     salterello   }
IV. rrrd   } x2
V.   2[3] t piva x2; 2 scossi, 1 doppio

Legiadra

Concordances: Pa. Compare with I and II of *Colonnese*, I of [*Rostiboli*] *Gioioso*, and the finales of *Gratioso*, *Spero*, and *Colonnese*.

Remarks: Entitled *Lizadra* in the music.

I. No mensural sign in either source; transcribed as in *Colonnese*, which it closely resembles, in an effort to match the music with the choreography (16 *tempi* of *saltarello*). However, adjustments are necessary in both the Pg and Pa versions: see n. 1.

II. No mensural sign in either version, but choreography suggests *bassadanza*.

III. None of the choreographic descriptions in the different versions is very clear. If there are only 2 *scossi* (see NY) and one *tempo* of German *saltarello* in what is presumably *quadernaria misura*, there appears to be twice as much music as steps. The notation, on the other hand, does not seem to suggest a transcription of ○ = ♪ . (See the variant version of Pa in n. 5.)

IV. No mensural sign in either version, but both choreography and music seem to indicate *bassadanza*. The first 3 notes seem to be superfluous; cf. the end of III in Pa's version, which leads directly to the second bar of IV. The absence of a division line between III and IV (in both sources) suggests that both sections are repeated, and the choreography—while vague—seems to confirm this.

V. No mensural sign; corresponds to the *piva* section in *Gratioso*, *Spero*, and *Colonnese*. Differs in Pa (see n. 9). The scribe first wrote a version identical with the first 3 bars of Pg, but with *minimae* and *semiminimae*, then cancelled it. The rewritten version (transcribed here in triplets), connects better with the last 3 bars, transposed up a fifth. In both versions there is a discrepancy in bars 1–3 with the choreography, which calls for 2 *tempi*. Compare with the final sections of *Spero*, *Gratioso*, and *Colonnese*, all of which have 3 *tempi* of *piva*.

Notes on the music:

1) Pa begins here. The missing notes in bars 4 and 8 of Pg are supplied after *Colonnese*, and the repeat numeral changed from 3 to 2 (as in Pa), to provide 17 bars of music, one extra bar for an introduction and *movimento* with which to initiate the *saltarello*.

2) *Semibreves* G, E in Pa; cf. *Colonnese*, bar 8.

3) D instead of a rest in Pa, followed by additional D and *semibreves* F, E.

4) Orig.: *minimae* instead of *semiminimae*.

5) Variant version in Pa (the 2 last notes are *minimae*):

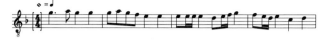

6) Superfluous *semibrevis* C omitted.

7) B♮ may be intended. It is not clear what function the Bb in the signature may have had in Pa's transposed variation.

8) Orig.: 2 *semibreves* instead of *minimae* (also in Pa).

9) Variant version in Pa:

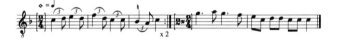

PART III

CRITICAL APPARATUS

Biographical Notes

THE following notes were originally compiled to help me keep track of the various names mentioned in Giovanni Ambrosio's Autobiography. Because of its utility as background information regarding Guglielmo's patrons—their dates, families, and interrelationships—I have decided to include these sketches as a guide for the reader. My main biographical source was the extraordinary twelve-volume work compiled by Pompeo Litta, *Famiglie celebri di Italia*, published over six decades beginning in 1819 by P. E. Giusti, Milan. Much of the reporting is narrative and it teems with piquant and violent detail.[1] Further information has been obtained from the *Dizionario biografico degli italiani* (Rome, 1960–), the *Enciclopedia italiana di scienze, lettere ed arti* (Rome, 1949), Abati-Olivieri Giordani, *Memorie*, Eiche, 'Alessandro Sforza', Southern, 'Prima Ballerina'. (There are some inconsistencies among the sources regarding birth and other dates.)

The Sforzas of Milan and Pavia

FRANCESCO SFORZA 1401–1466
Illegitimate son of Muzio Attendolo of Cotignola, he was known as Sforza and was the founder of that family. He was a great condottiere and served, among others, the Estes of Ferrara and the Viscontis of Milan. After his defence of Milan he married, in 1441, Bianca Maria Visconti (1422–68), heir to the Duchy of Milan. In 1450 he became the first Sforza Duke of Milan and proved to be a good ruler. Francesco Filelfo recited the oration at his funeral. He was the father of numerous children, including Polissena (who married Sigismondo Malatesta), TRISTANO, SFORZA SFORZA (SFORZA II), GALEAZZO, IPPOLITA, SFORZA MARIA, LUDOVICO, and Elisabetta.

TRISTANO SFORZA c.1422–1477
Illegitimate son of FRANCESCO. In 1455 he married BEATRICE D'ESTE (daughter of NICCOLÒ III, Duke of Ferrara) in Milan. Domenico da Piacenza was present at the wedding and danced with Tristano's stepmother, the Duchess Bianca Maria Visconti Sforza.

---

[1] Angene Feves, in her paper 'Caroso's Patronesses' (*Proceedings of the 9th SDHS Conference* (Riverside, Calif., 1986), 53), states: 'Litta and his associates in the project gathered as much information as they could about all the members of important Italian families, from the founding of the family to the time of publication, or the extinction of the family line. They went to the genealogical records and surviving members of the families, to investigate family legends as well as family trees. Sometimes these listings of family members are minimal, and sometimes they are accounts that would make soap opera plots seem pale in comparison. Perhaps the biographical details contained in the Litta volumes are precise and accurate, and perhaps they are expanded with backstairs gossip or censored by family pride . . .'.

SFORZA SFORZA (SFORZA II) 1433/5–1491/2

Illegitimate son of FRANCESCO. Head of the Borgonuovo branch of the Sforza family. (His son became lord of the neighbouring Castel San Giovanni in Piacenza's Val Tidone.) Sforza II was the recipient of a copy of *Il libro dell'arte del danzare*, the original of which Cornazano had dedicated to his sister IPPOLITA. He fought alongside Tiberto Brandolino and the Angevins against the Aragons in Naples.

GALEAZZO MARIA SFORZA 1444–1476

Son of FRANCESCO. Recipient of Guglielmo's *De pratica* (1463). Count of Pavia, in 1466 he became Duke of Milan and two years later he married (by proxy at the death of his first wife) Bona of Savoy. A great lover and patron of the arts, he was considered a corrupt and cruel ruler. He was assassinated in 1476 (see Ilardi, 'The Assassination'). Of his ten children, Bianca Maria (1472–1510) married the Emperor Maximilian after the death of his first wife, Marie of Burgundy. Another daughter, Anna, married ALFONSO D'ESTE of Ferrara (ISABELLA D'ESTE's brother). An illegitimate son, Carlo, was the father of Angela Sforza, who married ERCOLE D'ESTE, the son of SIGISMONDO. Galeazzo's heir, Giangaleazzo (Giovan Galeazzo, 1469–94), inherited the title of Duke at the age of 7, and married Isabella of Aragon (daughter of IPPOLITA SFORZA and ALFONSO II of Naples) in 1490. He was a ruler in name only and is said to have been murdered by his uncle, LUDOVICO SFORZA.

IPPOLITA SFORZA 1445–1488

Daughter of FRANCESCO. Married ALFONSO OF ARAGON, Duke of Calabria, later Alfonso II, in 1465. Cornazano dedicated his *Libro dell'arte del danzare* to her. Reputed to have been a brilliant and cultivated woman. Testimonials to her accomplishments in music and dancing can be found in Cornazano's treatise and in Giovanni Ambrosio's letter to Ippolita's mother, Bianca Maria Visconti Sforza.

SFORZA MARIA SFORZA 1451–1479

Son of FRANCESCO. His betrothal to ELEONORA OF ARAGON was subsequently rescinded. He was appointed Duke of Bari by the King of Naples in 1464.

LUDOVICO SFORZA (IL MORO) 1452–1508

Son of FRANCESCO. Named Duke of Bari by FERRANTE OF ARAGON after SFORZA MARIA's death. Banished from the Duchy of Milan after GALEAZZO's death, he was invited to return as regent in 1479, largely ignoring GALEAZZO's widow Bona and the 9-year-old Duke, Giangaleazzo. (He officially became Duke only in 1494 at Giangaleazzo's death.) In 1491 he married ISABELLA D'ESTE's sister BEATRICE. He was a patron of the arts and is considered to have been a clever political ruler. He died a prisoner in France.

The Sforzas of Pesaro

ALESSANDRO SFORZA 1409–1473
Illegitimate son of Muzio Attendolo and Lucia da Torsano (Torsciano). Following his father's death and mother's marriage, he and his brother FRANCESCO SFORZA were raised in Ferrara and educated with NICCOLÒ D'ESTE III's children. Throughout their lives the brothers continued to maintain a close bond. Alessandro was a military leader; he fought under Francesco, who made him a governor in the Marches. He helped the Aragons in Naples (after 1454) against the Angevins, thus ensuring the crown for FERDINAND I. The King held him in high esteem and promised his niece Camilla in marriage to Alessandro's son. Alessandro himself married COSTANZA VARANO in 1445 and became lord of Pesaro. After Costanza's death in 1447, Alessandro married SVEVA COLONNA OF MONTEFELTRO, the virtuous but plain sister of FEDERICO OF MONTEFELTRO. Sveva attempted suicide more than once, and Alessandro tried to murder her on at least one occasion. This unhappy marriage ended with Sveva being dragged, literally, to a convent, where she took the veil; she died in 1478. In his later years, Alessandro himself became deeply religious. He remained Guglielmo's patron to the end of his life.

COSTANZA (DA) VARANO c.1428–1447
Daughter of Piergentile da Varano, Marchese of Camerino, whose family is first heard of in the thirteenth century. Costanza's mother, Elisabetta Malatesta, was the only daughter of Galeazzo Malatesta, lord of Pesaro, and Costanza was able to bring this title as part of her dowry. At 14 she recited verses in Latin to Bianca Maria Visconti Sforza. Married to ALESSANDRO SFORZA in 1445, she died giving birth to her son COSTANZO.

RODOLFO (DA) VARANO d. 1463 or 1464
COSTANZA VARANO's brother. A military leader, he served FRANCESCO SFORZA, who, it seems, took a kindly interest in him. Rodolfo married CAMILLA D'ESTE (illegitimate daughter of NICCOLÒ III, lord of Ferrara) in 1444. He became lord of Camerino in December 1443, together with his cousin Cesare, with whom he ruled in harmony until his death or murder twenty years later.

GINEVRA SFORZA 1440–1507
Illegitimate daughter of ALESSANDRO SFORZA. She married into the noble Bentivoglio family of Bologna (which was later brought to ruin by Pope Julius II). Her first husband was Sante Bentivoglio, and at his death she married his brother Giovanni. She represented her father at COSTANZO SFORZA's wedding in Pesaro in 1475, two years after ALESSANDRO's death.

BATTISTA SFORZA 1446–1472
Daughter of ALESSANDRO SFORZA. She married FEDERICO OF MONTE-FELTRO in 1460. A well-loved and cultured woman who was also famous for her political capacities.

COSTANZO SFORZA 1447–1483
Son of ALESSANDRO SFORZA. A soldier, courtier, and man of letters. Considered to be a splendid and diligent prince. Married Camilla of Aragon, daughter of ELEONORA (ALFONSO I's illegitimate daughter) in 1475. (The wedding took place in Pesaro with magnificent entertainments.) Costanzo left no heirs when he died (or was murdered), but Camilla adopted his two illegitimate sons. One of them, Giovanni, became lord (and tyrant) of Pesaro and Lucretia Borgia's first husband. He was succeeded by his brother Galeazzo, who was, it seems, a good prince. On Galeazzo's death (c.1515), the line of the Pesaro Sforzas came to an end.

The Montefeltros and Duke Federico of Urbino

GUIDANTONIO 1403–1443
Descendant of the Montefeltro family, which prospered in the Marches from the twelfth century or earlier. His second wife was Caterina Colonna, mother of SVEVA COLONNA OF MONTEFELTRO, who was FEDERICO OF MONTEFELTRO's half-sister and ALESSANDRO SFORZA's second wife.

FEDERICO 1417 or 1422–1482
Illegitimate son of GUIDANTONIO OF MONTEFELTRO. He became the model for the Renaissance prince: soldier, patron of the arts, collector, music lover. Count and then Duke of Urbino, he erected a splendid palace. He was on good terms with the Aragonese court in Naples where, in 1474, shortly before becoming Duke, he was made a Knight of the Ermine. Federico's first marriage in 1437 to Gentile Brancaleone was without issue. Gentile died in 1456 and four years later he married BATTISTA SFORZA (ALESSANDRO's daughter). Federico fathered many children, among whom were: Giovanna (illegitimate), who married Giovanni della Rovere; Agnese, Vittoria Colonna's mother; Guidobaldo, who married the brilliant and virtuous Elisabetta Gonzaga. Guidobaldo became Duke of Urbino after Federico's death, but was frail and died without heirs in 1489. The marriage of Elisabetta (Isabetta), another daughter of Federico and Battista, to ROBERTO MALATESTA in 1475 represented a bond of peace between the two families. Staunch patron of Guglielmo/Giovanni Ambrosio.

The Malatestas of Rimini

SIGISMONDO MALATESTA 1417–1468

Lord of Rimini. After the death of his first wife, GINEVRA D'ESTE, he married Polissena, FRANCESCO SFORZA's daughter. He was a great patron of the arts and an excellent soldier. His cousin Galeazzo Malatesta, lord of Pesaro, was the father of Elisabetta Malatesta, the mother of COSTANZA VARANO, ALESSANDRO SFORZA's first wife.

ROBERTO MALATESTA 1442–1482/3

Illegitimate son of SIGISMONDO (later legitimized by the Pope). He was a capable soldier and fought for ALFONSO I of Naples. By duplicity he was able to obtain the lordship of Rimini after procuring the murders of his stepmother and stepbrother. His rule is considered a political disaster. After eleven or twelve years of marriage, Roberto died and his widow Elisabetta (Montefeltro) became a nun. In 1502 she was abducted by Cesare Borgia after his pillage of Urbino but she was released in exchange for two of his soldiers. The Malatesta Signory in Rimini, which had originated in the thirteenth century, came to an end in 1528 when Roberto's son Pandolfo was expelled from Rimini, which then became part of the Papal States.

The Aragons of Naples

ALFONSO I 1396–1458

Held the titles of King of Aragon (V), of Catalonia (IV), of Sicily and Sardinia, and was King of Naples from 1442 to 1458. His wife was Maria of Castille. Among his illegitimate children were MARIA, ELEONORA, and FERRANTE (FERDINANDO I).

MARIA OF ARAGON d. 1449

Illegitimate daughter of ALFONSO I. She married LEONELLO D'ESTE in 1444.

ELEONORA OF ARAGON

Illegitimate daughter of ALFONSO I. Her daughter, Camilla Marzano of Aragon, married COSTANZO SFORZA of Pesaro in 1475.

FERRANTE (FERDINANDO I) 1424–1494

Heir of ALFONSO I. Duke of Calabria and then King of Naples (1458–94). His children by his first marriage were ALFONSO II, Duke of Calabria; Federico (1452–1504); and the two sisters to whom Guglielmo/Giovanni Ambrosio taught dancing—[E]Leonora (1450–93, betrothed first to SFORZA MARIA and later married to ERCOLE I D'ESTE), and Beatrice (1457–1508, who married Matthias Corvinus and became Queen of Hungary).

ALFONSO II 1448–1495

FERRANTE's son, and Duke of Calabria. He married IPPOLITA SFORZA.
Their daughter, Isabella (of Aragon) married her cousin Giangaleazzo Sforza,
Duke of Milan. Two other children, illegitimate, were Sancha, Princess of
Squillace (who married Goffredo Borgia) and Alfonso, Duke of Bisceglie,
Lucretia Borgia's second husband.

The Estes of Ferrara

The following genealogical table shows how the Estes of Ferrara intermarried
with the Sforzas, Gonzagas, Malatestas, da Varanos, Borgias, and Aragons.
An asterisk indicates those weddings at which Guglielmo/Giovanni Ambrosio
was present, as well as others referred to in Chs. 1–3.

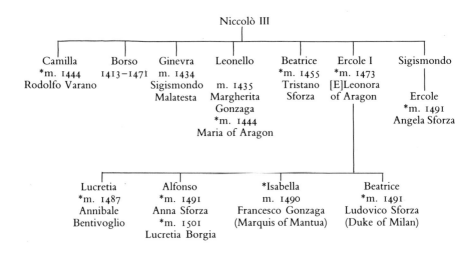

Glossary of Dance, Music, and Humanistic Terms

THE following definitions and explanations are by no means exhaustive; they correspond to the meanings of words and expressions as they are employed in *De pratica* and in the introductory chapters. In some cases several different interpretations are given, because the term, as used, is many-faceted. The Glossary gives definitions and/or explanations for: (1) words left in Italian when English equivalents are problematical; (2) words that are translated into an archaic English equivalent; (3) specific choreographic terms (including steps), translated and not; (4) specific musical terms, translated and not; (5) additional choreographic terms referred to in the critical notes. The step descriptions are based on information gleaned from all the fifteenth-century dance-treatises. However, these are, for the most part, only passing mentions, and it therefore remains impossible to determine whether they offer clues to how a step was regularly performed, or whether instead they are ornamented variations, regional or artistic alternatives, late (or early) forms, or possible indications of a new style. (See, for example, the variety of *meze volte* (half-turns).) While the duration of each step is known, thus making it possible to match choreography and music, the actual performance of the steps is still very much open to interpretation. All head-words in the Glossary are in Italian because it is there that the difficulty exists. The first relevant occurrence of any word appearing in the Glossary is marked in the Italian and English texts by an asterisk. Alternative spellings found in Pg and Pa (as well as variations due to genders and number) are included in parentheses. Abbreviations used: *pl.* (plural), *s.* (singular), *adj.* (adjective), *adv.* (adverb), *n.* (noun), *v.* (verb).

accidentale: fortuitous, accidental. Guglielmo also uses it to mean the opposite of natural or essential (see his first Rejoinder). Hence, artful, artificial, man-made (see also *artificiosamente* and *sottilita*). In the treatises of Domenico and Cornazano it also signifies an ornament.

aire (aiere, aira): air; a person's manner. For Guglielmo, one of the principal elements of the art of the dance: an ornament consisting of a rising movement applied to particular steps (see his 'Chapter on Air'). The term can also be interpreted as style, or quality, as in Giovanni Ambrosio's chapter on 'Recognizing a Good Dancer' (App. II). According to L. Lockwood, *Music in Renaissance Ferrara* (Oxford, 1984), 72, '*aere* was a term much used in this period for characteristic types of melodies as well as for the expressive qualities associated with them . . . [e.g.] *aere veneziane*'.

alta dança. Mentioned by Cornazano in relation to the *saltarello*. Literally, 'high dance', probably because of its characteristic springs. It contrasted with the *bassadanza* ('low dance'), which was performed more slowly and with the feet close to the ground.

artificiosamente, *adv.* (**artificioso**, *adj.*): skilfully; with artistry; the opposite of natural.

B molle and **B quadro**. The signatures—B♭ and B♮—of the *B molle* (soft) and *B durum* (hard) systems. See *chiave*.

ballo (**balli**, *pl.*). In fifteenth-century Italy a generic term for any sort of dance. Also a specific dance type, possibly created and certainly perfected by Domenico da Piacenza, characterized by changes of metre and tempo (*misura*). The four *misure* of which a *ballo* can be composed are: *bassadanza*, *quadernaria*, *saltarello*, and *piva*. Some *balli* are based on themes and call for pantomimic gestures. While some of the *balli* in *De pratica* are for four, six, or eight dancers, most are for a couple or a trio. The dancers perform abreast, in a line one behind the other, in squares, triangles, and longways sets. *Balli* were occasionally referred to as *balletti* (V, S, NY), the terms being interchangeable. *Ballo* also indicates an entertainment devoted to dancing, as a ball, though not as in a nineteenth-century context.

bassadanza (**bassadança**; **bassedanze**, **bassadançe** *pl.*). Literally, 'low dance' (see *alta dança*). In fifteenth-century Italy, an independent dance type. The choreographies of the more than forty extant *bassedanze* were composed largely by Guglielmo Ebreo/Giovanni Ambrosio, in lesser measure by Domenico da Piacenza, and by a handful of others. Most of the *bassedanze* are for a couple or a trio (there are also some for four and for eight), and the dancers are either abreast or in a line one behind the other. Circular *bassedanze* were performed in at least two allegorical spectacles, one to the singing of a chanson, the other to instrumental accompaniment (Ch. 3). The Italian *bassadanza* differs from the anonymous French-Burgundian *basse danse* of the same period in that the latter was performed by only couples or trios, it was processional (there being no *meza volta*), and, most important, it followed a rigid scheme of steps (*Reverence, branle, 2 simples*, 1, 3, or 5 *doubles*, 3 backward *reprises*), its length determined by a fixed arrangement of *mesures*. As Otto Gombosi has said,

While in France the *bassedanse* became more and more a mere social entertainment, in Italy even the society dance remained an art form . . . The French style was characterized by an utterly strict formalism contrasting with the freedom of the Italian style . . . The increasing formalizing of the [French *bassedanse*] sequences makes quite impossible a creatively artistic disposition of the spatial medium . . . In spite of their obviously common origin, the Italian and French styles differ from each other as the youthful Renaissance differs from the declining Middle Ages.

('About Dance and Dance Music in the Late Middle Ages', *Musical Quarterly*, 27 (1941), 289–305 at 303 and 305.)

The *bassadanza* can also be one of the sections of a *ballo*. It is the slowest of the four *misure*, and its mensural sign (C) and notation suggest a modern transcription in compound duple time ($\frac{6}{4}$ $\downarrow$. $\downarrow$.). According to Domenico, the *bassadanza*, which he considered 'the Queen of the *misure*', should begin on the up-beat; that is, the soprano player starts while the dancer makes a preparatory movement. The tenor enters on the down-beat as the dancer's step takes the weight. *Bassedanze* were danced to music based on tenor melodies, notated for the most part in *semibreves* or *breves*. Usually one or two melodies were improvised around the tenor. See, among others, Crane, *Materials*, Crane, 'Derivation', Bukofzer, 'Polyphonic Basse Dance', Heartz, '15th-Century Ballo', Southern, 'Basse-Dance Music in some German Manuscripts of the 15th Century' in Jan La Rue *et al.* (eds.), *Aspects of Medieval and Renaissance Music* (New York, 1966), 738–55; 'Some Keyboard Basse Dances of the Fifteenth Century', *Acta musicologica*, 35 (1963), 114–24; and *The Buxheim Organ Book* (Musicological Studies, 6; Brooklyn, NY, 1963), and Ch. 4 n. 35.

canto (**canti**, *pl.*): song; musical sound (see *suono*; *voce*). According to Tinctoris, *Terminorum, Cantus* is 'music . . . made up of a large number of individual sounds, and is either a single melody or a part-song'. It also means side.

chiave, *s.*, *pl.*: musical clef(s) or signature(s). The *chiavi* (*pl.*) of *B molle* (B♭) and *B quadro* (B♮) undoubtedly refer to the two systems known later as *cantus mollis* and *cantus durus*, which developed out of the hexachord theory. The three hexachords were *naturale*—beginning on C; *durum* (hard)—beginning on G; *molle* (soft)—beginning on F, with a B♭. The *cantus mollis*, where the B♭ was essential, was composed of the *molle* and *naturale* hexachords, whereas the *cantus durus*—with its B♮—included the *durum* and *naturale* hexachords. See 'Mode', 'Musica Ficta', and 'Solmization' in *New Grove* as well as K. Berger, *Musica Ficta* (Cambridge, 1987), and A. Hughes, *Manuscript Accidentals: Ficta in Focus 1350–1450* (American Institute of Musicology, Musicological Studies and Documents, 27; 1972).

cithara. In fifteenth-century Italy this was still a generic term for a plucked string instrument and was also used specifically to indicate a harp or lyre. Occasionally it referred to a bowed instrument such as a viola da braccio. Also an ancient Greek instrument similar to a lyre, but with a flat, shallow sound chest. The legendary instrument of Apollo. (Also spelled *kithara*.)

concordanti: concordant. In *De pratica*, *concordante voci* or *concordato suono* seems to suggest musical accompaniment. (See *concordantie*.)

concordantie: concordances; accordant sounds; harmonies (i.e. sounds which are agreeable to the ear, rather than harmony as chordal structure distinguished from melody and rhythm); music. In Guglielmo's time, the terms *concordantia* and *consonantia* were often used interchangeably, not only in their generic meaning but to indicate the three perfect musical *concordances/consonances* then recognized: the fourth, the fifth, and the octave.

concordato (**ben**): (well) tuned.

consonantia (**consonanza**; **consonanze**, *pl.*): consonance, concordance; an agreement of voices or sounds (harmony). Parrish in Tinctoris, *Terminorum*, translates the entry *concordantia* as 'A consonance is a blending of different pitches which strikes pleasantly on the ear, and which is either perfect or imperfect.' See *concordantie*.

continenza (**continenze**, **continencie**, **contenenze**, *pl.*). The fifteenth-century Italian *continenze*, with which many *bassedanze* begin, may well be similar to the French/Burgundian *branle* (a kind of 'setting' or 'swaying' step on, or to, the left and right; see *Borges*, App. II, Crane, *Materials*, and Brainard, *The Art of Courtly Dancing*). Two *continenze*, with or without a *riverenza*, could make up the 'honours' of a dance. They usually appear in pairs and, in Domenico's choreographies at least, are performed on alternate feet. They do not travel and in *De pratica* are done 'on' or 'upon' the foot (like *riprese*). N describes them as 'plospelg treten', 'treading the bellows (of an organ)' (Brainard, *Nürnberg*). According to Domenico and Cornazano, each *continenza* should last a half-*tempo*, so that two *continenze* are performed in one bar of music. More prevalent in *bassedanze* than in *balli*, they often seem, in long dances, to indicate the end of a 'dance phrase'. Cornazano (V, 7^r) adds that when performing two *continenze* (or *riprese*), they should always be 'differentiated from each other, that is, big and [then] little . . . or vice versa'.

contrapassi. Not mentioned as such by either Domenico da Piacenza (Pd) or Guglielmo Ebreo (Pg, Pa), but present in Cornazano's treatise (V) and included in NY, FN, FL, M, and S. According to Cornazano, three *contrapassi* (literally, counter-steps) were to be performed in two *tempi* (bars of music), and they seem to be the equivalent of Domenico's and Guglielmo's three *doppii* 'on [with, or upon] the same foot' (see Lo Monaco and Vinciguerra, 'Il passo doppio').

dinanzi (**dinanti**, **di nanci**). In the choreographies, in front of; forward; before. Also the equivalent of *sopra*: above; in the lead position; on the left side.

dolce: sweet, pleasant, gracious; sweet-sounding. In the fifteenth-century a universal adjective for describing the quality and effects of music.

dolceze: sweetnesses. *Dulcedo*, and its opposite, *subtilitas*, was a basic concept in the poetry and musical aesthetics of the Middle Ages. 'Sweet sounds' tended to be associated with natural (instinctive, sensual) qualities, like the simplicity of a melody, wheras 'subtleties' (*sottilita*)—the artistic creations of man—implied a rationally constructed polyphony. (See N. Pirrotta, '*Dulcedo e subtilitas* nella pratica polifonica franco-italiana al principio del Quattrocento', in *Musica tra Medioevo e Rinascimento* (Turin, 1984), 130–41.)

doppij, *pl.* (**doppii**; **doppio**, *s.*): double steps. According to Domenico da Piacenza and Cornazano, the *doppio* should last one *tempo* (bar). Cornazano's description of the *bassadanza* (V, 10^r) as divided into four parts—the up-beat with its 'surging movement', followed by three steps—may be a description of a *doppio* in that *misura*. When discussing *Maniera* (V, 3ᵛ–4ʳ), he specifies that the second step is short, and that the third step ends the *doppio*. The *doppio* is the basic step-unit in the other *misure* where, according to Domenico, it was ornamented by a *frapamento* (in *quadernaria*), a little *salto* (in *saltarello*), or performed very fast (*piva*). Sequences of two, three, or four *doppii*, each *doppio* beginning 'on', 'with', or 'upon the same foot' (rather than with the usual alternating of left and right feet) seem to be the equivalent of *contrapassi*.

festa: Florio gives 'feast . . . banquet . . . shew'. According to the context, it is translated as festivity, entertainment, celebration, reception, or banquet.

frapamento (Pd) (**frappamenti** (V), *pl.*). A step ornament which is not mentioned in *De pratica*, though widely used (see Pd and V). Not to be confused with the French *frappement*. *Frappe* and *frappatura* in Renaissance Italy meant fringe or embroidery, as *frappa* still does today. Florio also adds: cut, trick, boast, vaunt, i.e. an ornament. Although it could grace *sempii*, *riprese*, and *volte tonde*, it is most often mentioned with *doppii* in *quadernaria misura* and in *saltarello todesco* (German *saltarello*). While Domenico says the *quadernaria* step is a *doppio* with a *frapamento*, Cornazano described the step as two *passi sempii* and a little *ripresa* (see below, *quaternario*). It is not known if this particularly performed *ripresetta* resembles or not a *frapamento*.

galone (**gallone**): side, flank; edging or trimming (border). See *ripresa in galone*.

harmonia: harmony. According to Florio, 'melody; accord in music'. Tinctoris, *Terminorium*, defines it as 'a certain pleasantness caused by an agreeable sound', adding that melody is the same as harmony and that harmonic music is that which is performed by the human voice.

inanze (**inanti**, **inanci**, **inanzi**, **innanti**). See *dinanzi*.

in su (**insu**): upon. In *De pratica* the step-units which travel—*doppii*, *sempii*, and *saltarello* steps—are performed *con* (with) the left or right foot. Steps which are usually performed on the spot (or to the side)—*continenze*, *riprese*, *volte*, and *riverenze*—are made *su* or *insu* (on or upon) the foot. However, when *insu* is used of a sequence of *doppii* performed 'on' or 'upon the same foot' (rather than with alternating feet), this seems to be the equivalent of *contrapassi*. Also used (NY) to indicate the direction the dancer is to advance when separating from his/her partner. *Insu* and *ingiu* ('upwards', 'downwards') correspond to travelling to (or from) the head or foot of the hall.

largho (**larghe**): large, wide, ample; slow.
liberale (**scienza** or **arte**): liberal (science or art). A noble pursuit, intellec-

tual rather than manual; the opposite of *arte meccanica*, a craft or technical skill.

liverea (**liverei**, *pl.*): livery. Also a masked, costumed entertainment; a costume for a 'masque'; a masker (Battaglia and Squarotti, *Grande dizionario*). In *De pratica* it seems to signify a set or company ('mummery') of 'masques' or maskers.

mainiera (**mayniera**): manner; fashion, style. Guglielmo's chapter on Manner defines it as 'shading', a way of turning the body while dancing, an essential step adornment. For Cornazano, (V, 3ᵛ–4ʳ), *maniera* is a rising up on the second short step of a *doppio* and a lowering of the body on the third and final step. (Compare this with Guglielmo's Chapter on Air.)

mascare (**maschere**, *pl.*): masks; maskers; 'masques' (see *moresca*).

melodia: melody, tune; harmony (see *harmonia*); sweet singing.

meza volta (**meça volta**): half-turn. According to Cornazano, the *meza volta* was to last one *tempo* or bar (Domenico's indication of a half *tempo* is almost certainly an error), but in only two *balli* are steps specified. (*Ingrata* has a *meza volta* performed with two *sempii*; *Voltati in ça Rosina* uses a *doppio*. Both examples are in *quadernaria misura*.) Whereas Domenico almost always refers to 'a' *meza volta*, Guglielmo, perhaps significantly, avoids the article (except once in *Pellegrina*) although he uses it for the *volta tonda* (full-turn). (This translation silently includes the article.) The general omission in *De pratica* may indicate that 'dare *meza volta*' was meant as a verb ('to half-turn') and that the turning was performed without the specific time-value of a step. In most choreographies the *meza volta* seems to be made at the end of a *doppio* (taken with the right foot), during the up-beat (*vuoto*) before the following step (usually a *ripresa* on the left foot). In S this is referred to as a *ripresa in volta* (turning *ripresa*). There are also several examples (NY and Fol) of these 'up-beat' half-turns performed with a *salto* (a hop or leap). Most of Guglielmo's *meze volte* are made *on* or *upon the right foot* (the right foot, presumably, pivoting), the equivalent of what Domenico calls a *meza volta to the right side*. The *scorsa* (probably a kind of running step) could replace a *doppio* in a *meza volta* (Pd, fo. 3ʳ).

misura (**misure**, *pl.*): measure. In *De pratica*, *misura* has several meanings:

1. one complete unit or measure of a particular mensuration (Exercises III and IV);

2. rhythm; as time or timing; as in 'measured' music or dancing (i.e. 'measured' according to the correct division of the notes—or rhythm); in other words, playing and dancing in time (Chapter on Measure);

3. metre; as mensuration—tempus and prolation (Exercise V);

4. the four dance types in a *ballo*—bassadanza, quadernaria, saltarello, piva —each with its own mensuration, relative tempo, and characteristic steps. The steps of one *misura* could be performed to the music of another *misura*;

5. *chiave* (Rule I);

6. measurement, regulations, the proper rules; for example, those determining the composition of four voices (Rule IV) or the characteristics of steps in a particular dance type (Exercises III and IV);

7. quantity ('in such measure', Rule IV);

8. due amount, moderation ('her bearing should have the proper measure'—Rules for Women).

moresca (morescho; moresche, *pl.*). Literally, something Moorish. In fifteenth-century Italy *moresche* were musical, mimed, or danced interludes performed during banquets and plays. They portrayed allegorical, heroic, exotic, and pastoral scenes and were danced by courtiers and dancing-masters in costume. (See Ch. 3 for more details and examples.)

movimento (movimenti, *pl.*): movement. *Movimento corporeo* (Body Movement) was one of the basic principles of fifteenth-century dance. (See Guglielmo's chapter.) A *movimento* was also a 'natural' (basic) step-unit with which both the *bassadanza* and *saltarello* were to begin. This step or movement also appears in the main part or coda of many *balli* where, in Cornazano's words, it indicates 'a most virtuous question and answer between the man and lady'. In *De pratica*, Guglielmo retains the term *movimento* in only some of Domenico's *balli*, substituting *scosso* (shake) in the others as well as in his own. According to Domenico, the *movimento* should last a half *tempo* (bar), while for Cornazano there is no specific timing. Unfortunately, nothing more specific is known about the *movimento/scosso* except that it was to be ornamented with a rising motion (Pg, 8^r).

natural(e): natural; basic (essential), as in *passi naturali*. The opposite of *artificiale*, the artistic creations of man. Related to *dolceza*: simple, instinctive, sensual.

passi, *pl.* (**passo,** *s.*): steps.

pieno (piena): full; whole; perfect. Guglielmo (and, more often, Domenico) also uses the term for the 'strong'—as opposed to the 'weak'—beat in music, or to indicate what in modern terminology would be the down-beat. (See *vuoto*.)

pifare, pifferi. In the fifteenth century this was a generic name for wood-wind instruments. More specifically, the term referred to double-reed instruments, i.e. shawms, particularly when *pifferi* appeared together with *tromboni* (sackbuts). Shawms are the instruments most often depicted in fifteenth-century Italian dance iconography.

piva: a pipe or bagpipe; a rustic dance popular in fifteenth-century Italy; also, the fastest *misura* in a *ballo*, twice as fast—theoretically, at least—as the *bassadanza* (see Pd and V). Made up primarily of 'nimble and swift' *doppii* (V), it appears most often in the finale of a *ballo*. Two of Giovanni Ambrosio's *balli*, *Amoroso* and *Petit Riense*, are choreographed entirely in *piva misura*.

Cornazano (V) calls the *piva* '*cacciata*' (chase), the daughter of the *quadernaria*, and despite its 'lowly' and pastoral origins describes courtiers dancing it on festive occasions, the man ornamenting it with turns, capers, and jumps. For a discussion of its mensuration and transcription see Ch. 4. (Also see Ch. 3; V, fos. 5–6 and 34ᵛ; Cornazano, *Proverbi*.

piva todescha: German *piva*. Guglielmo uses this term to indicate *piva* steps performed in *quadernaria misura*, specifically two *piva doppii* danced to one *tempo*, or bar, of *quadernaria* music.

quaternario (quadernaria): quaternary. Unlike the other *balli misure*, the *quaternario* was not an independent dance type in fifteenth-century Italy. However, *Gelosia* and *Rosina* are *balli* which are exclusively in *misura quadernaria*. The prolation sign which is used in the notations is always C, and it corresponds to four beats per bar or *tempo* (4/4). In *quadernaria misura* (theoretically one-sixth faster than *bassadanza misura*), steps and music should begin on the down-beat. According to Domenico, the *quadernaria* step is a *doppio* with a *frapamento*, while Cornazano (who equates it with German *saltarello*) describes it as 'dui passi sempii et una ripresetta batuta detro el sicondo passo in traverso', a difficult phrase to translate because of various possible interpretations: 'two *passi sempii* and a little *ripresa* beaten (performed) behind (after) the second step cross-wise'. Besides this basic step, a few choreographies also use *sempii, riprese, continenze*, and *volte* in *quadernaria misura*.

ripresa (represa, rimpresa, *s*.; **riprese, rimprese**, *pl*.). A step to the side, as can be deduced from choreographies like *Cupido*, where the dancers separate from each other with one *ripresa*, or—as in *Mercantia*—with six, done to opposite sides. Like the *meza volta, volta tonda, riverenza*, and *continenza*, none of which travels, it should be performed, according to Guglielmo, *on* or *upon* the foot, rather than *with* the foot, as in *sempii, doppii, saltarello*. Each *ripresa* lasts one *tempo* (bar of music). Usually performed in pairs, Cornazano exhorts the dancer to vary their size. See *meza volta, volta tonda*, and *quaternario*, as well as *riprese in galone*.

riprese in galone: *riprese* performed while the dancer is advancing or retreating. It therefore seems likely that the basic *ripresa* to the side becomes a 'flanking' or diagonal step forwards or backwards. Domenico uses the expression 'riprese . . . in traverso . . . sul gallone senestro' (*riprese* done across, athwart, or transversely on the left flank or side). Guglielmo uses *riprese in galone* only once, preferring the term *riprese (in) portogalese* (see below), terms which seem interchangeable. (Compare *Damnes*, Pd and *Daphnes*, Pg.)

riprese (rimprese) in portogalese (riprese portogalese, portugalese): Portuguese *riprese*. See *riprese in galone*. In Giovanni Ambrosio's *Fiore de Vertu* (App. II), the choreography calls for 'three *rimprese* in *portogalese* in *bassadanza misura* beginning with the right foot, that is *in galone*'.

riverenza (**reverenza, riverencia; riverenze,** *pl.*): bow, curtsy. A basic step-unit which should be performed, according to Domenico and Cornazano, in one *tempo* (bar). The only references to its mode of performance are found in Pa, NY, and S, where there are several indications for a '*riverenza* down to the ground', perhaps the same as Giorgio's *piena* (full) *riverenza*. It is not known if these instructions were the exception or the rule, or if they also applied to the lady. A *riverenza* was made 'on' or 'upon' a foot, referring, apparently, to the foot or leg which moves. While most choreographies call for a *riverenza* made with the left foot, there are some dances (see, for example, NY, FN, Pd) in which a *riverenza* with the right foot is also used.

saltarello (**saltarelli,** *pl.*). According to extant musical sources, the *saltarello* was danced in Italy from at least the fourteenth century. In Guglielmo's time it was an independent dance type which was performed, primarily by couples, in village, town, and court festivities, often for hours on end (see Ch. 3). Scenes on fifteenth-century Italian wedding chests and contemporary engravings suggest that turning under the arm, promenading in closed position and, for the man, leg thrusts and kicks as well as hands on hips, were characteristic features. Cornazano (V) refers to the *saltarello* as 'the most merry dance of all, called *alta dança* by the Spanish'. (Indeed, in the early sixteenth century it was often synonymous with galliard.) *Saltarello* is also one of the *misure* of a *ballo*, theoretically one-third faster than the *bassadanza*, and almost always notated in compound duple (6/8). Like the *bassadanza*, it should begin on the up-beat, and Cornazano tells us that the three tenors included in his treatise are suitable for both *misure*. The *saltarello misura* step-unit, according to Domenico, is a *doppio* with a '*salteto*' (probably a hop; see *salto*). Cornazano confirms this (the *saltarello* 'consists only of *passi doppii*'), adding that it is ornamented 'by the rising up of the second short step which falls between one *tempo* and another'.

saltarello todescho (**todesco**): German *saltarello*. Guglielmo uses the term in *Iove* as an equivalent of Domenico's *saltarello in quadernaria*. (See also Giorgio's opening German *saltarello* in *Gelosia*.) Here and in four other *balli* it indicates *saltarello doppii* performed in *quadernaria misura*. One *saltarello doppio* danced to one *tempo* (bar) of *quadernaria* music produces a slow *saltarello* since the *quadernaria misura* is slower (theoretically, one-sixth slower) than the *saltarello misura*. Guglielmo substitutes *saltarello todesco* for *piva* in two of Domenico's *balli* (*Gelosia* and *Presoniera*). In *Spero* Guglielmo begins with four *doppii* 'in German' which in this case seems to mean *quadernaria doppii* danced to *saltarello* music. Puzzling are the instances, in Guglielmo's *Principessa* and *Caterva*, of German *saltarello* in *bassadanza misura*. This may indicate, as Cornazano maintained, that the German *saltarello* was also a specific step (see *quadernaria*). In *Presoniera*, Guglielmo specifies that it be performed with 'a *passo doppio* and a *ripresa* for each *tempo* of *saltarello*'.

salto: spring, bound; hop; leap; jump. Domenico considered the *salto* a 'natural' (basic) step—lasting half a *tempo* (bar)—and he included many in his choreographies. Cornazano, perhaps because his treatise was designed for a lady, or because he was a courtier and poet and not a *ballerino* or choreographer, excluded the *salto* from his lists of both basic and ornamental steps. Giovanni Ambrosio, in his chapters on a dancer's attire, asserts that a short garment or cape should be worn when performing the requisite jumps (*salti*), flourishes, and full-turns (*volte tonde*).

scossi, *pl.* (**scosso, schosso**, *s.*). The term Guglielmo and his followers used to replace what Domenico and Cornazano referred to as *movimento*.

sempij, *pl.* (**sempi, sempii; sempio**, *s.*): simples, simple steps. Two *sempii* were to be performed in one *tempo* (bar), on alternate feet. The choreographies do have examples, though rare, of a single *sempio* as well as sequences of three *sempii*. In some of the versions of Guglielmo's and Domenico's choreographies in NY and V, the terms *passi di natura* ('natural steps') or *passetti, passettini* ('little steps', 'very little steps') are occasionally substituted for *passi sempii*. Performed for the most part going forwards (straight ahead or around in a turn), *sempii* are occasionally taken backwards.

sopra: above; before. In the choreographies the term also indicates the lead position which, if the dancers are abreast, is on the left. In *Mercantia* it means in front. (See *sotto*.)

sottilita, *pl.*, *s.*: subtleties, subtlety. From *subtilitas*, the opposite of *dulcedo*; a basic concept in the poetry and musical aesthetics of the Middle Ages. It seems likely that subtleties meant the artistic creations of man (rationally constructed polyphony, for example) as opposed to the sweet qualities (*dolceze*) which were more instinctive and natural and pertained to the senses.

sotto (**soto**): under, beneath. In the choreographies the term also indicates the secondary or lower position which, if the dancers are abreast, is on the right. In *Mercantia* its meaning is 'behind'. (See *sopra*.)

suon(o), (**son**), *n.*: sound; tune, melody; pitch; music; audible music. 'Sound is whatever is perceived, properly and by itself, by hearing' (Tinctoris, *Terminorum*). By placing *suono* as an alternative to *canto*, Guglielmo seems to suggest it means instrumental or played sound, as opposed to vocal music.

tempo: time (see also *misura*). In *De pratica* it has a number of meanings:
1. an instance or moment; time as in 'while, during, in the mean time';
2. time as related to space;
3. dancing *in time* and *counter to the time* of a particular *misura*;
4. duration; a unit (specified or unspecified) of time;
5. a *brevis*: '*tempo* and *brevis* mean one and the same thing' (Jacopo da Bologna, *L'arte del biscanto misurato*);
6. 'measured time', as *tempus*: 'the measuring of a melody, determined by considering the breve to consist of a definite number of semibreves. It is, of course, twofold, namely perfect and imperfect' (Tinctoris, *Terminorum*);

7. a specific musical and/or step-unit. In the choreographies one *tempo* is usually the equivalent (i) of a modern musical bar and (ii) of a *passo doppio* in a particular *misura*, e.g. *bassadanza*;

8. rhythm; the organization of tones into a rhythmic structure (Chapter on Measure).

tirandosi (tirinsi) in dietro (si tirano, si tira, se tireno indirieto, se ritiri in drieto). Depending on the choreographic context, this term (literally, to draw oneself back) means to go backwards (as in 'draw back three steps'), or to go back (as in 'draw back a *doppio*, come towards [your partner] a *doppio*, that is making a *volta tonda*'). See *tornare in drieto*.

tornare (tornino, torni, tornando, ritornando) in drieto (dietro): to go back; to go backwards. This term can indicate that the dancer should:

1. go back to his place, or to where he began the dance;

2. go, that is *advance*, towards the back (as opposed to the front) of the set or room before making a *meza volta* to face his partner;

3. go backwards while facing his partner (when there is no *meza volta* in the choreography).

According to different versions of the same choreography, it can also be synonymous with *tirandosi in dietro*. (See *Borges*, French *bassadanza*, in App. II.)

tuono: a mode; whole tone; a tune (melodic line).

turcha (turca): A long tunic-like garment with a high neck and long sleeves. Its name suggests a Turkish origin.

vadano (vaghano) al (in) contrario l'un dell'altro. Literally, 'go contrary to one another'. Translated in the choreographies as 'advance in opposite directions'.

virtute (virtu, virtude): virtue, excellence, quality; a skill or accomplishment. (Florio gives honesty, strength, grace, power, perfection, authority, etc.)

virtuoso: virtuous, worthy; diligent.

voci, *pl.* (**voce**, *s.*): voices; strains, music; singing. *Vox*, which Parrish translates as 'a tone', is—according to Tinctoris—'a (musical) sound produced either naturally or artificially'. When coupled with *suono* in *De pratica*, it seems to suggest sung, rather than instrumental, music.

volta, *s.* (**volte**, *pl.*): turn; time. See *meza volta*; *volta del gioioso*; *volta tonda*. Virtuoso *volte* for male dancers are mentioned by both Giovanni Ambrosio (in his chapters on the dancer's attire) and Cornazano (V, fol. 6^r).

volta del gioioso. Literally, the turn of the blithe. Etymology unknown. It would appear to be identical (or at least interchangeable) with the *volta tonda* in *bassadanza misura*, inasmuch as in different versions of three *bassedanze*— *Alessandresca*, *Venus*, and *Lauro* (FN, FL, NY), one or other of the terms (*volta tonda* (full-turn) or *volta del gioioso*) is used at the same point in the text. (Compare also *Iove*, Pg, and *Jupiter*, Pd.)

volta tonda: full-turn. In Domenico's treatise, the *volta tonda*—when performed in *bassadanza misura*—lasts two *tempi* (bars), being composed of two *sempii* and a *ripresa*, and it always begins with the right foot. As regards the *volte tonde* in *De pratica* and its various versions, Guglielmo's instructions—in his own choreographies as well as in his renditions of Domenico's dances—are to make the turn with 'two *passi sempii*, beginning with the right foot, and (then do) a *ripresa*'. If the *volta tonda* was made with two *sempii* only, it would last *one* rather than two *tempi*. It is not known if Guglielmo was using a new kind of *volta*, one which he preferred for the finales of his *bassedanze*, or whether his version of 'two *sempii* [followed in the text by a stroke, i.e. comma] and (then) a *ripresa*' is simply a scribal interpretation. Other types of *volte tonde* in *piva* and *quadernaria misure* often begin with the left foot and are composed of: four *passetti*; three *sempii*; a *doppio* and a *ripresa*; one or two *doppii* —this last an ending which Guglielmo used in many *balli* (see *tirandosi in dietro*). The *volte tonde* for male dancers described by Giovanni Ambrosio (Chapter on Dancing in Short Attire) may have been particular virtuosic jump-turns. See *volta del gioioso*.

v[u]oto: empty. Used in *De pratica* (and even more so in Domenico's treatise) for the 'weak'—as opposed to the 'strong'—beat, and to indicate what in modern musical terminology is called the up-beat. (See *pieno*.)

APPENDICES

⁊

ADDITIONS FROM THE GIOVANNI AMBROSIO
COPY OF *DE PRATICA*

Introductory Note to the Appendices

As stated in Ch. 1, the Giovanni Ambrosio treatise (Paris, Bibl. Nat., fonds ital. 476) is a word-for-word copy of Guglielmo's *De pratica*. Written presumably eleven or twelve years later, it is missing the dedicatory pages and the Ode, but includes additional chapters (Appendix I), choreographies and music (Appendix II), as well as the Autobiography (Appendix III), all of extreme interest and importance (see Ch. 1). Punctuation, scarce and capricious in the original, has been added to the translation as an aid to understanding. Capital letters have been corrected in the transcription and full stops added to the end of each chapter or choreography.

APPENDIX I

CAPITOLO DE DANÇAR LONGO

[24ʳ] Nota che uno che dançasse con uno vestimento longho elle di bisogno de ballare con gravita, & ballare con un'altra forma che non se fa de ballare con uno vestito corto perche dançando como che gisse con uno vestito corto non dirria bono. E[t] bisognia che tucti li suoi giesti & movimenti siano gravi & tanto suave tanto quanto che he debito che porta & per forma che quella *turcha o panno longho che porta indosso non savia agire movendo troppo in qua & in la E[t] siati acorti che bisognia grande actetudine, & gran misura & gran tempo a dançare^a con esso a uno panno longo che con lo corto arichiede dançare un poco piu gagliardo.

CAPITOLO DE DANÇAR CORTO

[24ᵛ] Sappiate chi dança con uno vestito | corto bisognia de dançare in altra forma che quella dello longo. Li se arichiede de fare salti & volte tonde & fioregiare con misura & con tempo & a quello abito del vestire corto sta bene affare questo E[t] se tu volessi gire con gravita chomo avemo dicto di sopre non dirria bono e[t] serria signale de non intendere.

CAPITOLO DE DANÇARE CON MANTELLINA

Ancora siate avisati^b che bisogna altra discriccione de dançare con una mantellina corta piu che con una turca, neanche con uno vestito, e[t] la cagione sie che la mantellina piglia vento ch'e como tu dai un salto o una volta la mantellina si arimove elle di bisogno che a certi giesti & a certi movimenti & a certi tempi tu piglie la tua mantellina per un lato e[t] a certi tempi se piglia per tucti doi li lati che he una signoria a vedere
[25ʳ] pigliare col tempo. E[t] quando questo non se | facesse alli tempi che bisogna serria signale de non intendere E[t] questo basti quanto al dançare secondo li panni che porta in dosso.

---

^a The word *senza* ('without') follows but is cancelled.
^b *avisati* is written twice.

On Dancing

CHAPTER ON DANCING IN LONG [ATTIRE]

Note that someone dancing in a long garment should dance with solemnity and in a different fashion than when dancing in a short garment, because dancing as if he were going about in a short garment would not be seemly. And all his gestures and movements should be grave and as refined as his attire requires, and of an apt fashion, because the *turca or long robe that he is wearing would not work with too much moving here and there. And be aware that great ability and great [sense of] time and measure are necessary for dancing in a long robe since a short garment requires dancing a little more vigorously.

CHAPTER ON DANCING IN SHORT [ATTIRE]

Remember that whoever dances in a short garment must dance in a different fashion than when he dances in a long one. He is expected to perform jumps and full-turns and flourishes[1]—in time and measure—and for this a short garment is suitable. And if you wished to go about with solemnity, as we have said above, it would not be seemly, and would be a sign of little skill.

CHAPTER ON DANCING WITH A CAPE

Note further that another sort of dancing is required when wearing a short cape as opposed to a *turca* or even a [short?] garment. And the reason is, the cape catches the wind, so that as you do a jump or a turn, the cape swings about. And with certain gestures and movements, and with certain rhythms, you need to hold your cape by an edge, and with [other] rhythms you have to hold both edges, which is a lordly thing to see when done in time. And if this is not done when the rhythms require it, it is a sign of little skill. And let this suffice as to dancing according to how one is attired.

[1] See Ch. 1 n. 36 and Ch. 2 n. 55.

EXPERIMENTO DE COGNOSERE UN BONO DANÇATORE

Fate sonare de quactro o cinque ragione stromenti o veramente *pifare o organi o liuto o arpa o tamburino con fiauti o qualuncha stromento se sia. E[t] fateli sonare a uno per uno e[t] fateli sonare un ballo. E[t] che ongnuno sone quello ballo, & che ongnuno sone da per se. Elle di bisogno che dança sun quell'aira che sonaranno li stromenti benche elli soneno un ballo, ongnuno sonara con l'aira sua quantunca che sonassero un ballo midesimo, li pifare sonaranno in un'aira l'organo in un'aira l'arpa in un'altra aira el tamburino in un'altra aira. E[t] tucti sonaranno un ballo midesimo. Sappiate che cului |
[25ᵛ] che dança gli e bisognia de ballare con quell'aira & con quella misura & con quel tempo che sonaranno li dicti sonatori, cioe dançandolo ongnun da per se. E[t] s'el dançatore dançasse sempre con un'aira & benche dançasse a misurato & a tempo & non essendo comforma all'aira de li dicti sonatori el suo dançare seria imperfecto & e signale de non intendere.

APPENDIX II

[36ᵛ] ## BASSADANÇA FRANCESE CHIAMATA BORGES IN DOI

Imprima doi sempii & cinque doppii cominciando col pe sinestro & poi facciano doi sempii cominciando col pie sinestro & poi tornino in dirieto con tre sempii cominciando col pe dricto e[t] doi continencie sul pie sinestro & poi vagano annance con doi sempii & un doppio cominciando col pie sinestro & poi tornino in dirieto con tre sempii cominciando col pe dricto & doi continencie sul sinestro.

[50ʳ] ## BALLO CHIAMATO VOLTATI IN ÇA ROSINA IN TRI

[50ᵛ] Imprima doi doppii in misura quadernaria, & poi dagano una volta tonda pur con | doi doppii in misura quadernaria cominciando col pe sinestro & poi se parta quello di meço

EXERCISE FOR RECOGNIZING A GOOD DANCER

Get four or five kinds of instruments to play, such as *shawms, organs, lute, harp, pipe and tabor, or whatever other instrument there is. Have them play one by one, and have them play a *ballo*, and [get] each one to play that [same] *ballo*, each one playing by itself. The [dancer] must dance to that air[2] that the instruments play. For even though they are playing one [and the same] *ballo*, each one will play with his own air. [And] although they are playing the same *ballo*, the shawms will play in one air, the organ in one air, the harp in another air, the [pipe and] tabor in another air, but all will play one and the same *ballo*. Remember that the dancer must dance with that air and with that measure and with that rhythm that the said players are playing; that is, dancing each one on its own. And if the dancer always dances with one air, even though he dances with measure and in time but does not follow the air of the said players, his dancing will be imperfect and show little skill.

Choreographies and Music

FRENCH *BASSADANZA* FOR TWO CALLED *BORGES*[3]

First do two *sempii* and five *doppii* beginning with the left foot and then do two [more] *sempii* beginning with the left[4] foot and then go back with three *sempii* beginning with the right foot[5] and do two *continenze* [beginning?] on the left foot and then go forward with two *sempii* and a *doppio* beginning with the left foot and then go back with three *sempii* beginning with the right foot and do two *continenze* [beginning?] on the left.

BALLO FOR THREE CALLED *VOLTATI IN ÇA ROSINA*[6]

First do two *doppii* in *quadernaria misura*, and then make a *volta tonda* with two more *doppii* in *quadernaria misura* beginning with the left foot and then the man in the middle

---

[2] It is not clear what Giovanni Ambrosio intends here for 'air'. Professor Nino Pirrotta and others have suggested to me that the term may refer to the quality, intrinsic essence, style, or 'voice' of the single instrument.

[3] *Borges* (Bourgeois?) is the final *bassadanza* in Pa and follows *Caterva*. A similar choreography, called *bassa franzesse*, is included in NY.

[4] This should probably be the *right* foot.

[5] Here, and a little later in the dance, Giorgio substitutes three French *riprese* (*démarches*?) for the three *sempii* going back.

[6] 'Turn this way Rosina' was a very popular dance (see Ch. 2 n. 55). The NY version is for two men and a lady.

& vagha con doi sempii e[t] un doppio partendose col pe sinestro e[t] poi se ferme &
le donne facciano il simile, & in quel tempo del doppio quello di meço daga meça volta
al contrario delle donne & poi vagano al contrario l'uno di l'altro con doi tempi di
saltarello & poi se voltino & facciano doe rimprese & poi facciano una volta tonda con
un doppio e[t] poi quactro continencie sul pe sinestro e[t] poi vagano incontro l'uno
all'altro con doi sempii & un doppio & poi se tireno in dirieto, con un doppio cominciando col diricto e[t] poi dagano una volta tonda cominciando col pe sinestro & una
rimpresa sul dricto e[t] poi facciano una riverencia fino im terra & poi se levino &
facciano quatro continencie in sul pe sinestro & poi l'omo piglie la donna da la mano
diricta & vaga con quactro tempi di piva al tondo e[t] poi piglie l'altra donna da la
[51ʳ] mano sinestra & faccia il simile & poi se | movano tucti tre & vagano in piva ala guisa
d'una bissia tanto che l'omo rimanga al luocho suo cioe in meço.

BALLO CHIAMATO FIORE DE VERTU IN QUACTRO

Imprima quactro doppii im misura quadernaria. & nell'ultimo doppio li homini dagha-
no meça volta in sul pe dricto & arimanghano al contrario delle donne & poi hongnuno
piglie la donna sua per mano diricta & vadano con quactro tempi di piva al tondo e[t]
poi vaghano al contrario l'uno di l'altro con doi tempi di saltarello cominciando col pe
sinestro e[t] poi dagano meça volta sul sinestro & poi facciano doe rimprese & doi
continencie sul ͨ sinestro & poi vagano in contro l'uno al'altro passando per meço li
homini dalle donne con quactro tempi di saltarello cominciando col pie sinestro & poi
facciano una riverencia sul pe sinestro & poi vengano in contro l'uno all'altro con tre
[51ᵛ] rimprese in portogalese | in misura de bassadança cominciando col pe diricto cioe in
galone tanto che le donne se aritrovino al luoco loro & li homini facciano el simile &
poi dagano tucti quactro una volta tonda cominciando col pe diricto & una rimpresa
sul diricto & una riverencia sul sinestro & poi ongnuno piglie la donna sua con la mano
diricta con quactro tempi di piva & poi hongnuno se vada ala donna de l'uno & del
altro & vagano al tondo con quactro tempi di piva & ongnuno se vada a ritrovare la
donna sua ͩ puro al tondo con quactro tempi di piva, tanto che gli omini se trovino al
lu[o]co suo & li homini facciano un scosso e[t] le donne glie arispondano & poi se
tireno indirieto con un doppio & poi dagano una volta tonda cominciando col pe
sinestro.

ͨ *sul* is added in the margin in a similar hand.
ͩ Orig.: *suna*; n partially cancelled.

sets off and advances with two *sempii* and a *doppio* starting with the left foot and then he stops and the ladies do the same, and at the same time as the [ladies'] *doppio*[7] the man in the middle makes a *meza volta* [facing] the opposite direction to the ladies and then [all] advance in opposite directions with two *tempi* of *saltarello* and then turn and do two *riprese* and then make a *volta tonda* with a *doppio* and then do four *continenze* [beginning?] on the left foot and then advance towards one another with two *sempii* and a *doppio* and then draw back, with a *doppio* beginning with the right, and then make a *volta tonda* beginning with the left foot[8] and a *ripresa* on the right and then make a *riverenza* down to the ground and then rise and do four *continenze* [beginning?] upon the left foot and then the man takes the lady by the right hand and goes around with four *tempi* of *piva* and then he takes the other lady by the left hand and does the same and then all three move and go in *piva* [*misura*] in serpentine fashion so that the man finishes in his place that is in the middle.

BALLO FOR FOUR CALLED FIORE DE VERTU[9]

First do four *doppii* in *quadernaria misura*; and during the last *doppio* the men make a *meza volta* upon the right foot and finish [facing] in the opposite direction to the ladies and then each man takes his lady by the right hand and goes around with four *tempi* of *piva* and then [all] advance in opposite directions with two *tempi* of *saltarello* beginning with the left foot and then make a *meza volta* on the left and then do two *riprese* and two *continenze* [beginning?] on the left and then advance towards one another, the men passing between the ladies, with four *tempi* of *saltarello* beginning with the left foot and then make a *riverenza* on the left foot[10] and then advance towards one another with three Portuguese *riprese* in *bassadanza misura* beginning with the right foot,[11] that is *in galone*, so that the ladies finish in their places and the men do the same[12] and then all four make a *volta tonda* beginning with the right foot and a *ripresa* on the right and a *riverenza* on the left and then each man takes his lady by the right hand with four *tempi* of *piva* and then each man goes to the other's lady and goes around with four *tempi* of *piva* and each man goes back to his own lady [going] around again with four *tempi* of *piva*, so that the men finish in their places and the men do a *scosso* and the ladies reply and then [all?] draw back with a *doppio* and then make a *volta tonda* beginning with the left foot.

---

[7] See *Bassedanze*, n. 18.

[8] According to Giorgio's version, this *volta tonda*, like the previous one, is made with a 'turning *doppio*'.

[9] Flower of Virtue. This is the only extant choreographic description for this *ballo*, for which no music exists.

[10] A *meza volta* (and two *riprese*?) seems to be missing before the *riverenza*.

[11] Because of the steps that come before and after, this should probably read 'left foot'.

[12] It is not clear from the description if the four dancers are to finish facing each other or side by side in their starting positions, in which case the men—or ladies—must make a *meza volta*.

BALLO FRANCESE CHIAMATO AMOROSO IN DOI

Imprima octo tempi di piva cominciando col pe sinestro & poi l'omo se parta da la
[52ʳ] donna | con doi sempii & un doppio & tre sempii cominciando col pe sinestro & poi
l'homo se ferma & venga la donna appresso l'omo facendo il simile, Ancora l'homo se
parta da la donna & faccia quactro tempi de piva cominciando col pe sinestro & poy se
ferme & poi la donna vada appresso l'omo: facendo il simile ancora se parta l'omo da
la donna facendo doi sempii & un doppio cominciando col pe sinestro & ancora doi
sempii & un doppio cominciando col pe diricto & una riverencia fino in terra sul
sinestro & poi vaga al tondo con quactro tempi di piva & poi se ferme & poi la donna
vada actrovare l'homo & faccia il simile.

BALLO CHIAMATO PETIT RIENSE IN TRI FRANCESE

Imprima sedice tempi di piva & poi se fermino & poi el primo se parta con q[u]actro
[52ᵛ] tempi di piva & poi se ferme el secondo glie vada appresso facendo il simile | el terço
glie vada puro appresso facendo el simile. Ancora el primo se parte con un doppio
cominciando col pe sinestro el secondo faccia il simile el terço faccia puro el simile el
primo faccia una riverencia a quello di meço & quello di meço glia risponda & quello
ultimo faccia una riverencia a quello di meço & poi facciano tucti tre insieme una
riverencia & poi se tireno in dirieto con un doppio al contrario l'un di l'altro & poi
vengano in contro l'uno all'altro con un doppio cominciando col pe diricto & poi
facciano doe rimprese l'una sul sinestro & l'altra sul dricto & poi dagano una volta
tonda tucti tre insieme in sul pe sinestro.

FRENCH *BALLO* FOR TWO CALLED *AMOROSO*[13]

First do eight *tempi* of *piva* beginning with the left foot and then the man leaves the lady with two *sempii*[14] and a *doppio* and three *sempii* beginning with the left foot and then the man stops and the lady comes up to the man doing the same. Again the man leaves the lady and does four *tempi* of *piva*[15] beginning with the left foot and then he stops and then the lady goes up to the man doing the same; the man leaves the lady again doing two *sempii* and a *doppio* beginning with the left foot and then two more *sempii* and a *doppio* beginning with the right foot and a *riverenza* on the left [foot] right down to the ground and then [he] goes around with four *tempi* of *piva* and then [he] stops and then the lady goes up to the man and does the same.[16]

FRENCH *BALLO* FOR THREE CALLED *PETIT RIENSE*[17]

First do sixteen *tempi* of *piva* and then stop and then the first [dancer] sets off with four *tempi* of *piva* and then stops; the second goes up to him doing the same; the third goes up to him as well doing the same. Again the first sets off with a *doppio* beginning with the left foot; the second does the same; the third does the same as well; the first makes a *riverenza* to the one in the middle and the one in the middle returns it and the last one makes a *riverenza* to the one in the middle and then all three make a *riverenza* together and then draw back with a *doppio* in opposite directions to one another and then come towards one another with a *doppio* beginning with the right foot[18] and then do two *riprese*, one on the left and the other on the right, and then all three make a *volta tonda* together upon the left foot.

---

[13] Loving; a sweetheart. The Giorgio (NY) *baleto* by the same name provides interesting differences and is more detailed, particularly the ending. It is not clear if a 'French *ballo*' was a particular dance type. However, *Amoroso* and *Petit Riense* are the only *balli* entirely in *piva misura*, suggesting that the 'French *ballo*', in contrast to the *bassadanza*, may have been just that—a fast dance in *piva misura*.

[14] *Passi di natura* ('natural steps') are substituted for *sempii* throughout the Giorgio version.

[15] Giorgio has three *tempi* of *piva* and one *passo di natura*, which fits the music exactly.

[16] See Giorgio's finale in NY. A synthesis of his choreography is included with the musical transcription.

[17] Little Nothings. According to Crane, *Materials*, 92, both this title and *Petit Vriens*—the title given in the music—are similar to that of the French/Burgundian *basse danse*, *Le petit roysin*. (See also *Balli*, *Petit Rose* and n. 66.)

[18] See *Bassedanze*, n. 47.

VOLTATI IN ÇA ROSINA

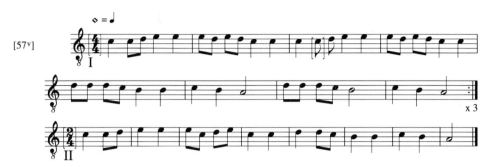

[57ᵛ]

x 3

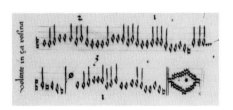

CHOREOGRAPHY

Giovanni Ambrosio (Pa)

I. mis quad [1] dddd ssd ssd
            [2] 2 t saltarello rr
                vt(d [d) or r?] cccc
            [3] ssdd vt([d])r R cccc

II. 4 t piva x2; [8 t?] piva 'in a snake'

Voltati in ça Rosina

Remarks: The melody is based on a popular tune that survives in several polyphonic compositions and a keyboard setting. It appears in the refrain of the anonymous frottola 'Poi che 'l ciel e la fortuna' (modern edition in Pirrotta, *Music and Theatre*, 98–9), in a quodlibet by L. Fogliani, and in Nicolò Pifaro's 'Per amor fata solinga'; for these and other settings see Luisi, *Apografo miscellaneo marciana*, examples 59–74. A keyboard version entitled 'Margaritum' is found in a Venetian manuscript of *c.*1520 edited by Jeppesen in *Balli antichi veneziani*.

I. The choreography specifies *quadernaria misura*. There is a discrepancy of one step-unit in the second and third playings.

II. The proportion sign ⏀ indicates a change from *quadernaria* to *piva*. The music presumably continues at the same tempo but the steps go twice as fast, one *piva doppio* per bar. Played once, this section is sufficient for 4 *tempi* of *piva* done twice. Pa does not indicate the number of *tempi* for the *piva* 'snake' figure, nor is additional music supplied. The NY version specifies 8 *tempi*, which would require another playing of this section.

AMOROSO

[58ᵛ]

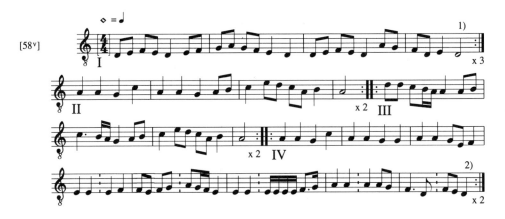

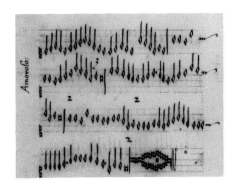

CHOREOGRAPHY

Giovanni Ambrosio (Pa)

I. 8 t piva
II. ss d sss x2
III. 4 t piva x2
IV. ssd ssd R, 4 t piva x2

Giorgio (NY)

I. 12 t piva
II. pp, 1 t piva, ppp x2
III. 3 t piva, p x2
IV. pp, 1 t piva, ppp R, 3 t piva, p x2

Amoroso

Remarks: *Amoroso* is one of the few known fifteenth-century French choreographies with music that is neither a *basse danse* nor a *pas de Brabant*. According to the NY version, the entire *ballo* is in *piva misura*, transcribed here, for easier reading only, in 4/4 rather than 2/4 ($\circ = \phi$).

I. The choreography in NY, which specifies 12 *tempi* of *piva* (rather than Pa's 8), corresponds to the playing of this section 3 times. Eight *piva doppii* require changing the repeat numeral to '2'.

III. Lacks half a bar for Pa's choreography, but fits the NY version.

IV. Pa has 9 step–units for the 8 bars of music (plus one beat from the last note). The dotted barlines follow the NY description, which fits the music exactly.

Notes on the music:
1) Orig.: *semibrevis*.
2) Orig.: *brevis*.

PETIT VRIENS

[58ᵛ]

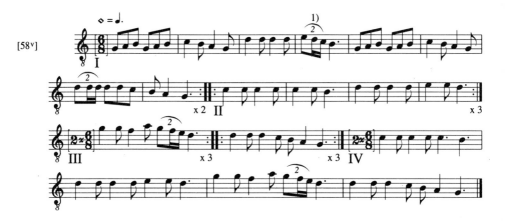

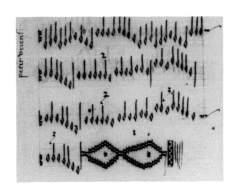

Giovanni Ambrosio (Pa)

I. 16 t piva
II. 4 t piva x3
III. 1 doppio x3; R x3(4?)
IV. dd rr vt

Petit vriens

Remarks: The choreography gives the title as *Petit Riense*.

I–II. The choreography specifies *piva misura*. For easier reading I have preferred a transcription in 6/8 rather than one in 2/4 overrun with triplets.

III. The notation does not change, but the choreography now appears to have *quadernaria* steps to *piva* music, thus requiring a different barring. See the endings of *Spero*, *Legiadra*, *Gratioso*, *Colonnese*, and [*Rostiboli*] *Gioioso*. In the second part, the choreography can be interpreted as indicating 3 or 4 *riverenze*.

IV. There is a discrepancy between the choreography—which calls for 5 or 6 *tempi* (depending upon how the *volta tonda* is performed, presumably with one *doppio* in this case)—and the music, which is 4 bars. It may be that *quadernaria riprese* performed in *piva misura* last only a half-*tempo* each, while the *doppio* remains one *tempo*. (See Pg's 'saltarello in piva fashion' in *Ingrata*, and Pd's *Tesara*.)

Note on the music:

1) This figure fits more easily into 2/4 time but does not seem to be an error.

EL GIOIOSO

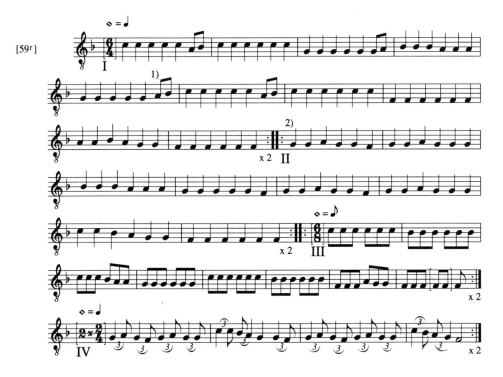

[59r]

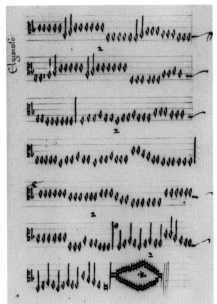

CHOREOGRAPHY

Guglielmo (Pg)

I.   rr ss dd rr ss dd x2
II. rr ss ddd vt(ssr) x2
III. 16 t saltarello
IV. 2 scossi d x2; [2 scossi] d;
     2 scossi d

[*Rostiboli*] *Gioioso*

Concordances: Found as a French/Burgundian *basse danse* in Brussels MS 9085 (*Le Manuscrit dit des basses danses*, ed. Closson) and in Toulouze, *L'Art et instruction de bien dancer*. For other concordances, see Heartz, 'A 15th-Century Ballo'.

Remarks: Entitled *El gioioso* in the music. According to Heartz (369–70), the tune was probably in 'D minor' and he suggests that in Pa it is incorrectly transcribed in 'F major'.

I–II. The step sequence suggests *bassadanza misura*.

III. ₵ indicates a proportional increase in speed and a change of *misura* to *saltarello* (specified in the choreography). It is not known if Pa intended the sign to be read in diminution, halving the value of the *semibrevis*, which would make the *saltarello* twice as fast as the *bassadanza*, and not one-third faster, as stated in Pd. There are only 7½ bars (repeated) for 16 *tempi* of *saltarello*. I have added 2 quavers and moved the final note to before, rather than after, the division line.

IV. O indicates a change of *misura*, probably to *piva*, since this section follows a scheme used in several *balli* by Guglielmo (*Spero, Colonnese, Gratioso, Legiadra*), all of which end with 2 *scossi* and one or 2 *doppii*. The steps are apparently performed in *quadernaria misura* to *piva* music, which is transcribed in 2/4 with triplets. Pg omits the second 2 *scossi*, creating a discrepancy with the music. However, NY specifies them in both the 2- and the 3-dancer versions of the *ballo*.

Notes on the music:
1) Superfluous *semibrevis* rest omitted.
2) Superfluous F omitted.

APPENDIX III

Giovanni Ambrosio's Autobiography[1]

I, GIOVANNI AMBROSIO OF PESARO, WAS PRESENT AT ALL THE FOLLOWING
FESTIVITIES OF EMPERORS, KINGS, MARQUISES, AND GREAT LORDS, AND I WAS
ALSO PRESENT AT MANY OTHER FESTIVITIES OF CITIZENS OF WHICH I WILL
MAKE NO MENTION

[1] First I was present at the nuptials of the Marquis Leonello [d'Este] who took [to wife Maria,] the daughter of King Alfonso [of Aragon], and the court festivities lasted for a month, and great jousts and great balls took place [Ferrara, 1444]. And the lord Messer Rodolfo [da Varano] took me with him and then he was betrothed to[2] Lady Camilla [d'Este; Leonello's sister].

[2] Moreover, I was present in Camerino when the lord Messer Alessandro [Sforza] was betrothed to Lady Costanza [da Varano]. And the Count of Urbino [Federico of Montefeltro] was there and a fine celebration took place [December 1444]. And up in the hall there was a servant who had killed masses of people[3] and the lord Messer Alessandro ordered that he be hung. And as they were going to the gallows to hang him that blessed soul, Lady Costanza, sent after him and she did not want him to be hung, and she granted him his life.

[3] I was also present in Pesaro when the lord Count Francesco [Sforza] and Lady Bianca [Maria Visconti Sforza] came to Pesaro [1447] and the lord Messer Alessandro [Sforza] and Lady Costanza [da Varano Sforza] honoured them most nobly and great festivities took place.

[4] Moreover, I went to Ravenna to buy grain and news arrived there of a victory won by the Signory [Francesco Sforza defeated the Venetians at Caravaggio in 1448], and a very great celebration took place. And naturally it behoved me to go and dance. A prize was offered and it was given to me; and another, similar to that, was given to the lady who danced with me. And I carried that prize up the mast of the ship.[4] And the prize was a beautiful silk handkerchief, a little ring, and a purse.

---

[1] The Italian text is given in Gallo, 'L'autobiografia'. See there for the dating of the events, for the numbering of the entries, and for most of the additional information in square brackets. Throughout the Autobiography, the verb *fare* (to make, to do) is used to indicate the 'taking place', offering, preparing, arranging, performing, giving, and serving of a repast, festivity, *moresca*, etc., and is so translated.

[2] The verb *sposare* (to marry or to betroth, Florio) is used here, rather than the usual *nozze* (nuptials). Since in entry [11] *sposare* refers to betrothal, apparently the case in [2] as well, it is possible that here too it means the same.

[3] In the phrase 'un fameglio che taglio parecchie macci de centi', the last three words, as they appear here, do not mean anything. My translation is based on a reading of the words as 'massi de genti'.

[4] At jousts, according to Tuohy, 'Studies' (ch. 7), prizes were the most expensive items budgeted for, their value varying according to the occasion. Most were in the form of cloth for clothing (the word *palio* originally meant a robe and came to mean a prize for a race). Giovanni

[5] I was also present when the lord Messer Alessandro [Sforza] took his other wife [Sveva Colonna of Montefeltro], and a fine wedding pageant and a fine celebration took place [Pesaro, 1448].

[6] Moreover, I was present at the nuptials of Messer Sante del Bentivogli[o], when we accompanied Lady Ginevra [Alessandro Sforza's daughter], and the festivities lasted three days [Bologna, 1454]; and I never saw finer repasts or finer refreshments or greater ceremony. And the platters of boiled meat, that is, the capons, were in [the form of] his device.[5] And, moreover, around the tables there were peacocks whose feathers and spread tails seemed like curtains in that hall.

[7] I was also present at the nuptials of [Giovanna,] the daughter of Virgilio Malvezzi, who married into the Piattesi family of Ferrara [Bologna, 1454].

[8] Moreover, I was present at the nuptials of the Count of Urbino [Federico of Montefeltro], who took to wife [Battista,] the daughter of the lord Messer Alessandro [Sforza; Urbino, 1460].

[9] I was also present in Forlì with Messer Domenico [da Piacenza] at the nuptials of the lord of Forlì [Pino Ordelaffi], who took to wife [Barbara Manfredi,] the daughter of the lord of Faenza, and a noble celebration took place [1462].

[10] Moreover, I was present when Duke Francesco [Sforza] made his entry into Milan and was made Duke [1450]. And the jousts and the dancing and the great festivities lasted a month. And I saw two hundred knights dubbed. And I understood Giovanni of Castel Nova [Castelnuovo?][6] and Giovanni Chiapa to say to the lord Messer Alessandro [Sforza][7] that ten thousand people sat down to table when the trumpet sounded and all of them were in the court.[8]

[11] Moreover, I was present when a most noble celebration took place when the Duchess of Calabria [Ippolita Sforza] was betrothed in Milan [1455].[9] And I understood the lord Messer Alessandro [Sforza] to say that the festivities cost 63,000 ducats.[10] And I was present with Messer Domenico [da Piacenza] and we performed *moresche* and many *balli*.[11] And many ambassadors from all the provinces were there.

[12] I was also present at a great celebration in Milan when the Duke [John] of Clèves came, when the Pope [Pius II] went to Mantua [1459]. And Duke Francesco [Sforza] did him the greatest honour, and on every occasion he was accompanied in

Ambrosio is here, as elsewhere, too condensed to provide unambiguous meaning. Did he climb the mast and tie his handkerchief there, or was it from the mast that he retrieved the prize? On St George's day in Ferrara, the *palio* was hung on a stake. On another occasion there was a child on top of a mast, and when the challenge was won, a ring was given as a prize (Tuohy).

[5] J. Gage, *Life in Italy at the Time of the Medici* (London and New York, 1968), 141, cites the banquet given in honour of Eleonora of Aragon by Cardinal Riario in 1473 (see Ch. 3 n. 30), during which 'a capon in gelatine forming the coat of arms of the Cardinal' was served.

[6] Could this be Giovanni Bentivoglio of entry [14]?

[7] Here, and in entry [11], it is not at all clear from the original Italian if the 'hearsay' is being said by, or to, Alessandro. It is also conceivable in this instance that it is being said by, or to, all three. For reports based on hearsay, see Ch. 1 n. 39.

[8] This may mean 'in the courtyard', i.e. within the castle walls. Compare with entries [27] and [30].

[9] For Ippolita's marriage, see entry [17].

[10] For the value of ducats, see Ch. 2 n. 41.

[11] The original is *fare* [to make or do] *moresche e molti balli*. It is unclear whether *fare* means to choreograph and/or perform, and whether *balli* refers to the specific dance type or to dances in general. See also [26].

the dance by the entire court. And he stayed three days. The first day he wore a cloak that was reckoned at 60,000 ducats[12] and it was covered entirely with pearls and jewels. The second day he wore a gold chain with a large jewel which was worth a great fortune. The third day he dressed in the Italian fashion and all the garments he wore belonged to Duke Francesco.

[13] I was also present at a most noble festivity in Milan of a German lady who came there with five ladies-in-waiting on her way to the Pope [Pius II] in Mantua [1459]. And Duke Francesco [Sforza] gave her Lord Messer Alessandro [Sforza] to keep her company there in Milan.

[14] And, moreover, I was present at the nuptials of Messer Tiberto Brandolino, who took to wife [Cornelia Manfredi,] the sister of the lord of Imola [Imola, 1458]. And we also went to Bologna and he took [Antonia Bentivoglio,] the sister of Messer Giovanni dei Bentivogli, as his daughter-in-law, and we brought her to Castel Novo [Castelnuovo, Forlì?] and we took part in very great festivities. And in Parma one of his swordsmen, brawling, thrust his sword at one of his chamber grooms, who died on the spot, and his head was speedily cut off.

[15] I was also present in Milan with Lord Costanzo [Sforza] at a very great celebration when Duke Francesco [Sforza] was made lord of Genoa [1464]. And Papi made a great dragon and a great balloon [which floated] in the air and sent forth fire and birds, and everyone was delighted by it all.

[16] Moreover, I was present in Milan at a very great celebration, and I was with the lord Messer Alessandro [Sforza] when Duke Francesco [Sforza] went to Mantua to see the Pope [Pius II; 1459]. And we were more than sixty ships, what with the bucentaurs[13] and galleons and barges, all covered with velvet and tapestries, and with flags full of gold trimming. And the lord Messer Alessandro had to cover two of them all in silk.

[17] I was also present in Naples at the nuptials of the Duke of Calabria [Alfonso of Aragon], and a most noble celebration took place and, above all, the finest repast that I ever saw [1465]. I remained with His Majesty the King for two years and saw fine celebrations and fine repasts prepared. With every dish of the repast there was a castle, and likewise there was a horse, and likewise a dove with gold streamers, and these things were all of sugar and were in the middle of the dish of sweetmeats. And when half the repast was over, the leavings were open to all comers, as is the custom in this place.

[18] Moreover, I was present in Padua at the nuptials of one of Messer Andrea Dandro's [sic][14] sons [Girolamo Dandolo], who took [to wife Endea Malatesta,] the daughter of Lord Galeazzo of Pesaro, and a most noble celebration took place [1459]. And, moreover, the entire Council of Venice was present and never was there a more gracious sight than to see all the gentlemen proceed two by two up the square of Padua

[12] Tuohy, 'Studies' (18–20) points out that 'Price evaluation . . . seems to have been a polite and fairly normal practice for princes . . .'. Estimating the value of gifts, for example, provided 'considerable scope for inaccuracy as well as flattery' and was 'essential in order to gauge the degree of magnificence'. See also entry [30].

[13] Venetian state barges.

[14] Andrea Dandolo was a military and political leader whose noble family, particularly important in the 12th to 14th cc., gave Venice four doges.

with those long robes of crimson velvet, and of black velvet as well, which reached the ground. And this was when they accompanied the bride to the church, and the square was a vision of paradise.

[19] I was also present at the nuptials of Duke Galeazzo [Maria Sforza], who took [to wife Bona of Savoy,] the Duchess who came from France [Milan, 1468]; and the Count of Urbino [Federico of Montefeltro] and many other lords were there.

[20] Moreover, I was present in Venice when the Emperor [Frederick III] came, and the festivities that took place were the most noble that I ever saw in all my lifetime [1469]; in particular, the galleys, barges, bucentaurs, all covered with tapestries; and they went to meet the Emperor with pipes and trumpets [shawms and sackbuts]. And the Signory arranged dancing one evening and I organized a most noble entertainment of a livery [set] of masques[15] with new *balli*. And on that evening I was knighted. And in all Christendom there never took place a finer celebration or a finer repast.

[21] I was also present another evening at the house of the Priuli[16] in Venice, and the Emperor [Frederick III] came there and a most noble repast took place [1469].

[22] Moreover, I was present at the nuptials of [Federico Gonzaga,] the son of the Marquis of Mantua, [and Margaret of Bavaria,] where, for pleasure, there were two Germans who ran a fair and honest race[17] and one of them fell dead. And many barrels of wine were placed in all the streets so that everyone might refresh his mouth [Mantua, 1463]. And this suffices.

[23] I was also present at a fine celebration which took place in Urbino where the family alliances of Lord Roberto [Malatesta] were consolidated when he took [as his betrothed] the most Illustrious Lady Elisabetta, daughter of the most Illustrious lord [Federico of Montefeltro], Count of Urbino [1471]. And I prepared a fine livery [set] of masques, and other fine ones were also performed. And worthy repasts took place, and as a remembrance I was sick abed for eight days.

[24] Moreover, I was present in Pesaro when the most Illustrious lord, Messer Alessandro [Sforza], arranged many very grand Carnival festivities. And in particular he offered a repast which was the most noble and well-ordered that was ever offered in Christendom. And he offered this repast to his citizens and it took place on Shrove Tuesday [1471]. Anyone wishing to write it all would be long a-writing; but we will write a few particulars. The said repast lasted from morning till after the twenty-second hour of the evening,[18] and some eighteen courses were served, and a salad went with every four courses. And all the roasts were covered in gold. More than a thousand pounds of sweetmeats and marzipan were thrown upon the table, so that there were ladies who carried [off] twenty pounds of sweetmeats. And the floor of the hall was entirely covered in sweetmeats. And then there was dancing, and liveries of maskers came and they bore great flames upon their heads which were wounds of love. The

---

[15] See *liverea* in Glossary.

[16] The Priuli, a noble family dating back to 1110, gave Venice three doges.

[17] The original reads 'che per piacere foro doi todeschi che cursero a ferri puliti'. 'A ferri puliti', according to Crusca, and Battaglia and Squarotti, *Grande dizionario*, was a 15th-c. idiom meaning 'open; unfeigned'. Using the same sources, it is also possible to interpret the phrase as: the two Germans 'contended with clean [naked, unbated, unsheathed?] arms [swords, lances, knives, etc.]'. Presumably the 'for pleasure' refers to that of the onlookers.

[18] The first hour of the 24 was calculated as starting either at sundown or at dawn, and so varied according to the season.

evening when the festivities came to an end, the Illustrious lord [Alessandro], with his own hands, presented all the ladies one by one with a grand new torch and a glass goblet full of sweetmeats. And there were a hundred ladies or thereabouts and they were accompanied to their homes to the sound of pipes [shawms] with great ceremony and with great mirth. FINIS.

[25] I was also present in Urbino when the most Illustrious lord [Federico of Montefeltro,] Count of Urbino, did very great honour to the lord Don Al[f]onso [d'Avalos; 1460]. And he arranged two days of Carnival festivities and liveries of masques and a great deal of dancing took place.

[26] I was also present in Pavia with Duke Francesco [Sforza] and with Lady Bianca [Maria Visconti Sforza] and a most noble celebration took place there [1460]. And I was told that I had to perform a fine *moresca*. And this I did. And a fine repast took place, and during that repast they were presented with a large cage of hammered silver and enamel with a woodlark inside which sang.

[27] Moreover, I was present at a great reception that Duke Francesco [Sforza] gave in Milan for the arrival of an ambassador of the King of France [Louis XI; 1460]; and many gentlewomen of Milan were invited to it and a great deal of dancing took place. And that day a man walked on a rope and danced with clogs on his feet. And the rope was as high as the cathedral of Milan, and he danced to the sound of pipes [shawms]. And so many were the people who stood watching that they were reckoned eighty thousand souls, and all were [with]in the court.

[28] And, moreover, I was present at the port of Pesaro when the lord Messer Alessandro [Sforza] arranged dancing and a fine entertainment, and there were many ladies from Pesaro there [1469]. And on that evening there was a Greek who had himself bound hands and feet; and he had himself put into a sack with a crossbow. Then he had three people tightly fasten the opening of the sack, and he had himself put into a boat and thrown into the sea. Two crossbow shots and suddenly out he came with the crossbow loaded, and he shot a green finch and came to no harm. FINIS.

[29] I was also present at the nuptials of Messer Carlo [Manfredi] of Faenza, who took to wife the daughter of the lord Messer Rodolfo [da Varano] of Camerino [1471]. And the court festivities lasted for three days and great jousts took place and great gifts were offered. And there were so many gifts that the lord did not want to accept them because they began to weary him. And the bride arrived on horseback in great pomp and the lord went to meet her and married her on horseback. And when the lord went to meet her a fair company of citizens and of ladies of the court, dressed in velvet and cloth of silver, went with him. And here a fine lot of dancing took place and some fine *moresche* were performed. Moreover, such was the magnanimity of this lord that he presented coin and cloth for clothing worth 500 ducats to those of his household who had been long in his service.[19] And during the festivities there was a tumbler upon a very high rope, and he fell down and smashed to pieces and died at once.

[30] Moreover, I was present in Naples when His Majesty the lord King [Ferdinando I of Aragon (Ferrante)] did great honour to the ambassador of the Duke of Burgundy

---

[19] According to Tuohy, 'Studies', ch. 4, a prince needed to dress his court suitably if he wished to appear magnificent. (His own apparel reflected his wealth and status: see [12].) For weddings —and other special occasions—new clothes were provided for all those of his 'household' who would appear in public. See entry [30].

[Charles the Bold], and never in all Christendom was there grander pomp than took place then [1474[20]].

First, each and every one of the lords and gentlemen of the realm offered a repast and this repast lasted from the morning till the evening. And then, after the repast, every one of them offered him presents: some offered coursers and some jewels and some mules and some one thing and some another.

The repast of the Duke of Calabria [Alfonso of Aragon] went this way. The aforesaid repast was organized the evening of Shrove Tuesday and began at the second hour after sunset and lasted until the morning Angelus. And all the platters that came with every course were covered with silver castles and with life[-like] peacocks and roe deer. And that meat seemed real enough to eat. And, moreover, on the aforesaid platters [there were] lambs and eagles reproduced in silver. Never was such magnificence seen, and I was dumbfounded to see such magnanimity. Now came a fish course, now came a meat course and all sorts of salads; that is, galantine of fish, galantine of meat, and white galantines and red galantines and green galantines and all sorts of galantines. And when it was close upon midnight and Lent was about to begin, all meat was taken away. And then came many large fish prepared in many ways. I will be brief; long would be the writing if I were to recount everything. And then in the middle of the repast the Duke of Calabria and Don Federico [of Aragon, his brother,] came with a mummery of maskers dressed in the French fashion; that is, in cloth of gold down to the hem with an ermine flounce. One sleeve was of gray damask—embroidered—and it almost touched the ground. And French dances were performed there during the repast itself with Lady [Ippolita Sforza,] Duchess [of Calabria], and with Lady [E]Leonora [of Aragon, her sister-in-law]. And then the Duke of Calabria presented [the Duke of Burgundy's ambassador with] seven large coursers, and there were two of them entirely covered in gold; and he was [also] given a lance with fifty rubies or else diamonds [set] round about, beginning at the tip of the lance; and each was reckoned at 10 ducats and the lance was worth 500 ducats. And then, from word to deed, the Duke of Calabria disrobed and gave those garments of gold cloth to the drummers. And this was the Duke of Calabria's repast.

This was the hunt of the Astroni,[21] the finest that ever took place in Naples [1474?], and mark everything well: More than twenty thousand persons were present at the hunt and there were more than five thousand hunters. And one hundred twenty-three animals were caught, so that His Majesty the lord King [Ferrante] and the Duke of Calabria [Alfonso of Aragon] were tired of killing so many animals, and they gave permission to everyone to kill the aforesaid animals; and one hundred ten boars and nine very large stags and three large wolves and two roe deer died. And in the morning all the game was put on to one hundred twenty-three mules with flowers and herbs, and they went throughout Naples with all the dogs and all the hunters sounding their horns. And never was such lordliness and such finery seen, and it was as if the heavens had opened, such was the noise of the dogs and of the horns played by the hunters. And this was the hunt, as is recounted.

This was the finest joust that ever took place in Naples many years ago [1474?], and it was held in the saddlery, and mark well: All those lords came very richly [clad] and

---

[20] See Ch. 2 and n. 40 for doubts about the accuracy of Gallo's dating.
[21] The Astroni family had their own game preserve.

in array, with many paraments, and they made a great breaking of lances; and it was a lordly thing to see the shafts of those lances fly through the air. And there were many thousands of people watching. And there were four champions defending their championship.[22] And Don Federico [of Aragon] won the prize for the joust. And when the ambassador of the Duke of Burgundy took leave of His Majesty the lord King, Messer Carlino, ambassador of the Duke of Milan at the time, gave—or rather, presented—three fine coursers and three fine gerfalcons; and he presented this present on behalf of the Duke of Milan [Galeazzo Maria Sforza?], and this took place in the middle of the courtyard of Castello Nuovo. And he was dressed in silver cloth with a doublet of crimson satin. And all the grooms and household servants and lads were dressed in velvet, and likewise wore short silver doublets. And when they entered that courtyard it was such a lordly sight to see them advance that everyone commented on it.

And when the aforesaid ambassador took his leave from His Majesty the lord King, he gave many chains to the King's gentlemen [to wear about their necks]; and the Duchess of Calabria [Ippolita Sforza] and the King's daughter [probably Eleonora or Beatrice] gave the ambassador many presents. Long would be the writing if I intended to report all the presents which were given to him and the things that came to pass, inasmuch as the value of the presents given to him was reckoned at 15,000 ducats. And these were the presents.

---

[22] '. . . quactro tavoliere che tenevano tavole' is another problematic phrase, particularly since Crusca is incomplete and the Battaglia dictionary has not yet reached the letter 'T'. According to Tuohy, 'Studies', 202, *tavolieri* and *tegnire tavoli* meant the 'defenders' in a joust, hence the translation given. (Is it also possible that *tavolieri* were marshals who kept account of the joust?) Tuohy also explains that 'holding tables' was a chivalric allusion to King Arthur's table.

BIBLIOGRAPHY

APEL, WILLI, *The Notation of Polyphonic Music 900–1600* (Cambridge, Mass.: Mediaeval Academy of America, 1953).

ABATI-OLIVIERI GIORDANI, ANNIBALE DEGLI, *Memorie di Alessandro Sforza signore di Pesaro* (Pesaro: Gavelli, 1785).

ATLAS, ALLAN W., *Music at the Aragonese Court of Naples* (Cambridge: Cambridge University Press, 1985).

BATTAGLIA, S., and SQUAROTTI, G. B., (eds.), *Grande dizionario della lingua italiana*, 14 (A–R) vols. (Turin: UTET, 1960–).

BAXANDALL, MICHAEL, *Painting and Experience in Fifteenth Century Italy* (Oxford: Oxford University Press, 1972).

BIANCHI, DANTE, 'Tre maestri di danza alla corte di Francesco Sforza', *ASL* 89 (1962), 290–9. Dated and unreliable.

BITTARELLI, A. A., *Camerino* (Camerino: Mierma, 1985).

BRAGAGLIA, ANTON GIULIO, *Danze popolari italiane* (Rome: ENAL, 1950).

BRAINARD, INGRID, *The Art of Courtly Dancing in the Early Renaissance* (West Newton, Mass.: I. G. Brainard, 1981). Contains a great deal of personal interpretation.

—— 'The Art of Courtly Dancing in Transition: Nürnberg, Germ. Nat. Mus. MS. 8842, a Hitherto Unknown German Source', in Edelgard E. DuBruck and Karl Heinz Göller (eds.), *Crossroads of Medieval Civilization: The City of Regensburg and its Intellectual Milieu* (Medieval and Renaissance Monograph Series, 5; 1984), 61–79.

BUKOFZER, MANFRED, 'A Polyphonic Basse Dance of the Renaissance', in *Studies in Medieval and Renaissance Music* (New York: Norton, 1950), 190–216.

CALDWELL, JOHN, 'Early Keyboard Tablatures and Medieval Dance Theory', in *Atti del XIV Congresso della Società Internazionale di Musicologia: Trasmissione e recezione delle forme di cultura musicale*, ed. A. Pompilio, D. Restani, L. Bianconi, F. A. Gallo, 3 vols. (Turin: Edizioni di Torino, 1990), iii. 681–6.

CALMO, ANDREA, *Le lettere di Messer Andrea Calmo* (1563), ed. V. Rossi (Turin: Loescher, 1888).

CASTELLI, PATRIZIA, 'La kermesse degli Sforza pesaresi', in Castelli *et al.*, *Mesura et arte*, 13–33.

—— 'Il moto aristotelico e la "licita scientia": Guglielmo Ebreo e la speculazione sulla danza nel XV secolo', in Castelli *et al.*, *Mesura et arte*, 35–57.

—— Mingardi, Maurizio, and Padovan, Maurizio (eds.), *Mesura et arte del danzare. Guglielmo Ebreo da Pesaro e la danza nelle corti italiane del XV secolo* (Pesaro: Gualtieri, 1987).

CASTIGLIONE, BALDASSARE, *The Book of the Courtier* (1528), tr. G. Bull (Harmondsworth: Penguin Books, 1967, repr. 1976).

CLOSSON, ERNEST (ed.), *Le Manuscrit dit des basses danses de la Bibliothèque de Bourgogne* (Brussels, 1912; fac. repr. Geneva: Minkoff, 1975).

CORNAZANO, ANTONIO, *Proverbi di messer Antonio Cornazano in facetie* (fac. of 1865 edn., Bologna: Forni, 1968).

CRANE, FREDERICK, 'The Derivation of Some Fifteenth-Century Basse-Danse Tunes', *Acta musicologica*, *37* (1965), 179–88.

—— *Materials for the Study of the Fifteenth Century Basse Danse* (New York: Institute of Medieval Music, 1968).

CRUCIANI, FABRIZIO, *Teatro nel Rinascimento Roma 1450–1550* (Rome: Bulzoni, 1983).

DE MARINIS, TAMMARO, *Le nozze di Costanzo Sforza e Camilla d'Aragona celebrate a Pesaro nel 1475* (Florence: Vallecchi–Alinari, 1946).

EICHE, SABINE, 'Towards a Study of the "Famiglia" of the Sforza Court at Pesaro', *Renaissance and Reformation*, 9 (1985), 79–103.

—— 'Alessandro Sforza and Pesaro: A Study in Urbanism and Architectural Patronage', Ph.D. thesis (Princeton, NJ, 1982).

FRANKO, MARK, *The Dancing Body in Renaissance Choreography* (Birmingham, AL: Summa, 1986). Information on Italian dance is unreliable.

GAGE, JOHN, *Life in Italy at the Time of the Medici* (London: B. T. Batsford Ltd., and New York: G. P. Putnam's Sons, 1968).

GALLO, F. ALBERTO, 'L'autobiografia artistica di Giovanni Ambrosio (Guglielmo Ebreo) da Pesaro', *Studi musicali*, 12 (1983), 189–202.

—— 'Il "ballare lombardo" (circa 1435–1475)', *Studi musicali*, 8 (1979), 61–84.

—— 'La danza negli spettacoli conviviali del secondo quattrocento', in *Spettacoli conviviali dall'antichità classica alle corti italiane del '400* (Rome: Nuova Coletti Editore, 1982), 261–7.

GOMBOSI, OTTO, 'About Dance and Dance Music in the Late Middle Ages', *Musical Quarterly*, 27 (1941), 289–305.

—— *Compositione di Messer Vincenzo Capirola* (Société de musique d'autrefois: Neuilly-sur-Seine, 1955).

GREGOROVIUS, FERDINAND, *Lucrezia Borgia* (1874; Italian edn. Bologna: Avanzini e Torraca, 1968).

HEARTZ, DANIEL, 'The Basse Dance. Its Evolution circa 1450 to 1550', *Annales musicologiques*, 6 (1958–63), 287–340.

—— 'Hoftanz and Basse Dance', *JAMS* 19 (1966), 13–36.

—— 'A 15th-Century Ballo: *Rôti Bouilli Joyeux*, in Jan La Rue et al. (eds.), *Aspects of Medieval and Renaissance Music: A Birthday Offering to Gustave Reese* (New York: Norton, 1966), 359–75.

ILARDI, VINCENT, 'The Assassination of Galeazzo Maria Sforza and the Reaction of Italian Diplomacy', in Lauro Martines (ed.), *Violence and Civil Disobedience in Italian Cities: 1200–1500* (Berkeley, Calif.: University of California Press, 1972), 72–103.

INGLEHEARN, MADELEINE, and FORSYTH, PEGGY, *The Book on the Art of Dancing. Antonio Cornazano* (London: Dance Books Ltd., 1981). I do not always agree with the translation. The reader is urged to consult the original.

—— 'A Little-Known Fifteenth-Century Italian Dance Treatise', *Music Review*, 42 (1981), 174–81.

JEPPESEN, KNUD (ed.), *Balli antichi veneziani/Old Venetian Dances* (Copenhagen: Wilhelm Hansen, 1962).

KINKELDEY, OTTO, 'Dance Tunes of the Fifteenth Century', in D. G. Hughes (ed.), *Instrumental Music: A Conference at Isham Memorial Library* (Cambridge, Mass.: Harvard University Press, 1959), 3–30 and 89–152.

—— 'A Jewish Dancing Master of the Renaissance', in *Studies in Jewish Bibliography . . .*

in Memory of Abraham Solomon Freidus (New York: The Alexander Kohut Memorial Foundation, 1929). Repr. as *A Jewish Dancing Master of the Renaissance: Guglielmo Ebreo* (Brooklyn, NY: Dance Horizons, 1966). Dated, but interesting, as Kinkeldey was the first in the field.

LAWLER, LILLIAN B., *The Dance in Ancient Greece* (Middletown, Conn.: Wesleyan University Press, 1964).

LOCKWOOD, LEWIS, *Music in Renaissance Ferrara* (Oxford: Oxford University Press, 1984).

LITTA, POMPEO, *Famiglie celebri di Italia* (Milan: P. E. Giusti, 1819–83).

LO MONACO, MAURO, and VINCIGUERRA, SERGIO, 'Il passo doppio in Guglielmo e Domenico. Problemi di mensurazione', in *Guglielmo Ebreo*, 127–36.

LOPEZ, GUIDO, *Festa di nozze per Ludovico il Moro, nelle testimonianze di Tristano Calco, Giacomo Trotti ed altri* (Milan: De Carlo, 1976).

LUISI, FRANCESCO, *Apografo Miscellaneo Marciano. Frottole canzoni e madrigali con alcuni alla pavana in villanesco (Edizione critica integrale mss. marc. it. cl. IV, 1795–1798)* (Venice: Fondazione Levi, 1979).

LUZIO, ALESSANDRO, and RENIER, RODOLFO, *Mantova e Urbino: Isabella d'Este ed Elisabetta Gonzaga* (Turin and Rome, 1893; repr. Bologna: Forni, 1976).

MAGNANI, RACHELE, *Relazioni private fra la corte sforzesca di Milano e casa Medici 1450–1500* (Milan: San Giuseppe, 1910).

MARROCCO, W. THOMAS, *Inventory of 15th Century Bassedanze, Balli & Balletti* (New York: Congress on Research in Dance, 1981).

MARTINES, LAURO, *Power and Imagination* (Baltimore: The Johns Hopkins University Press, 1979; repr. 1988).

McGEE, TIMOTHY J., 'Dancing Masters and the Medici Court in the 15th Century', *Studi musicali*, 17 (1988), 201–24.

MINGARDI, MAURIZIO, 'Gli strumenti musicali nella danza del XIV e XV secolo', in Castelli *et al.*, *Mesura et arte*, 113–55.

MOTTA, EMILIO, 'Musici alla corte degli Sforza', *ASL* 4 (1887), 29–64.

—— *Nozze principesche nel quattrocento* (Milan: Fratelli Rivara, 1894).

OSTHOFF, WOLFGANG, *Theatergesang und darstellende Musik in der italienischen Renaissance*, 2 vols. (Tutzing: Hans Schneider, 1969).

PADOVAN, MAURIZIO, 'Da Dante a Leonardo: la danza italiana attraverso le fonti storiche', *La danza italiana*, 3 (1985), 5–37.

—— (ed.) *Guglielmo Ebreo da Pesaro e la danza nelle corti italiane del XV secolo (Atti del Convegno Internazionale di Studi, Pesaro 16/18 luglio 1987*; Pisa: Pacini, 1990).

—— 'Guglielmo Ebreo da Pesaro e i maestri del XV secolo', in Castelli *et al.*, *Mesura et arte*, 77–86.

PALISCA, CLAUDE V., *Humanism in Italian Renaissance Musical Thought* (New Haven and London: Yale University Press, 1984).

PESCERELLI, BEATRICE, 'Una sconosciuta redazione del trattato di danza di Guglielmo Ebreo', *Rivista italiana di musicologia*, 9 (1974), 48–55.

PELLEGRIN, E., *Supplement [of La Bibliothèque des Visconti et des Sforza . . .]* (Florence: L. S. Olschki, and Paris: F. de Noble, 1969).

PIRROTTA, NINO, '*Dulcedo e subtilitas* nella pratica polifonica franco-italiana al principio del Quattrocento', in *Musica tra Medioevo e Rinascimento* (Turin: Einaudi, 1984), 130–41.

—— *Music and Culture in Italy from the Middle Ages to the Baroque* (Cambridge, Mass.: Harvard University Press, 1984).

—— and Povoledo, Elena, *Music and Theatre from Poliziano to Monteverdi*, tr. K. Eales (Cambridge: Cambridge University Press, 1982).

POLIDORI CALAMANDREI, E., *Le vesti delle donne fiorentine nel quattrocento* (Rome: Multigrafica Editrice, 1973).

PONTREMOLI, ALESSANDRO, and LA ROCCA, PATRIZIA, *Il ballare lombardo* (Milan: Vita e Pensiero, 1987).

ROSSI, VITTORIO (ed.), *Un ballo a Firenze nel 1459* (Milan: Istituto Italiano d'Arti Grafiche, 1885).

SAVIOTTI, ALFREDO, 'Una rappresentazione allegorica in Urbino nel 1474', *Atti e memorie della R. Accademia Petrarca di Scienze, Lettere ed Arti in Arezzo*, I (1920), 180–236.

SMITH, A. WILLIAM, 'Studies in 15th-Century Italian Dance: *Belriguardo in due*; A Critical Discussion', in *Society of Dance History Scholars Proceedings* (1987), 86–105. Contains much questionable interpretation.

—— 'Una fonte sconosciuta della danza italiana del Quattrocento', in *Guglielmo Ebreo*, 71–84.

SOLMI, EDMONDO, 'La Festa del Paradiso di Leonardo da Vinci e Bernardo Bellincione', *ASL* I (1904), 75–89.

SOUTHERN, EILEEN, 'A Prima Ballerina of the Fifteenth Century', in A. D. Shapiro (ed.), *Music and Context: Essays for John M. Ward* (Cambridge, Mass.: Harvard University Press, 1985).

—— 'Basse-Dance Music in some German Manuscripts of the 15th Century', in Jan La Rue *et al.* (eds.), *Aspects of Medieval and Renaissance Music* (New York: Norton, 1966), 738–55.

—— 'Some Keyboard Basse Dances of the Fifteenth Century', *Acta musicologica*, 35 (1963), 114–24.

—— *The Buxheim Organ Book* (Musicological Studies 6; Institute of Medieval Studies: Brooklyn, NY, 1963).

SPARTI, BARBARA, 'The 15th-century *Balli* Tunes: A New Look', *Early Music*, 14 (1986), 346–57.

—— 'Stile, espressione e senso teatrale nelle danze italiane del '400', *La danza italiana*, 3 (1985), 39–53.

—— 'Style and Performance in the Social Dances of the Italian Renaissance: Ornamentation, Improvisation, Variation, and Virtuosity', in *Society of Dance History Scholars Proceedings* (1986), 31–52.

SPENCER, JOHN R. (ed. and tr.), *Leon Battista Alberti 'On Painting'* (New Haven, Conn., and London: Yale University Press, 1966).

TARTINI, G. M. (ed.), 'Ricordi di Firenze 1459', in *Rerum italicarum scriptores*, ed. L. A. Muratori, 27, pt. I (repr. Città di Castello, 1907).

TINCTORIS, JOHANNES, *Terminorum musicae diffinitorium* (c.1495); tr. and annotated by Carl Parrish (London and New York: The Free Press of Glencoe, 1963).

TOSCANINI, WALTER, 'Notizie e appunti sui maestri di ballo ebrei nel '400', *Il Vasari*, 18 (1960), 62–71.

TOULOUZE, MICHEL (publisher), *L'Art et instruction de bien dancer* (Paris, c.1488; fac. edn. London, 1936; repr. New York: Dance Horizons, and East Ardsley, Wakefield: Scholar Press, Ltd., 1971).

TUOHY, THOMAS J., 'Studies in Domestic Expenditures at the Court of Ferrara (Artistic Patronage and Princely Magnificence)', Ph.D. thesis (Warburg Institute, 1982).

VERONESE, ALESSANDRA, 'Una societas ebraico-cristiana in *docendo tripudiare ac cantare* nella Firenze del Quattrocento', in *Guglielmo Ebreo*, 51–8.

WARD, JOHN, 'The manner of dauncying', *Early Music*, 4 (1976), 127–42.

WHALLEY, J. I., and KADEN, V. C., *The Universal Penman* (London: H.M. Stationery Office, 1980).

WILSON, D. R., *Domenico of Piacenza (Paris, Bibliothèque Nationale, MS ital. 972)* (Cambridge: The Early Dance Circle, 1988).

WINTERNITZ, EMANUEL, *Leonardo da Vinci as a Musician* (New Haven, Conn.: Yale University Press, 1982).

WOODWARD, WILLIAM H., *Vittorino da Feltre and Other Humanist Educators* (Cambridge: Cambridge University Press, 1897; repr. Teachers College, Columbia Univ., 1963/1970).

YATES, FRANCES A., *The Art of Memory* (Chicago: University of Chicago Press, 1966).

ZAMBRINI, FRANCESCO (ed.), *Trattato dell'arte del ballo di Guglielmo Ebreo pesarese* (Bologna, 1873; repr. Bologna: Forni, 1968).

Page numbers in italics indicate Glossary definitions, choreographic descriptions and music of the dances, and pertinent chapters or sections in Guglielmo's treatise. All references to pages in the treatise are to both the Italian and the English texts.

air (*aire*) 11 n. 25, *96*, *97*, 116, 117, *217*, 234, 235 and n. 2
  airy, 104, 105
Alberti, Leon Battista 9 n. 21, 10 and n. 23, 11 n. 25, 12 n. 26, 15–16 n. 39, 44 n. 58, 69 n. 20
allegory 7 n. 14, 37, 54–5, 56 and n. 30, see also *moresche*
Alexandresca 37 n. 38, *126*, *127*, *128*, *129*, 227
Amoroso 58 n. 43, 67, 223, *238*, *239*, *242—3*
Anello 160, 161, 162, 163
Angelosa (Tangelosa) 14 n. 36, 58 n. 43
antiquity, influence of, on 15th-century dance 3 n. 1, 9 n. 21, 10, 11, 54 n. 22, 55, 56 n. 30
  references to, in *De pratica* 86–9, 172–7
  see also instruments; Jews, Old Testament
anti-semitism, see Jews; violence
Aragons of Naples 212, 213, 214, *215–16*
  Alfonso I, King of Naples 215, 248
  Alfonso II, Duke of Calabria 4, 20 n. 59, 23, 25, 29, 37, 212, 215, 216, 250, 253
  Beatrice 31, 32, 215, 254
  Camilla 25, 32 n. 21, 38, 42, 55–6, 213, 214, 215
  (E)Leonora 31, 32 n. 20, 37, 38 n. 42, 56 n. 30, 212, 215, 216, 249 n. 5, 253, 254
  Federico 37–8, 54, 215, 253, 254
  Ferdinand I, King of Naples (Ferrante) 25, 31, 32, 37, 212, 213, 215, 250, 252, 253, 254
  Isabella 31 n. 19, 51–2, 55 nn. 24 and 26, 212, 216
  Maria 27, 215, 216, 248
Arbeau, Thoinot 12
Aristotle 11 nn. 23 and 25, 172, 173
audiences, see dance, art of, spectators' reactions
Autobiography, see Giovanni Ambrosio

ballerino, see dancing-masters
ballo, balli 7 n. 14, 12, 15, 29, 48–9, 51, 61 n. 51, 64–5, 67–8, 69–70, 71–2, 104, 105, 112, 113 n. 3, *218*
  balli tunes 3, 4, 13, 15, 63–72, 179, *181–207, 240—7*

balls 27 n. 12, 47–8, 49, 51, 52, 56, 218, 248
  the dancing space, halls, arrangements 51 n. 10, 53 n. 18, 55 and n. 29, 56–7 and n. 32
  see also festivities
banquets (repasts) 37, 47, 49, 55–6 and n. 30, 223, 249 and n. 5, 250, 251, 253
bassadanza, bassedanze 7 n. 14, 51, 61 n. 51, 104, 105, 118, 119, *218–19*, 220
  in allegories and *moresche* 54 n. 21, 55
  composition of 12, *106*, *107*
  in *De pratica* (and copies) 12, 15, 18, *126–45, 234, 235*
  misura 64–72, 100, 101, 169 n. 115, *182–9*, *192–207*, 246–7
  step 97 n. 9, 220–1
  tenors 4 and n. 8, 7 n. 14, 13, 58 n. 43, 63 nn. 2 and 4, 65–6, 72 and n. 35, 106, 107, 219, 225
basse danse (dance) 3 n. 1, 7 n. 14, 12 n. 28, 15 and n. 37, 151 n. 66, *218–19*, 220, 234, 235, 239 n. 17, 247
beats (up-beat, beating time) 66 and n. 13, 72, 92, 93, 100, 101, 102, 103, 117, 144, 145 and n. 51, 168, 169 and n. 115, 187, 219, 223, 225, 228
Belfiore 158, 159
Belreguardo 18 n. 54, 19 n. 57, 49 and n. 6, 58 n. 43, 67, 72 n. 34, *164*, *165*, 179, *184–5*
Bembo, Pietro 39 n. 47
Bentivoglio, family 37
  Annibale 32 n. 22, 53 n. 17, 54 n. 21, 216
  Giovanni 213, 249 n. 6, 250
  Sante 120, 121, 129 n. 9, 213, 249
Boccaccio, *The Decameron* 61 and n. 49
body, for dancing 53, 84, 85, 88, 89, 94, 95, 96, 97, 98, 99, 104, 105, 106, 107, 108, 109
  see also air; grace; manner; moderation; movement and gesture
Bologna 24, 32 n. 22, 37, 54 n. 22, 58, 120, 121, 249, 250
  see also Bentivoglio
Bona of Savoy 32 n. 22, 42, 212, 251
Bono, Pietro 38 and n. 42
Borges 227, 234, 235

Borgia:
　Pope Alexander VI 53
　Cesare 16, 53, 54 n. 20, 215
　Goffredo 216
　Lucretia 53, 55 n. 26, 59, 214, 216
bow, see *riverenza*
Brandolino, Tiberto 49 and n. 4, 212, 250
Bruni, Leonardo 11 n. 23, 57 n. 38
Burgundy:
　ambassador to Charles the Bold, Duke of
　　37 and n. 40, 47, 51 n. 8, 252–3, 254
　Marie of 212

caccia, see hunt
Calmo, Andrea 43 n. 55
Camerino 24, 26 and nn. 3 and 5, 120, 121,
　213, 248
　see Varano
campeggiare 99 n. 11
Cangé, J. P. G. Chastre de 8 and n. 17
Canzone a ballo, see Medici, Lorenzo de'
Caravaggio 34 n. 29
Caroso, Fabritio xvii, 12, 49 n. 5
Castiglione, Baldassare and *The Book of the
　Courtier* 38 n. 42, 39 and n. 47, 41,
　54 n. 20, 61
Caterva 71 n. 29, 143 nn. 44 and 47, *144*, *145*,
　169 n. 115, 225
Cennini, Cennino 99 n. 11
chansons, dancing to 7 n. 14, 55 and n. 25,
　203
　see also singing, dancing to
Chiaranzana 49 and n. 5
chiave *104–5*, 218, *219*
choreographies, dances in *De pratica* *124–71*,
　234, *235*, *236–9*
choreography (dance composition) 7 n. 14,
　12, *104*, *105*, *106*, *107*
cloth, clothing, see dress
Colonna, Sveva, see Montefeltro
Colonnese 39 n. 45, 67, 70 n. *a*, 71 n. 26, 72
　and n. 34, *150*, *151*, 201, 203, *204—5*,
　207, 245, 247
continenza, continenze 64, 77, 96, 97 n. 9, 108,
　109, 127 n. 4, 180, *220*
contrapasso 72, 131 n. 16, 155 n. 79,
　157 n. 83, 165 n. 102, 183, 185, 186, 187,
　190, *220*, 221
Cornazano, Antonio, and his treatise 4,
　6 n. 8, 12, 13, 17 n. 48, 20 n. 59,
　31 n. 18, 58 and n. 43, 212, 226
　on the dance (steps etc.) 97 n. 9, 99 n. 11,
　　217, 220, 221, 222, 223, 224, 225, 226,
　　227
　on dance and music 63 n. 4, 64–7, 69, 71,
　　72, 180, 185, 187, 189, 197
　other works 20 n. 59, 54 n. 20, 58

costumes, see dress
Crivelli, Taddeo 59 n. 45, 60 pl. 15
Cupido *132*, *133*, 224

dance, the art and science of 3, 9–10, 11–12,
　88–123
　born from and related to music 9–10, 88,
　　89, 92, 93, 94, 95, 106, 107, 108, 109,
　　112, 113, 114, 115
　for the chaste, well-proportioned, noble,
　　etc. 90, 91, 98, 99, 114, 115
　those excluded from and enemies of 90, 91,
　　98, 99, 114, 115, 120, 121, 122, 123
　exercises 12, 15, *100–3*, 118, 119, *234*, *235*
　expressivity 3 n. 1, 11 n. 24, 88, 89, 106,
　　107
　principles, basic 3, 11–12, 84, 85, *92–9*,
　　114–18, 119; see also air; manner;
　　measure; memory; movement;
　　partitioning the ground
　spectators' appraisement and reactions 53
　　and n. 17, 94, 95, 96, 97, 104, 105, 106,
　　107, 110, 111, 112, 113
　for the young woman 12, 108, 109, 110,
　　111
　see also Domenico, theory; grace;
　　humanistic thought and influences;
　　moderation; ornamentation; virtuosity
dance music, see *ballo, balli* tunes; *bassedanze*
　tenors; chansons; instruments for
　dancing; singing
dance notation 12 n. 28
dance theory, see dance, the art of; Domenico,
　theory
dancing in 15th-century Italy:
　circles dances 54 n. 21, 55, 59,
　　60 pls. 15–16
　dancing schools 35–6, 58 and n. 44
　on private occasions 58, 59, 61
　status of 9–11, 21, 44, in humanist
　　education 57, 68–9
　rope dancing 47, 252
　women and girls 4, 8 pl. 3, 12, 32 n. 20,
　　35, 38, 46 pl. 10, 47 pl. 11, 48 and pl. 12,
　　49, 51–3, 55, 59 and n. 44, 60 pls. 15–16,
　　61 and nn. 48 and 51, 116, 117, 174, 175,
　　248, 253
　see also balls; chansons; dancing-masters;
　　instruments for dancing; *moresche*; singing
dancing-masters and *ballerini* 12, 14, 20,
　31 n. 18, 54, 61 n. 51, 120, 121
　performing with a young girl 38, 48, 53
　　and n. 17
　role and activities 15, 29, 31, 32 n. 22,
　　35–6, 37, 38, 39, 41
　status 9–10, 20, 21, 29, 31, 32 and n. 22,
　　35, 39, 41–5

see also Domenico da Piacenza; Giuseppe
  Ebreo; Lavagnolo, Lorento; Moses of
  Sicily; Pierpaolo
Dandolo, family 250 and n. 14
Daphnes 19 n. 57, 136, 137, 138, 139, 224
De pratica (Paris, Bibliothèque Nationale,
  Guglielmo Ebreo, fonds ital 973) vii,
  2 pl. 1, 5 pl. 2, 6, 7 and n. 15, 8 pl. 3,
  8–13, 19, 20–2, 73–207
  see also antiquity; ballo, balli tunes;
    choreographies; dance, art and science of;
    De pratica, copies; Domenico of Piacenza;
    humanistic thought and influences; music;
    orthography; Pagano of Rho; poems;
    women
De pratica, copies 6, 9, 16–21
  comparison of 16–21, 72, 103 n. 13,
    127 nn. 3, 4, and 6, 220, 227
  Florence, Biblioteca Medicea Laurenziana
    16, 18, 20, 36, 42 n. 51
  Florence, Biblioteca Nazionale Centrale 16,
    17, 18, 20, 21, 36, 42 n. 51, 72, 203
  Foligno, Biblioteca Jacobilli 19, 20, 21, 222
  fragments, Florence and Venice 18; see also
    Nuremberg
  lost copies 16–17, 21, 27, 35 n. 31, 39, 42
  Modena, Biblioteca Estense 16, 17, 18, 19,
    21, 65 n. 12
  New York Public Library (Giorgio) vii, 16,
    17, 18, 19, 20, 21, 36, 58 n. 43, 72, 183,
    190–1, 200–1, 203, 207, 222, 225,
    239 nn. 14–16, 241, 242–3, 247
  Paris, Bibliothèque Nationale (Giovanni
    Ambrosio, fonds ital 476) vii, 9 n. 18,
    14–15, 19, 21, 75–6, 79, 225, 231–54; see
    also Giovanni Ambrosio, Autobiography,
    and musical innovations
  Siena, Biblioteca Comunale 16, 17, 18, 19,
    20, 21, 49 nn. 5 and 6, 51, 58 n. 43,
    64 n. 9, 65 n. 12, 72, 192–3, 222, 225
Domenico da Piacenza 3–4, 17 n. 49, 26 n. 2,
  34 n. 29, 43, 211, 218
  his dances and their music 7 n. 14, 13 and
    n. 30, 37 n. 38, 43, 49 and 51 n. 6,
    58 n. 43, 64 n. 6, 67–8 and n. 19, 69 and
    n. 23, 72 and n. 34, 245
  his dances and tunes in De pratica 12, 13,
    21, 67, 124 n. e, 126, 127, 130, 131, 134,
    135, 136–7, 138, 139, 140, 141, 146, 147,
    150, 151, 152–66, 167, 182–99
  and Guglielmo 6, 23, 27, 29, 88, 89, 90, 91,
    249
  on steps 180, 220, 221, 222, 223, 224, 225,
    226, 228
  his theory 12, 64–6, 68–9, 72, 219
  his treatise 3 and n. 3, 4, 9 n. 18, 11, 12,
    19, 21

doppio, doppii 64, 71, 72, 92, 95, 96, 97 and
  n. 9, 98, 99 and n. 11, 108, 109,
  155 n. 79, 161 n. 95, 169 n. 115, 180,
  220–1, 223, 224, 225, 227, 228
dress (cloth, clothing) 10 pl. 4, 28 pl. 5,
  30 pls. 6–7, 37, 40 pls. 8–9,
  50 pls. 13–14, 52 n. 11, 59 and n. 47,
  248 n. 4, 250, 251, 252 and n. 19, 253,
  254
  and dancing (and costume) 7, 8 pl. 3, 14,
    46 pl. 10, 47 pl. 11, 48 pl. 12, 51 n. 10,
    52, 53, 54, 56 n. 32, 57, 60 pls. 15–16,
    232, 233
ducats, worth of 13 n. 31, 20 n. 59, 38 and
  nn. 41–2, 249, 250 and n. 12, 252, 253,
  254
  see also expenditure; magnificence;
    reckoning
Duchesco 146, 147, 148, 149

Emperors, see Frederick III; Maximilian
Este of Ferrara 3–4, 27 and n. 6, 38 n. 42, 52,
  159 n. 85, 165 nn. 101 and 103, 211, 212,
  216
  Alfonso 52, 55 n. 26, 212, 216
  Beatrice (wife of Tristano Sforza) 4, 211,
    216
  Beatrice (sister of Isabella) 32 n. 22, 52,
    61 n. 48, 212, 216
  Borso 20 n. 59, 34 n. 30, 59, 60 pl. 15, 216
  Camilla 27, 213, 216, 248
  Ercole I 31 n. 19, 37, 38 n. 42, 56 n. 30,
    215, 216
  Ercole (son of Sigismondo) 52, 53, 212,
    216
  Ginevra 215, 216
  Isabella 25, 32 n. 22, 38, 42, 52, 59, 212,
    216
  Leonello 27, 33 n. 26, 120, 121, 165 and
    n. 103, 215, 216, 248
  Lucretia 32 n. 22, 53 n. 17, 54 n. 21, 216
  Niccolò 27 and n. 6, 211, 213, 216
  Sigismondo 212, 216
exercises, for dancing, see dance, the art and
  science of
expenditure 15, 16 n. 39, 34 n. 30, 56, 57
  see also ducats; magnificence; reckoning
expressivity, see dance, the art and science of

Faenza 249, 252
Feltre, Vittorino da 57
fermata, see signa congruentiae
Ferrara 3, 4, 23, 24, 25, 27, 32 n. 22,
  38 n. 42, 42, 55 n. 26, 56 nn. 30 and 32,
  57, 120, 121, 159 n. 85, 165 nn. 101 and
  103, 213, 248, 249
  see also Este

festivities 36–8, 39, 47–9, 51–3, 54–7, 58, 59, 61, 120, 121, 221, 248–54
  Festa del Paradiso 51 n. 10, 52, 55 n. 26
  see also balls; *moresche*
Ficino, Marsilio 11 n. 25
Figlia Gulielmina 7 n. 14
Filarete, Antonio 10 n. 23, 12 n. 26
Filelfo:
  Francesco 13 and n. 31, 211
  Mario (Giovanni Mario) 9, 13 and n. 31, 38 and n. 42, 39 and n. 47, 172–7
Fiore de vertu 224, *236, 237*
Firenzuola 7 n. 14, 59 and n. 46
Flandesca 13 n. 30, *140, 141*
Florence 24, 25, 32 n. 22, 35–6, 41–2, 48–9, 50 pls. 13–14, 52 n. 11
  see also Medici
flourishes 14 and n. 36, 43 n. 55, 233
  see also ornamentation
Forlì 24, 29, 249, 250
France:
  Kings of: Henry IV 49 n. 5; Louis XI, ambassador of 23, 31, 47, 252; Louis XII 7
  see also Bona of Savoy; French dances
Frederick III, Holy Roman Emperor 25, 34 and n. 30, 47, 251
French dances 15, 37, 52, 218, *234, 235, 238, 239* and nn. 13 and 17, 243, 247, 253

Gaffurio (Gafurius), Franchino 10 n. 23, 69 n. 20
Galli, Angelo 11 n. 25
Gallo, F. Alberto xv, 16 n. 40, 26 n. 4, 29 n. 17, 31, 37, 79, 124 n. *e*, 147 n. 54, 159 n. 85, 165 n. 103, 248 n. 1, 253 n. 20
Gelosia 20, 51, 64 n. 6, 71 n. 26, *162, 163, 190–1,* 224, 225
Genevra 37 n. 38, *128, 129, 130, 131*
Genoa 24, 31, 250
German:
  dances 52, 118, 119
  Germans in Italy 58, 250, 251
  saltarello (saltarello todescho) 66 n. 13, 70 n. *b,* 71–2, 143 n. 46, 161 n. 95, 169 nn. 113 and 115, 182–3, 188–9, 190–1, 197, 200–1, 202–3, 224, *225*
gesture, *see* body; movement
Ghiberti, Lorenzo 10 n. 23
Gioioso, see *Rostiboli gioioso*
gioioso, see *volta tonda*
Gioliva 138, 139
Giorgio, and his treatise (NY) 17 and n. 49, 18, 19–20, 21
  see also *De pratica,* copies, New York

Giovanni Ambrosio:
  Autobiography 15, 23, 37, 79, 121 and n. 4, 231, *248–54*
  musical innovations 15, 19, 67, 70 and n. 25, 183, 187, 191, 199, 201, 203, 207
  see also De pratica, copies (Paris); Guglielmo Ebreo
Giuseppe Ebreo 18, 25–6, 35–6, 41
Gonzaga, family 32 n. 22, 33, 45 n. 59
  Chiara 32 n. 22
  Elisabetta 32 n. 22, 214
  Federico 13 n. 31, 23, 32 n. 22, 37, 251
  Francesco 216
  Margaret of Bavaria 23, 32 n. 22, 37, 251
  Margherita 216
Gozzoli, Benozzo 48, 50 pls. 13–14
Gratioso 18 n. 54, 67, 70 n. 25, 71 n. 26, 72, 153 n. 69, *166, 167, 168, 169,* 201, *202–3,* 205, 207, 245, 247
grace 53 and n. 17, 55, 56, 59, 61, 84, 85, 96, 97, 98, 99, 116, 117
  see also body; moderation; movement and gesture
Guarini, Guarino (Guarino da Verona) 57
Guglielmo Ebreo 6, 26 n. 2
  and Bianca Maria Sforza 29, 31–3, 212
  birth 25–6
  and brother Giuseppe 25–6, 35–6, 41
  career 26–7, 29, 31–3, 34–5, 36–8, 41–3, 120, 121, 248–54
  conversion 13–14, 23, 33–4
  and Domenico da Piacenza 6, 23, 27, 29, 88, 89, 90, 91, 249
  and Galeazzo Maria Sforza 5 pl. 2, 6, 9, 20, 23, 25, 32, 35, 36, 38, 44; and his heirs 42–3
  and Isabella d'Este 25, 38, 42
  knighthood 25, 34 and nn. 29–31, 35 and n. 31, 251
  last years 25, 42–3
  and Lorenzo de' Medici 25, 35 n. 30, 36, 38, 41–2
  marriage 23, 33
  musical innovations, *see* Giovanni Ambrosio
  Ode, in honour of 172–7
  patrons 16–17, 20, 21, 26, 27 and n. 8, 29, 31, 32, 33, 34, 35, 37, 38, 39, 41, 42, 43, 44, 80–1, 120, 121, 213, 214; *see also* Medici, Lorenzo; Montefeltro, Federico; Sforza, Alessandro; Sforza, Costanzo; Sforza, Francesco; Sforza, Galeazzo Maria
  social position 31, 32, 33, 34–5, 37, 38, 39, 41, 42–5
  son, Pierpaolo 25, 39, 41 and nn. 48–9

as teacher, choreographer, composer, and performer of dances 12, 29 and n. 14, 32 n. 20, 38, 43, 44, 248, 249, 251, 252
his treatises, see *De pratica*; *De pratica*, copies

hearsay, *see* reckoning
humanistic thought and influences in *De pratica* 9–12, 44 n. 58, 68–9 and n. 20, 77, 78, 79
humanists:
on dance 57
their treatises 9 n. 21, 10 n. 23, 11 and n. 25, 12 n. 26, 57 n. 38
see also Alberti, Leon Battista; Bruni, Leonardo; Cornazano, Antonio; Feltre, Vittorino da; Ficino, Marsilio; Filelfo, Francesco and Mario; Guarini, Guarino; Manetti, Gianozzo; Pius II (Aeneas Piccolomini); Trissino, Giangiorgio; Vergerio, Pierpaolo
hunt (*caccia, cacciata*) 47, 54 n. 22, 66 n. 13, 224, 253

illuminations, *see* miniatures
improvisation, *see* instruments, performance; ornamentation; virtuosity
Ingrata 64 n. 8, 69 n. 23, 72 n. 34, 78 n. 5, 158, 159, 160, 161, 194–5, 222, 245
instruments, musical:
in antiquity 86, 87, 88, 89, 219
for dancing 8 pl. 3, 15, 46 pl. 10, 47 pl. 11, 48 pl. 12, 49, 51, 53, 54 and n. 21, 60 pl. 15, 63 n. 2, 72 n. 35, 92, 93 and n. 3, 108, 109, 219, 234, 235
performance 63 n. 2, 65 n. 11, 68, 71, 72 n. 35
pipe and tabor 53 n. 17, 54, 63 n. 2, 234, 235
the player(s) 55 n. 29, 56, 58, 72, 100, 101, 102, 103, 104, 105, 112, 113, 114, 115, 118, 119, 219, 234, 235
shawms and sackbuts (*piffari*) 46 pl. 10, 49, 51, 53, 55, 60 pl. 15, 63 n. 2, 223, 234, 235, 251, 252
see also chansons; singing, dancing to
intermedi, see moresche
Iove (Jupiter) 18 n. 50, 20, 67 and nn. 14–15, 69 n. 23, 152, 153, 154, 155, 188–9, 225, 227

Jews:
in 15th-century Italy 26 n. 2, 33 and nn. 25–6, 34, 35, 55, 58 and n. 44; conversion of 34 n. 29, 36; community of Pesaro 55; Jewish dancing-masters 17 n. 49, 25–6, 58 and n. 44

in Old Testament, in *De pratica* 88, 89, 172, 173, 174, 175
see also Judah Leon
jousts (tournaments, mock battles) 32 n. 20, 47, 49, 54, 56 and n. 30, 122, 123, 248 and n. 4, 249, 252, 253–4 and n. 22
Judah Leon 34 nn. 29–30

knighthood and orders 34 and nn. 29–30, 35 n. 31, 39, 52 n. 14, 88, 89, 249, 251
Knight of the Ermine 39, 214
Knight of the Golden Spur 3–4, 34, 35 n. 31, 39
Order of Malta 34 n. 29

Lauro 36, 49 n. 6, 227
Lavagnolo, Lorenzo 32 n. 22
Legiadra 64 n. 6, 67, 70 n. *a*, 71 n. 26, 72 and n. 34, 76, 148, 149, 201, 203, 205, 206–7, 245, 247
Leonardo da Vinci 9 n. 21, 11 n. 25, 29 n. 17, 36, 43, 52, 55 n. 26
Leoncello 18 n. 54, 43, 49 and n. 6, 51, 58 n. 43, 67, 164, 165, 186–7
liberal, art (science) 10, 44 n. 59, 69, 86, 87, 90, 91 and n. 7, 114, 115, 221–2
libraries:
in 15th-century Italy 4, 7 and nn. 13 and 15, 16, 20–1 n. 60, 27 and n. 7, 39
in France 7–8
see also *De pratica*, copies
Lorenzo de' Medici, *see* Medici
Lucian 3 n. 1, 11 n. 25, 12

magnificence, policy of 15, 56 and n. 33, 57, 249, 250 n. 12, 252 and n. 19, 253, 254
Malatesta, family 215
Elisabetta 213, 215
Galeazzo 26 n. 3, 213, 215, 250
Roberto 13, 25, 32 n. 22, 38, 39, 214, 215, 251
Sigismondo 48, 50 pl. 13, 211, 215, 216
Manetti, Gianozzo 10 n. 23, 57 n. 38
manner (*maniera*) 11 and n. 25, 64 n. 8, 97 n. 9, 98, 99, 116, 117, 222
Mantegna, Andrea 27, 45 n. 59
Mantua 23, 24, 31, 32 n. 22, 33 n. 26, 37, 48, 56 n. 32, 249, 250, 251
see also Gonzaga
Marchesana 58 n. 43, 64 n. 6, 67 n. 16, 78 n. 5, 156, 157, 198–9
masques, see *moresche*
Maximilian, Emperor 52, 59 n. 48, 212
measure (*misura*) 11 n. 25, 12 n. 26, 64–71, 92, 93, 94, 95 and n. 5, 100, 101, 102, 103, 104, 105, 106, 107, 108, 109, 111, 112, 113, 114, 115, 116, 117, 222–3, 232, 233, 234, 235

measure (*cont.*):
see also mensuration; *misure*; proportion; rhythm; *tempo*; timing
Medici, de', family 6 n. 12, 36 n. 37, 59 n. 47
Cosimo 48, 49 n. 3
Lorenzo 13 n. 31, 33, 48, 50 pl. 14; *Canzone a ballo* 59 and n. 47, 60 pl. 16; dances by 18, 36, 49 n. 6; and Giuseppe Ebreo 36; and Guglielmo/Giovanni Ambrosio 16–17, 25, 35 n. 30, 36, 38, 41–2, 44
Marie 49 n. 5
memory 11 and n. 25, *94, 95*, 114, 115, 116, 117
mensuration and mensural signs 64–71, *102, 103* and n. 13, 179, 182–207, 219, 222, 224, 226, 246–7
Mercantia 21, 67 n. 14, 72 n. 34, *166, 167, 196–7*, 224, 226
meza volta 64 and n. 5, 127 n. 7, 180, 187, 218, *222*
Mignotta 127 n. 4, *130, 131*
Milan 4, 6 n. 12, 13 n. 31, 23, 24, 25, 29, 31, 32, 33, 35, 36, 42–3, 51–3, ,61 n. 48, 120, 121, 176, 177, 211, 249, 250, 251, 252
see also Sforza, Francesco; Sforza, Galeazzo Maria; Sforza, Giangaleazzo; Sforza, Ludovico; Visconti
miniatures and miniaturists 2 pl. 1, 3 n. 3, 5 pl. 2, 6 and n. 10, 7 and n. 13, 8 pl. 3, 10 pl. 4, 14, 20, 39, 55 n. 27, 59 and n. 45
misure, the four (in a *ballo*) 64–72, 100, 101, *102, 103*, 104, 105, 108, 111, 179–80, 182–207, 218, 222, 223, 224, 225, 236, 237, 240–7
see also *bassadanza*; choreographies; *piva*; *quadernaria*; *saltarello*
moderation, in the dance 96, 97, 108, 109
see also body; dance, art of; movement and gesture
Montefeltro, family 6 n. 12, *214*
Elisabetta 13, 25, 38, 39, 214, 215, 251
Federico, Count and Duke of Urbino 13 n. 31, 16, 21, 23, 25, 26, 32–3, 35 and n. 31, 36, 37, 38, 39, 40 pl. 9, 41, 42, 43–4, 120, 121, 213, 214, 248, 249, 251, 252
Guidobaldo 32 n. 22, 39 nn. 47–8, 214
Sveva Colonna 27 n. 11, 28 pl. 5, 39 and n. 45, 150, 151 and n. 62, 213, 214, 249
moresche (maskers, masques, Moorish) 29, 31, 37, 39, 48, 52, 53–7, 61 and n. 51, 118, 119, 222, *223*, 249, 251, 252, 253
Moses of Sicily 23, 25–6 and n. 1
movement, body, and gesture 3 n. 1, 11 and nn. 24–5, 41, 52, 53, 55, 72, 84, 85, 88, 89, 92, 93, 94, 95, 96, 97, *98, 99*, 102,

103, 104, 105, 106, 107, 108, 109, 110, 111, 116, 117, 218, 219, 223, 232, 233
see also body; grace; moderation; ornamentation; virtuosity
movimenti (*scossi*) 64, 72, 96, 97, 108, 109, 153 n. 74, 185, 186, 187, 194, 195, 197, 205, 207, 219, *223*
music, see *bassadanza* tenors; *ballo, balli* tunes; beats; chansons; *chiavi*; Giovanni Ambrosio, musical innovations; instruments; measure; mensuration; *misure*; music, in *De pratica*; notation, music; proportion; rhythm; singing; *tempo*; timing; voices
music, in *De pratica* 11, 13, 63–72, 92, 93, 94, 95, 100–19, 179–207, 234, 235, 240–7
dance born from and related to 9–10, 88, 89, 106, 107, 108, 109, 112, 113
the inventors of 86, 87
the power of 88, 89, 106, 107

Naples 24, 25, 31, 32, 34, 37, 39, 47, 52, 215–16, 250, 252–4
see also Aragons of Naples
notation(s), music 13, 14 n. 35, 15, 63–72, 179, 182–207, 240–7
see also dance notation; Giovanni Ambrosio, musical innovations: *signa congruentiae*
Nuremberg xv, 58, 220

ombreggiare, see manner
ondeggiare, see air
ornamentation, in dancing 12, 14 and n. 36, 43 n. 55, 52, 53, 64–5, 96, 97 and n. 9, 98, 99, 217, 221, 222, 224, 232, 233, 234, 235
orthography, punctuation 75–7, 78, 217, 231

Pagano of Rho vii, 6 and n. 10, 9, 13, 15, 20, 23, 67, 76, 77, 176, 177
Partita crudele 36 and n. 36
partitioning the ground, and spatial awareness 11, 12, 55, *94, 95, 96, 97*, 116, 117, 218, 226
Patienza 138, 139, *140, 141*
patronage 32 n. 22, 33 n. 34
see also Guglielmo Ebreo, patrons
Pavia 6, 7 and nn. 13 and 15, 13 n. 31, 20, 23, 24, 31, 212, 252
Pellegrina 19 n. 57, 51 n. 6, *134, 135*, 222
pellegrina 51 n. 6, 77 and n. 3, 80, 81, 116, 117, 120, 121, 122, 123
Pergola 51
Perugino 27
Pesaro 16 and n. 46, 23, 24, 25, 26 and nn. 1, 3, and 5, 27 and n. 7, 33, 34 n. 30, 37, 38, 55–6, 120, 121, 213, 214, 248, 249, 251, 252

see also Sforza, Alessandro; Sforza, Costanzo
Petit Riense (Vriens) 64 n. 6, 67, 151 n. 66,
   223, 238, 239, 244–5
Petit Rose 13 n. 30, 64 n. 6, 150, 151, 152,
   153
Petit Vriens, see Petit Riense
Petrarch 7 n. 15, 43
Phoebus 13 n. 30, 134, 135, 136, 137
Piacenza 4 and n. 7, 24, 58, 212
Piccolomini, Aeneas, see Pius II
Pierpaolo, see Guglielmo Ebreo, son
Pietosa 127 n. 4, 130, 131, 132, 133
Pisanello 11 n. 25
Pius II (Aeneas Piccolomini) 13 n. 31, 23, 31,
   33 n. 26, 48, 57 n. 38, 249, 250
piva 48 and pl.12, 51, 52, 54 n. 20, 55, 58, 61
   and n. 51, 64–72, 161 n. 95, 188, 189,
   190, 191, 192, 193, 194, 195, 200, 201,
   202, 203, 204, 205, 206, 207, 222, 223–4,
   239 n. 13, 240, 241, 242, 243, 244, 245,
   247
Pizocara 68 n. 19, 69 n. 23, 192–3
plague 36
Plato 3 n. 1, 11 n. 24, 172, 173
poems:
   in De pratica, and copies 9, 11, 12, 13, 19,
     80–5, 122, 123, 172–7
   and dancing 51, 58, 59
   see also Galli, Angelo; Medici, Lorenzo de',
     Canzone a ballo
popes, see Borgia, Alexander VI; Pius II
Presoniera 67 n. 14, 70, 71 nn. 26 and 31,
   105 n. 16, 154, 155, 156, 157, 161 n. 95,
   182–3, 225
Principessa 49 n. 6, 71 n. 29, 142, 143,
   225
proportion 12 n. 26, 64–5, 68–70, 179, 183,
   189, 193, 240, 241, 246, 247
punctuation, see orthography

quadernaria 64–72, 102, 103 and n. 13,
   169 n. 115, 183, 186, 187, 188, 189, 190,
   191, 194, 195, 196, 197, 198, 199, 201,
   203, 205, 207, 221, 222, 224, 225, 240,
   241, 245, 247

Ravenna 24, 37, 248
Reale 13 n. 30, 37 n. 38, 126, 127
reckoning (and hearsay) 15 and n. 39, 249,
   250 and n. 12, 253, 254
   see also magnificence
rhythm 88, 89, 93, 94, 95, 97, 197, 222, 227,
   233, 235
   see also misura; tempo; timing
Rimini 24, 26 n. 5, 38, 39, 215
   see also Malatesta

ripresa 64 and n. 6, 96, 97, 108, 109,
   137 nn. 31 and 34, 143 n. 44, 161 n. 95,
   180, 221, 224, 228
riverenza (bow) 15, 55, 64, 108, 109, 110, 111
   and n. 20, 180, 225
Rome 24, 33 n. 26, 34 n. 30, 45 n. 59, 53,
   56 n. 30, 59
Rosina, see Voltati in ça Rosina
Rostiboli gioioso 13, 14 n. 36, 15, 18 n. 54, 43
   and n. 55, 49 n. 6, 51, 58 n. 43, 67,
   69 n. 23, 70 n. a, 72, 146, 147 and n. 52,
   203, 205, 207, 246–7
Ruzante (Angelo Beolco) 43 n. 55

saltarello 18 n. 54, 46 pl. 10, 47 pl. 11, 48–9,
   51 and n. 7, 54 n. 20, 58, 61 and n. 51, 64
   and n. 7, 65–72, 96, 97, 100, 101, 102,
   103, 104, 105, 118, 119, 169 n. 115, 182,
   183, 184, 185, 188, 189, 190, 191, 192,
   193, 194, 195, 196, 197, 200, 201, 202,
   203, 204, 205, 206, 207, 217, 223, 225,
   246, 247
   see also German saltarello
Schifanoia, Palazzo 27 n. 6, 56 n. 32
scossi, see movimenti
scribes, and script 3 n. 3, 6, 9 and n. 20, 14
   and n. 35, 15, 17, 18, 19, 20, 39, 67,
   75–7, 179
   see also orthography; Pagano of Rho
sempio, sempii 64, 92, 93, 96, 97, 98, 99, 108,
   109, 127 n. 6, 131 n. 15, 135 n. 27,
   159 n. 87, 161 n. 95, 171 n. 116, 180,
   195, 222, 224, 226, 228, 235 n. 5,
   239 n. 14
Sforza, family 211–14
   Alessandro 11 n. 25, 13 n. 31, 16, 21, 23,
     25, 26–7, 28 pl. 5, 29, 31, 32, 33, 34 and
     n. 30, 35, 37 and n. 38, 38, 39, 42, 44,
     120, 121, 126, 127, 129 n. 9, 151 n. 62,
     213, 214, 215, 248, 249, 250, 251, 252
   Angela 52, 53, 212, 216
   Anna 52, 212, 216
   Battista 23, 27 n. 11, 28 pl. 5, 29 n. 16, 39,
     40 pl. 8, 214, 249
   Bianca Maria (wife of Emperor
     Maximilian) 52, 59 n. 48, 212
   Bianca Maria, see Visconti
   Carlo 52, 212
   Costanzo 16, 25, 27 n. 11, 28 pl. 5, 31, 32,
     38, 41–2, 43–4, 55–6, 213, 214, 215, 250
   Elisabetta 211
   emblems 5 pl. 2, 6 and n. 12
   Francesco 5 pl. 2, 6 n. 12, 13 n. 31, 20, 23,
     25, 26 n. 3, 27 n. 6, 29, 30 pl. 6, 31, 32,
     33, 34, 37 and n. 38, 42, 48, 120, 121,
     147 n. 54, 176, 177, 211, 212, 213, 215,
     248, 249, 250, 252

Sforza, family (*cont.*):
 Galeazzo (son of Costanzo) 214
 Galeazzo Maria 5 pl. 2, 6, 7 nn. 12, 14–15,
  9, 10 pl. 4, 13 n. 31, 20, 23, 25, 29 n. 17,
  31 n. 19, 32, 35 and n. 33, 36, 38, 42, 44,
  48–9, 50 pl. 13, 51, 59, 80, 81, 82, 83,
  211, 212, 251, 254
 Giangaleazzo 31 n. 19, 42–3, 44, 51–2,
  55 n. 24, 212, 216
 Ginevra 37 and n. 38, 128, 129 and n. 9,
  213, 249
 Giovanni 27 n. 7, 214
 Ippolita 4, 7 n. 14, 20 n. 59, 23, 25, 29, 31
  and nn. 18–19, 32 n. 20, 37, 51 n. 10,
  52 n. 11, 54 n. 22, 211, 212, 216, 249,
  253, 254
 Ludovico (il Moro) 5 pl. 2, 6 n. 12, 51–2,
  53 n. 16, 56 n. 32, 61 n. 48, 211, 212,
  216
 Muzio Attendolo 5 pl. 2, 6 n. 12, 211, 213
 Polissena 211, 215
 Sforza Maria 31 and n. 19, 211, 212, 215
 Sforza Sforza (II) 4, 211, 212
 Tristano 4, 211, 216
shading, body, *see* manner
Siena 54 n. 22
signa congruentiae 192, 193, 194, 195
singing, dancing to 7 and n. 14, 54 and n. 22,
  59
 see also chansons
Sobria 21, 67, 68 n. 19, 72 n. 34
Socrates 172, 173
 Socratic dialogue 12, *112–19*
soprano 72, 219
 see also voices
space, spatial awareness, *see* partitioning the
  ground
Spain 34
Spanish:
 dances 52, 147 n. 52, 225
 dancers 52, 53, 59
 dress 52, 61 n. 48
spectacles, see *moresche*
spectators, *see* dance, art of, spectators
Spero 51 n. 6, 67 and n. 15, 70 and n. 25, 71
  and nn. 26 and 31, 72, *168*, *169*, and
  n. *170*, *171*, *200–1*, 203, 205, 207,
  225, 245, 247
steps 64, 71–2, 77, 92, 93, 94, 95, 96, 97 and
  n. 9, 114, 115, 180, 217, 220–1, 222, 223,
  224, 225, 226, 227–8
 see also *bassadanza*; *continenza*; *contrapasso*;
  doppio; *meza volta*; *movimenti*;
  ornamentation; *piva*; *quadernaria*; *ripresa*;
  riverenza; *saltarello*; *volta tonda*
style, *see* air
syncopation(s) 104, 105 and n. 14

tempo, tempus 64, 66, 68, 70, 72, 92, 93, 94,
  95, 96, 97 n. 8, 98, 99 n. 10, 100, 101,
  104, 105, 106, 107, 131 n. 18, 145 n. 51,
  226–7
 see also mensuration; *misura*; rhythm; timing
tenor 72, 87 n. 4, 92, 93, 104, 105, 106, 107,
  219
 see also *bassadanza* tenors; voices
Tesara 64 n. 6, 68, 72, 161 n. 95, 245
theatrical dance, see *moresche*
timing, dancing in time 11, 64–5, 69, 70, 71,
  92, 93, 94, 95, 96, 97 n. 8, 98, 99 and
  n. 10, 100, 101, 102, 103, 114, 115, 116,
  117, 145 n. 51, *222*, *226*, 232, 233, 234,
  235
Tinctoris 14 n. 36, 69 n. 20, 93 n. 3,
  105 n. 14, 219, 220, 221, 226, 227
Toscanini, Walter vii, 4 n. 4, 17 n. 49,
  18 n. 52, 29 n. 17, 34 n. 29
tournament, *see* jousts
treatises:
 dance 3 and n. 1, 4, 6, 12 n. 27, 15 n. 37;
  see also *De pratica*, and copies;
  Cornazano, Antonio; Domenico da
  Piacenza; Nuremberg
 other (architecture, art, education, family,
  music, etc.) 10 nn. 22–3; 11 n. 24;
  12 n. 26; 16 n. 39, 57 and n. 38; *see also*
  Gaffurio; Tinctoris
Trissino, Giangiorgio 43
Trotto (Trotti), family 4
 Giacomo 7 n. 12, 51 n. 10, 52 n. 14,
  57 n. 37

Urbino 7 n. 14, 11 n. 25, 16, 20 n. 60, 23,
  24, 25, 26, 32 n. 22, 35, 38–9, 41 n. 49,
  54–5, 61, 120, 121, 214, 215, 249, 251,
  252
 see also Montefeltro

van der Weyden, Rogier 27 and n. 11,
  28 pl. 5
Varano (da), family 26 n. 3, 213
 Costanza 23, 26, 27, 28 pl. 5, 29 and n. 16,
  213, 215, 248
 Rodolfo 26 n. 3, 27, 28 pl. 5, 120, 121,
  213, 216, 248, 252
Venice 18, 24, 25, 34, 36, 37, 47, 58 n. 44,
  120, 121, 250 and n. 14, 251 and n. 16
Venus 36, 227
Verçepe 67, 72 n. 34
Vergerio, Pierpaolo 10 n. 23, 57 n. 38
violence:
 anti-semitism 33–4
 dance and 112, 113, 114, 115
 death, violent 251, 252; *see also* plague

murder 112, 113, 114, 115, 212, 213, 214, 215, 248, 250
plunder 7, 16
and power 35 and n. 33, 212, 213, 214, 215
virtuosity in dance 14, 43 n. 55, 52 and n. 13, 53 and n. 17, 55, 226, 228, 232, 233
Visconti, family 5 pl. 2, 6 n. 12, 7, 13 n. 31, 29, 211
  Bianca Maria 4, 7 n. 12, 20, 27 n. 6, 29, 30 pl. 7, 31, 32, 33, 34, 44, 211, 212, 213, 248, 252
voices, the four principal 86, 87 and n. 4, 106, 107 and n. 18, 227
Voltati in ça Rosina 15, 43 and n. 55, 64 n. 6, 69, 222, 224, *234, 235, 236, 237, 240–1*

volta tonda (*volta del gioioso*) 64 and n. 6, 127 n. 6, 159 n. 87, 180, 188, *227–8*, 232, 233, 237 n. 8

Weyden, *see* van der Weyden
women:
  in *De pratica* 8 pl. 3, 11, 12, 94, 95, 96, 97, 104, 105, 108, 109, 110, 111, 113 and n. 1, 116, 117, 120, 121, 174, 175, 176, 177, 248, 250, 251, 252
  in 15th-century Italy 4, 11 n. 23, 27 and n. 6, 33, 35, 42, 51–2 and n. 11, 55, 57, 59 and n. 44, 61 and n. 51, 212, 213, 214, 226
  see also dancing in 15th-century Italy; women's names under Aragons; Borgia; Burgundy; Este; Gonzaga; Malatesta; Montefeltro; Sforza; Varano; Visconti